D0937789

MULTICULTURAL UNDERSTANDING
OF CHILD AND ADOLESCENT PSYCHOPATHOLOGY

Multicultural Understanding of Child and Adolescent Psychopathology

Implications for Mental Health Assessment

THOMAS M. ACHENBACH
LESLIE A. RESCORLA

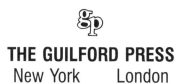

THE GUILFORD PRESS
New York   London

© 2007 The Guilford Press
A Division of Guilford Publications, Inc.
72 Spring Street, New York, NY 10012
www.guilford.com

Printed in the United States of America

This book is printed on acid-free paper.

Last digit is print number: 9 8 7 6 5 4 3 2 1

Library of Congress Cataloging-in-Publication Data

Achenbach, Thomas M., 1940–
  Multicultural understanding of child and adolescent psychopathology:
implications for mental health assessment / Thomas M. Achenbach,
Leslie A. Rescorla.
    p. ; cm.
  Includes bibliographical references and index.
  ISBN-10: 1-59385-348-3   ISBN-13: 978-1-59385-348-8 (cloth: alk. paper)
  1. Child psychopathology—Cross-cultural studies. 2. Adolescent
psychopathology—Cross-cultural studies. I. Rescorla, Leslie. II. Title.
  [DNLM: 1. Mental Disorders. 2. Adolescent. 3. Child. 4. Cross-Cultural
Comparison. 5. Psychopathology—methods. WS 350 A177m 2006]
  RJ499.M85 2006
  618.92′89—dc22

                                                            2006022956

About the Authors

Thomas M. Achenbach, PhD, Professor of Psychiatry and Psychology, is Director of the Center for Children, Youth, and Families at the University of Vermont Department of Psychiatry. He received his doctorate from the University of Minnesota and was a postdoctoral fellow at the Yale Child Study Center. Before moving to the University of Vermont, Dr. Achenbach taught at Yale and was a research psychologist at the National Institute of Mental Health. He has been a DAAD Fellow at the University of Heidelberg, Germany; an SSRC Senior Faculty Fellow at Jean Piaget's Centre d'Epistémologie Génétique in Geneva; Chair of the American Psychological Association's Task Force on Classification of Children's Behavior; and a member of the American Psychiatric Association's Advisory Committee on DSM-III-R. He has given over 230 invited presentations in 30 countries and has authored over 250 publications, including *Developmental Psychopathology*; *Research in Developmental Psychology: Concepts, Strategies, Methods*; *Assessment and Taxonomy of Child and Adolescent Psychopathology*; *Empirically Based Taxonomy*; *Empirically Based Assessment of Child and Adolescent Psychopathology* (with Stephanie H. McConaughy); and manuals for the *Child Behavior Checklist, Teacher's Report Form, Youth Self-Report*, and other standardized assessment instruments for adults as well as for children. The assessment instruments have been translated into 74 languages and their use has been reported in over 6,000 publications from 67 cultures. Dr. Achenbach's honors include the Distinguished Contribution Award of the American Psychological Association's Section on Clinical Child Psychology, the University Scholar Award of the University of Vermont, selection for the Institute for Scientific Information's Most Highly Cited Authors in the World Psychiatry/Psychology Literature, and election to fellowship status in four divisions of the American Psychological Association.

Leslie A. Rescorla, PhD, Professor of Psychology at Bryn Mawr College, was Director of the Clinical Developmental Psychology doctoral program for 20 years and Chair of the Psychology Department for 10 years, and has been Director of the Bryn Mawr School Psychology Certification Program since 1985. Dr. Rescorla is Director of the Child Study Institute of Bryn Mawr, which provides clinical services to children and families. She is also Director of the Bryn Mawr Early Childhood Programs, which include the Phebe Anna Thorne School for typically developing children and the Language Enrichment Program for children with language delays. Dr. Rescorla did a clinical internship at the Yale Child Study Center and then continued her clinical training at the Philadelphia Child Guidance Center and the Children's Hospital of Philadelphia. Before joining the faculty at Bryn Mawr in 1985, she was a research associate at the Yale Child Study Center and a lecturer at the University of Pennsylvania. Her honors include the McPherson Award for outstanding performance and service to Bryn Mawr College. Dr. Rescorla developed the Language Development Survey (LDS), a screening tool for identifying language delay in young children. She won the *Journal of Speech and Hearing Disorders* Editor's Award in 1989 for her paper introducing the LDS, and she has served as an Associate Editor for the *Journal of Speech and Hearing Research*. She has presented findings from her 15-year longitudinal study on late talkers at many national and international conferences as well as in numerous publications. Dr. Rescorla is a licensed clinical psychologist and a certified school psychologist. She maintains a clinical practice at the Child Study Institute, where she works with children and their families and consults with schools. In addition to her research on language delays in young children and in longitudinal patterns of school achievement, Dr. Rescorla conducts research on empirically based assessment of emotional and behavioral problems in children, adolescents, and adults. She has given many research presentations and training workshops on empirically based assessment, both in the United States and abroad.

Preface

Around the world, many forces are at work to bring people of different cultures together. These forces include both voluntary migration to seek new opportunities and involuntary migration to escape intolerable conditions. As people from different cultures encounter one another, the results vary enormously. One kind of positive result is the blending of diverse cultural characteristics into vibrant new combinations. Another kind of result is peaceful coexistence without much blending. Less positive results include chronic tensions between different groups and outbreaks of bloody strife.

Decisions about migration and about relations with other groups are usually made by adults. However, tens of millions of children must cope with the consequences of these decisions. The consequences for immigrant and minority children include immersion in educational, social welfare, and mental health systems that may be ill equipped to evaluate and help them. Unfortunately, prevailing theories of children's development and functioning that stem from only a handful of cultures may not be applicable to children from diverse cultures.

In this book we bring together findings from many cultures. Our purpose is to examine similarities and differences between cultures in the problems reported for children, the prevalence of such problems, the patterning of the reported problems, and the correlates of the problems. Comprehensive understanding of normal development and of its perturbations requires knowledge of cultural variations in children's problems. This understanding is especially urgent in these days of both cultural blending and cultural clashes.

Because *what* is known depends heavily on *how* it is known, we present multicultural aspects of psychopathology from two perspectives: the empirically based and the diagnostically based approaches. Both of these approaches have generated impressive amounts of international research. Although there are important differences between the empirically based and diagnostically based approaches, the two approaches need not be mutually exclusive. On the contrary, multicultural findings from both perspectives can contribute to new ways of understanding, assessing, preventing, and treating psychopathology.

This book is intended for all who care about children's behavioral, emotional, and social problems and their cultural variations. Because the book makes extensive use of research findings, readers would benefit from having some familiarity with the language of research in the behavioral sciences. However, the main issues, findings, and conclusions can be understood without such knowledge.

As will be evident from reading the book, researchers from many cultures have contributed to the knowledge base. We have been privileged to work with wonderful colleagues from amazingly diverse cultures. We have also been privileged to have exceptional collaborators in all aspects of our research and to have benefited greatly from comments on the manuscript by Drs. Hector Bird, Levent Dumenci, Masha Ivanova, Stephanie McConaughy, Barry Nurcombe, Michael Sawyer, and Frank Verhulst. We are especially grateful to Rachel Bérubé, who prepared the manuscript and its many changes with great care and patience.

Contents

MULTICULTURAL UNDERSTANDING
OF CHILD AND ADOLESCENT PSYCHOPATHOLOGY

CHAPTER 1

Why Should We Do Multicultural Research on Children's Problems?

For thousands of years, human cultures have followed amazingly diverse pathways. Yet, despite their diversity, human cultures also display some striking similarities. Just as Bach's Goldberg Variations express many intricate permutations of a single basic theme, so do human cultures express many permutations of certain basic themes. One basic theme concerns the birth and development of children. Another basic theme concerns intense emotions that need to be channeled, such as anger and sadness. Yet another basic theme concerns variations in how children respond to the challenges and opportunities they face as they grow up. Marked differences in language, religion, art, and social systems reveal fascinating cultural variations in how these themes are expressed. Research in different cultures reveals equally fascinating variations in childrearing practices related to these themes. Survival of the human species under incredibly varied conditions and the persistence of so many cultural variations attest to the adaptability of the species and to its delightful diversity.

Despite the successful survival of the species, there is nevertheless cause for concern about children whose developmental courses are not so successful. Over the past few decades, efforts have become more systematic to identify and help children whose behavioral and emotional problems impair their functioning. The most systematic efforts have occurred in economically developed cultures. However, a full understanding of children's behavioral and emotional problems and help for

1

such problems around the world require research and intervention efforts that include all kinds of cultures.

In this chapter we present the case for doing multicultural research on children's problems. The case for doing such research is based on the need for members of helping professions to care for children from diverse backgrounds. Findings from multicultural research can help us improve our ways of caring for children from different backgrounds. Multicultural research can also contribute to our understanding of the developmental course of psychopathology by identifying similarities and differences across cultures in the problems children manifest, in the prevalence and patterning of such problems, and in the correlates of the problems.

THREATS TO CHILDREN'S MENTAL HEALTH

Millions of children face grave threats to their mental health. War, famine, disease, genocide, malnutrition, abandonment, military conscription, and slavery threaten many children. Even in the more secure parts of the world, child abuse, family instability, exposure to violence, poverty, substance abuse, and parental psychopathology are common threats to children's well-being. In addition to environmental threats, various biological liabilities make children vulnerable to maladaptive deviations from healthy development.

Mental health professionals, school psychologists, health care providers, educators, and welfare workers are increasingly called upon to help children whose backgrounds are very different from their own. Some of the calls for help come from cultures that lack indigenous personnel. However, even where indigenous personnel are available, they often need to help refugee and immigrant children whose backgrounds differ greatly from their own. In pluralistic societies, increasing sensitivity to cultural differences among native-born groups also argues for multicultural approaches to helping children.

FROM DICHOTOMOUS CATEGORIES
TOWARD MULTICULTURAL THINKING

The world and its inhabitants are very complex. To deal with this complexity, people construct categories. These categories help to simplify information. However, categories may oversimplify reality in misleading ways. To avoid the potentially misleading effects of preconceived categories on our understanding of multicultural similarities and differences, it is helpful to highlight some common categorical distinctions. In the following sections we explore dichotomous categories that may interfere with our understanding of multicultural variations.

"We" versus "They"

Cultural differences may seem too complex to be understood in any coherent way. To cope with this complexity, people often view each other in terms of two categories that can be labeled as "we" versus "they." Throughout recorded history, people have found innumerable ways to distinguish the *we* from the *they*, whether by physical appearance, language, religion, nationality, tribe, occupation, or social status. Too often, the distinctions between we and they become justifications for bloodshed. We-versus-they distinctions have driven ethnic cleansing, genocide, holy wars, strife over differences in language, and many forms of harmful discrimination.

To outsiders, the differences between the *we* and the *they* in a particular conflict may seem trivial. Yet even minor differences lead to bloodshed. Ironically, the distinctions between the *we* versus the *they* can quickly change. Struggles between subgroups within larger groups can become as deadly as struggles between the larger groups. Civil wars can be as bitter and bloody as wars between nations. And doctrinal differences within particular religions can fuel struggles as fierce as those between religions.

The we-versus-they dichotomy often obscures the following basic fact: All humans are members of the same species. As members of the same species, all humans follow the same sequence of biological, cognitive, and linguistic development. Despite the developmental similarities, however, there are also important individual differences: Genetic and environmental influences can produce marked individual differences in developmental rates, in the endpoints that are achieved, in temperament, and in adaptive success within particular environments. Equally important, the microenvironments of children's families and neighborhoods, as well as the macrocultural environments in which children develop, differ widely with respect to the content, models, rewards, and punishments that affect what children learn.

To understand and ameliorate children's problems, we need to take account of both the consistencies characterizing the human species and the individual differences resulting from genetic and environmental factors, as well as group differences associated with cultural factors. No humans, including the authors of this book, are immune to the we-versus-they mindset. Nevertheless, we seek to present multicultural findings regarding children's problems from perspectives that take account of both human diversity and the common challenges people face in rearing their young. We use the term "multicultural" to include the term "cross-cultural," which implies comparisons of cultures that are assumed to be separate and distinct from each other. Our use of *multicultural* also includes cultural variations within countries as well as between countries.

The terms "cultural" and "multicultural" have a variety of meanings related to group differences in behaviors, attitudes, traditions, values, and ideals. Nationality, language, ethnicity, and other characteristics can be used to identify members of cultural groups. Most of the research reviewed in this book compares findings for groups of children who speak a particular language, share a particular nationality, and live within a particular country or other geographical entity, such as a commonwealth or a province within a country. In our comparisons of findings for problems reported for children from different cultural groups, use of the same standardized assessment procedures in all the cultural groups provides a basis for operationally defining multicultural variations in terms of the scores obtained by the different groups.

"The West versus the Rest" and Other Cultural Dichotomies

In an article subtitled "The Perilous Problems of Cultural Dichotomies in a Globalizing Society," Hermans and Kempen (1998) argued that conceptualization of cultural variations in terms of dichotomies interferes with understanding the increasing interconnections between cultures. An especially influential dichotomy is "the West versus the rest." According to this dichotomy, western cultures are characterized by individualism (Dumont, 1985), egocentricity (Shweder & Bourne, 1984), and primary control, whereby individuals are rewarded for influencing existing realities (Weisz, Rothbaum, & Blackburn, 1984). In contrast, non-Western cultures are characterized by wholism, sociocentricity, and secondary control, whereby individuals are rewarded for adapting to existing realities.

Another influential dichotomy is "individualism versus collectivism" (Triandis, 1989). This dichotomy highlights differences between (1) cultures in which personal goals have priority over the goals of collectives, versus (2) cultures in which people either make no distinction between personal and collective goals or they subordinate personal goals to collective goals.

Even if these dichotomies are merely viewed as the opposite ends of dimensions of cultural variation, Hermans and Kempen (1998) maintained that such dichotomies falsely represent "cultures as internally homogeneous and externally distinctive" (p. 1119). In responding to critics of their views, Hermans and Kempen (1999) argued against "the disproportionate use of category labels to characterize cultures ... [which] reduces cultures to things (reification) possessing traitlike attributes" (p. 840). In referring to reification, Hermans and Kempen were warning that categorical thinking tends to reify abstractions concerning cultures as if cultures were objects. For example, even if we find significant cross-cultural differences in responses to measures of individualistic versus collectivistic values, we should not assume that the values held by all members of one culture differ categorically from the values held by all members of another culture.

Avoiding Reification of Categories

In considering multicultural similarities and variations in child psychopathology, we occasionally use categorical labels to communicate particular views. However, by focusing on quantitative data obtained for large samples of children in multiple cultures and by highlighting differences within as well as between cultures, we seek to avoid the reification of cultural dichotomies and other categories. Because the findings inevitably depend on how data are obtained, we also compare conclusions based on data obtained from multiple sources and methods whenever possible.

Variations within and between Cultures

The term *culture* may seem to imply enduring characteristics of all members of one group that make them categorically different from all members of other groups. However, in referring to multicultural comparisons, we do not imply that all members of one cultural group share intrinsic characteristics that make them categorically different from all members of other cultural groups. Instead, we stress that culture is merely a convenient term for shared social conventions that are associated with characteristics such as nationality, ethnicity, and language. Culture may also refer to social conventions shared by people from a particular socioeconomic stratum (SES) if they differ much from people of other SES. However, the variations *within* cultural groups, both at a particular point in time and from one time to another, may be as important as the variations *between* cultural groups. The forces of globalization that are exposing members of each culture to multiple cultural influences may also intensify differences within each culture (Arnett, 2002).

EMIC AND ETIC VIEWPOINTS ON MULTICULTURAL RESEARCH

Multicultural researchers distinguish two viewpoints from which to describe behavior that occurs within a particular culture, as explained in the following sections.

The Emic Viewpoint

From the *emic* (pronounced ′ē-mik) viewpoint, behavior is studied from inside a particular cultural system in order to understand the meaning of that behavior within that system. The linguist Kenneth Pike (1954, 1967) coined the term *emic* by shortening the linguistic term *phonemic*, which refers to units of sound that speakers of a particular language recognize as components of words.

The Etic Viewpoint

From the *etic* (pronounced ′ĕ-tik) viewpoint, behavior is studied via standardized methods that are applicable to multiple cultures. Pike coined the term *etic* by shortening the linguistic term *phonetic*, which refers to linguists' systems for representing the total repertoire of sounds used in all human languages. Phonetic systems provide standardized methods of assessing sounds used in different languages, even though not all the sounds are used phonemically (i.e., are recognized as components of words) by speakers of each language. Analogously, etic approaches to multicultural research provide methods for assessing behavior in similar standardized ways in different cultures, even though the behaviors may not have identical meanings to members of each culture.

Emic and Etic Perspectives on Development and Psychopathology

Many classic studies of childrearing in particular cultures have applied emic perspectives (Whiting & Child, 1953). Using ethnographic methods, such studies richly describe children and parents within each culture. Although emic perspectives yield important pictures of individual cultures, comparisons of findings from multiple cultures require methods that can be used in all the cultures that are compared. In this book we compare findings obtained via standardized empirically based and diagnostically based assessment of children in many cultures. We thus approach the multicultural study of psychopathology from an etic viewpoint.

Applying Etic Assessment Procedures to Psychopathology

Most multicultural research on child psychopathology uses standardized assessment procedures. When assessment of children's problems is first attempted in a culture that lacks indigenous assessment instruments, translations of instruments that have been developed in other cultures are often used. If, despite the vicissitudes of translation, such instruments are found to work well in the culture, they can enable members of a particular culture to capitalize on procedures and knowledge developed in other cultures without having to start from scratch. The growing interdependence of cultures with respect to computerization, economics, science, and immigration both facilitates and necessitates multicultural transfers of many kinds of technology, including standardized procedures for assessing psychopathology. Etic assessment procedures facilitate systematic examination of both differences and similarities between cultures (Tanaka-Matsumi & Draguns, 1997). Equally important, such procedures provide an international language for communicating about children's functioning in many cultures.

Although we apply etic perspectives in this book, we recognize that emic perspectives are also needed for understanding child psychopathology in each culture. Emic perspectives can illuminate reasons for the cultural variations in children's problems that etic procedures identify. For example, to probe why gender differences for some kinds of problems are found in some cultures but not in other cultures, emic procedures may be very helpful.

EMPIRICALLY BASED AND DIAGNOSTICALLY BASED APPROACHES TO PSYCHOPATHOLOGY

Much of the multicultural research on child psychopathology has been generated by empirically based and diagnostically based approaches (Bird, 1996). These approaches differ in certain ways. Nevertheless, there are important points of contact between them that can enhance our understanding of psychopathology both within and across cultures. The particular aspects of the two approaches that are most relevant to this book concern the following tasks:

1. *Assessment*, which is the identification and measurement of the distinguishing features of individuals and of patterns of problems.
2. *Taxonomy*, which is the grouping of individuals and of patterns of problems according to their distinguishing features.

Both empirically and diagnostically based approaches need to identify the distinguishing features of individuals and of patterns of problems, and both need to group individuals and patterns according to their distinguishing features.

Empirically Based Assessment and Taxonomy

The word *empirical* stems from the Greek word *empeiria,* meaning experience (Mish, 1988, p. 408). The empirically based approach to assessment and taxonomy systematically draws on the experience of people who have knowledge of children's functioning in various contexts. These people include parents, teachers, and the children themselves. As detailed in Chapter 2, the empirically based approach obtains people's ratings of questionnaire items that describe specific problems. In developing empirically based assessment instruments, researchers obtain ratings on large samples of children, then cull and revise the problem items on the basis of findings and feedback from many raters. The problem items are also tested for their effectiveness in identifying children who need help. In order to derive taxonomic constructs, researchers statistically analyze ratings of large samples of children to identify patterns of problems that tend to occur together. These patterns of co-occurring problems are called *syndromes*, in the sense of things that occur together (from the Greek word *syndrome*, meaning "the act of running together"; Gove, 1971, p. 2320).

In effect, the empirically based approach uses a *bottom-up* strategy whereby children's problems are assessed in terms of data obtained from raters who see the children in various contexts. The assessment data are then analyzed statistically to derive taxonomic constructs. As an example, a syndrome of aggressive behavior problems has been found in many multivariate analyses of children's problems (e.g., Achenbach & Rescorla, 2001; Quay & Peterson, 1996). Chapter 2 details the syndromes and scales derived statistically according to the bottom-up approach. The bottom-up strategy differs from the strategy employed by the diagnostically based approach, which is described in the following section.

Diagnostically Based Assessment and Taxonomy

The diagnostically based approach stems from nosological models of psychopathology. The term *nosological* refers to classification of diseases (from Latin *nosos*, meaning disease; Gove, 1971, p. 1542). Diagnostically based models of psychopathology describe children's behavioral and emotional problems as symptoms of diseases or, more broadly speaking, of disorders. From the diagnostic perspective, taxonomies should consist of categories of disorders, whereas assessment should determine whether children meet sufficient criteria for particular disorders to be classified as having those disorders. The goal of diagnostically based assessment and taxonomy is thus to classify individuals according to specific categories of disorders. In the United States, the fourth edition of the American Psychiatric Association's (1994, 2000) *Diagnostic and Statistical Manual of Mental Disorders* (DSM-IV) is currently the dominant nosology for child psychopathology. The tenth edition of the *International Classification of Diseases* (ICD-10; World Health Organization, 1992) is also used in many countries, including the United States.

In contrast to the bottom-up strategy of the empirically based approach, the diagnostically based approach uses a *top-down* strategy whereby experts initially formulate diagnostic categories based on their clinical experience. These diagnostic categories can be viewed as taxonomic constructs. For each diagnostic category, the experts then choose criteria for determining whether a child has the disorder represented by that category. For example, one DSM-IV diagnostic category is designated as conduct disorder (CD). Those who formulated DSM-IV stipulated that, to meet criteria for CD, a child must manifest at least 3 of the 15 kinds of behavior problems specified as symptoms of CD. Chapter 3 details the diagnostic constructs and criteria that are most relevant to multicultural studies of child psychopathology using the top-down approach.

THE VALUE OF MULTICULTURAL RESEARCH ON CHILDREN'S PROBLEMS

There are several important reasons for doing multicultural research on children's problems. Multicultural research can advance understanding of adaptive and maladaptive functioning, can illuminate developmental aspects of psychopathology, and can help service providers around the world meet children's needs. To do multicultural research on cultural variations in the prevalence, patterning, and correlates of children's problems, it is necessary to use the same standardized methods to assess psychopathology in different cultures. Because empirically based and diagnostically based approaches are used so widely, another reason for doing multicultural research is to advance the dialogue between these different approaches. Such research will enhance our understanding of psychopathology in general, as well as of multicultural aspects in particular.

Understanding Adaptive and Maladaptive Functioning

By studying variations in functioning within and across multiple cultures, we can better understand factors associated with successful versus unsuccessful adaptation under various conditions. For example, certain factors may be associated with successful adaptation under a broad range of conditions both within and across cultures; other factors may be associated with unsuccessful adaptation under a broad range of conditions; still other factors may be associated with successful adaptation under some conditions but not under other conditions. Findings that are similar in multiple cultures can alert us to risk and protective factors that play similar roles across cultures. Conversely, findings that differ between cultures can alert us to risk and protective factors that may be more culture specific.

Illuminating Developmental Aspects of Psychopathology

Children develop within the microcultures of families and neighborhoods that are, in turn, affected by larger macrocultures characterized by particular languages, traditions, social structures, economies, values, and attitudes. Multicultural research on the development of psychopathology can reveal the degree to which associations between development and particular adaptational problems are similar or different in different macrocultures. Such research can also tell us which adaptive and maladaptive sequences are similar across multiple cultures and which ones are more culture specific. This information can provide a basis for understanding variations in the developmental course of psychopathology. In addition, developmental studies of psychopathology may be easier in cultures that offer better access to relevant participants and data than in less accessible cultures. If cross-culturally robust methodology is used, developmental findings from a few cultures may be generalizable to other cultures.

Helping Service Providers Help Children

Multicultural research on children's problems can help service providers by increasing their understanding of the variations within and between cultures and of the particular problems that may be more common in some cultural groups than others. Multicultural research can also help us develop and test assessment instruments for use with children from multiple cultures. If certain assessment instruments are found to be practical, cost effective, reliable, and valid in several cultures, then providers in other cultures may benefit from the research and development work done with those instruments in the initial cultures. If the instruments are used to assess representative samples of children in new cultures, it can be determined whether problems reported for children in the new cultures differ significantly from the problems reported for children in the cultures where the instruments were initially used.

If significant differences are found between the problems reported for representative samples of children from different cultures, these differences need to be considered when evaluating children from each culture. For example, if most children in a representative sample from Culture A are reported to have many more problems of a particular kind than most children from other cultures, knowledge of this finding can help providers distinguish between the high problem levels that characterize most Culture A children and the problems that may be more specific to a particular child from Culture A. Nevertheless, when evaluating a child, providers always need to evaluate all relevant characteristics of that child, no matter where he or she currently resides.

STRUCTURE OF THE BOOK

In Chapters 2 and 3 we present details of the empirically based and diagnostically based approaches to psychopathology, respectively. Chapter 3 also compares the two approaches with respect to their major points of contact and differences. Our presentations highlight the conceptual frameworks, methodologies, reliabilities, and validities of the relevant assessment instruments. They also highlight the taxonomic constructs on which the assessment instruments focus.

Chapters 4, 5, and 6 present multicultural research on empirically based scale scores, correlates of scale scores, and patterns of problems. Analogously, Chapters 7 and 8 present multicultural research on prevalence rates, correlates, and patterns of disorders defined in terms of diagnostic categories.

In Chapter 9, we compare findings from the empirically based and diagnostically based approaches. Chapter 10 then delineates challenges posed by the findings and strategies for meeting the challenges. In Chapter 11 we consider ways in which multicultural research contributes to understanding, assessing, preventing, and treating child psychopathology.

SUMMARY

Across the world, mental health professionals, school psychologists, health care providers, educators, and welfare workers must increasingly serve children from backgrounds that differ markedly from their own. In addition, growing recognition of the need to help troubled children is leading cultures that lack indigenous mental health assessment procedures to try procedures that have been developed elsewhere.

Multicultural differences are sometimes perceived in dichotomous terms, such as "we versus they" and "the West versus the rest." Such dichotomies may unduly mask the many differences between members of each culture as well as similarities between members of different cultures.

The term *culture* may seem to imply enduring characteristics of all members of one group that distinguish them from all members of other groups. However, individual differences among members of each cultural group may be as important as differences between cultural groups.

We outlined the *emic* perspective, which emphasizes the study of behavior from within a particular culture, and the *etic* perspective, which uses standardized methods to compare behavior across cultures. We also outlined the *empirically based* ("bottom-up") approach to psychopathology, which uses reports by multiple informants to derive and assess syndromes, and the *diagnostically based* ("top-down") approach, which conceptualizes children's problems as symptoms of disorders.

Multicultural research on children's problems can improve our understanding of adaptive and maladaptive functioning within and across cultures. It can also advance the developmental study of psychopathology and assist service providers in helping children.

CHAPTER 2

The Empirically Based "Bottom-Up" Approach to Psychopathology

As outlined in Chapter 1, the empirically based approach makes use of the experience of different kinds of informants to obtain data on children's problems in multiple contexts. In this book we focus mainly on data obtained from parents, teachers, and children themselves. However, empirically based assessment procedures are also available for obtaining data from clinical interviewers, psychological examiners, observers who record children's behavior in group settings such as classrooms, self-reports by adults from age 18 to over 90, and reports by people who know the adults who are being assessed (Achenbach, Newhouse, & Rescorla, 2004; Achenbach & Rescorla, 2001, 2003; Conners, Erhardt, & Sparrow, 1999; McConaughy & Achenbach, 2001, 2004).

The empirically based approach uses data from multiple informants to derive syndromes from statistical analyses of problems. The use of statistically derived syndromes to form taxonomic constructs contrasts with the diagnostically based top-down approach to psychopathology. The top-down approach forms taxonomic constructs based on experts' agreement on categories of disorders, for which the experts then formulate definitions in terms of symptoms and yes/no decision rules.

For purposes of exposition, we compare and contrast the bottom-up and top-down approaches in various ways; however, these different approaches are not mutually exclusive. Instead, because both approaches may advance our understanding of psychopathology, we work toward a synthesis of their contributions to understanding, assessing, preventing, and treating child psychopathology. In the present chapter we detail the rationale for empirically based assessment and its multicultural applications. We then present the methodology of the bottom-up approach, including various instruments, statistical procedures, samples that have provided the basis for particular taxonomic constructs, and samples on which norms are based. We also present empirically based syndrome scales, DSM-oriented scales, and psychometric properties of the scales, including internal consistency and reliability, plus correlations among ratings by various informants. Thereafter, we present an overview of validity findings. Chapter 3 details the diagnostically based approach and compares it with the empirically based approach. Although each approach spans a broad spectrum of problems, no approach or assessment instrument can be expected to include every problem that may possibly be relevant to evaluating children's functioning in every culture.

RATIONALE FOR THE EMPIRICALLY BASED APPROACH

Many diagnostic categories for adult psychopathology originated in the 19th century with Emil Kraepelin's (1883) system for classifying major disorders. Although the names and specific criteria for the categories have changed since the 19th century, many of the original categories for adult psychopathology still have counterparts in the DSM. However, most diagnostic categories for child psychopathology have a far shorter history. Until 1968, the prevailing DSM provided only the following two diagnostic categories for child psychopathology: *adjustment reaction of childhood* and *schizophrenic reaction, childhood type* (DSM-I; American Psychiatric Association, 1952). One rationale for the empirically based approach was to determine whether statistically derived patterns of co-occurring problems could provide a more differentiated picture of child psychopathology than was provided in the official nosology.

Early Empirically Based Efforts

In one of the earliest empirically based efforts, Jenkins and Glickman (1946) computed and inspected correlations among problems reported in clinic case records to identify clusters of co-occurring problems. Combinations of statistical and subjective criteria were used to select items for each cluster. Jenkins and Glickman identified five clusters that they designated as *Overinhibited, Unsocialized Aggressive, Socialized Delinquent, Brain-injured,* and *Schizoid.* Hewitt and Jenkins (1946) then found support for the first three clusters in correlations among problems that were reported in another sample of clinic case records.

In the 1960s, the advent of electronic computers facilitated the use of factor analysis to identify patterns of behavioral and emotional problems reported for children. Factor analyses and other multivariate analyses of different rating instruments revealed considerably more syndromes than were implied by the DSM-I categories of adjustment reaction of childhood and schizophrenic reaction, childhood type (e.g., Achenbach, 1966; Borgatta & Fanshel, 1965; Conners, 1970; Miller, 1967; Quay, Morse, & Cutler, 1966). Despite differences in the samples, informants, instruments, and analytic methods, reviews of these and subsequent studies revealed considerable convergence on several specific syndromes, plus two broad-band groupings of problems for which Achenbach (1966) coined the terms "Internalizing" and "Externalizing" (Achenbach & Edelbrock, 1978; Quay, 1979). Internalizing problems occur primarily within the self, such as depression, anxiety, and somatic problems without known medical cause. Externalizing problems, by contrast, involve conflict with other people and with social mores, such as fighting, lying, and stealing. The two broad groupings have also been called "overcontrolled" versus "undercontrolled" and "personality disorder" versus "conduct disorder" (Achenbach & Edelbrock, 1978; Quay, 1979).

Empirically Based Assessment Instruments

Some of the empirically based research efforts yielded assessment instruments designed to assess individual children for clinical services as well as for research purposes (e.g., Achenbach & Edelbrock, 1983; Conners, 1990; Miller, 1981; Quay & Peterson, 1987). Figure 2.1 illustrates the empirically based bottom-up approach to deriving syndromes via statistical analyses of associations among problem items. Table 2.1 outlines the steps involved in developing empirically based instruments for assessing child psychopathology.

Several empirically based assessment instruments have been developed according to steps such ass those outlined in Table 2.1 (e.g., Achenbach, 1991a, 1991b, 1991c; Achenbach & Rescorla, 2000, 2001; Conners, Sitarenios, Parker, & Epstein, 1998a, 1998b; Miller, 1981; Quay & Peterson, 1996). For other instruments, such as the Strengths and Difficulties Questionnaire (SDQ; Goodman, 1997) and the Behavior Assessment System for Children (BASC; Reynolds & Kamphaus, 1992, 2004), statistical methods such as factor analysis have also been

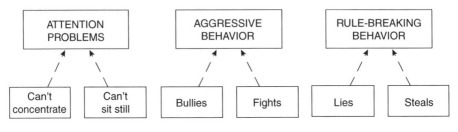

FIGURE 2.1. The bottom-up approach to deriving syndromes via statistical analyses of associations among problem items. Copyright T. M. Achenbach. Reprinted by permission.

used, but the arrangement of items into scales and the placement of items on scales were based on authors' judgments rather than on statistically identified associations. In this chapter we provide an overview of the empirically based instruments that have generated the most multicultural research. We also summarize additional instruments that have used some components of the empirically based approach and that have been used in multicultural research. In later chapters we present findings obtained with empirically based instruments that have been used in multiple cultures.

TABLE 2.1. Developing Empirically Based Instruments for Assessing Child Psychopathology

1. Assemble pool of items that describe children's problems.
2. Formulate instructions and rating scales appropriate for the informants (e.g., parents, teachers, children).
3. Pilot test and revise instruments based on informants' responses.
4. Use instruments to assess large clinical and epidemiological samples.
5. Do statistical analyses to identify syndromes of co-occurring problems.
6. Construct scales and profiles for scoring syndromes from the assessment forms.
7. Construct norms based on scores obtained by samples that are representative of relevant populations.
8. Test reliability and other psychometric properties.
9. Test validity in relation to external criteria.

INSTRUMENTS OF THE ACHENBACH SYSTEM OF EMPIRICALLY BASED ASSESSMENT

We start with empirically based assessment instruments that are components of the Achenbach System of Empirically Based Assessment (ASEBA).

Child Behavior Checklist

The Child Behavior Checklist (CBCL) is descended from an instrument designed to record problems reported in child psychiatric case records. Factor analyses of data obtained from case records with this forerunner of the CBCL yielded several statistically robust syndromes, plus broad-band groupings of problems for which the terms *Internalizing* and *Externalizing* were coined (Achenbach, 1966). Based on findings from the psychiatric case records, plus collaboration with psychiatrists, psychologists, social workers, and parents, the CBCL was developed to assess children's problems and competencies on the basis of reports by parent figures (Achenbach & Edelbrock, 1983; Achenbach & Lewis, 1971).

The CBCL has 21st-century editions for ages 1.5–5 (CBCL/1.5–5) and for ages 6–18 (CBCL/6–18; Achenbach & Rescorla, 2000, 2001). However, not enough multicultural research has been done with the CBCL/1.5–5 to warrant consideration in this book. The CBCL/6–18 has 118 specific problem items, plus 2 items for adding problems that are not specifically listed. Examples of CBCL/6–18 problem items include *Acts too young for age*; *Cruel to animals*; *Too fearful or anxious*; and *Unhappy, sad, or depressed*. The CBCL/6–18 also includes 20 items for assessing children's competencies in sports, other activities, organizations, jobs and chores, friendships, social relations, and school. On both forms of the CBCL, parent figures rate the problem items as *0 = not true (as far as you know)*; *1 = somewhat or sometimes true;* and *2 = very true or often true.* The CBCL/6–18 ratings are based on the child's functioning over the preceding 6 months. Both forms of the CBCL also have open-ended items for reporting illnesses and disabilities, the respondent's concerns about the child, and the best things about the child.

Teacher's Report Form

The 2001 edition of the Teacher's Report Form (TRF) is designed for ages 6–18 (Achenbach & Rescorla, 2001). An analogous form, the Caregiver–Teacher Report Form (C-TRF; Achenbach & Rescorla,

2000), is designed to obtain assessment data from day care providers and preschool teachers for ages 1½–5 years. However, because there has not been sufficient multicultural research with the C-TRF, we focus on the TRF.

Like the CBCL/6–18, the TRF has 118 specific problem items, plus 2 open-ended problem items, all of which are rated as 0, 1, or 2. Most of the TRF problem items have counterparts on the CBCL/6–18, but CBCL/6–18 problem items that are not assessable by teachers (e.g., *Nightmares*) are replaced with items that are more appropriate for teachers to rate (e.g., *Disrupts class discipline*). Ratings of TRF problem items are based on the child's functioning over the preceding 2 months. The CBCL/6–18 competence items are replaced on the TRF with items for assessing the child's academic performance and adaptive characteristics, including how hard the child is working, how appropriately the child is behaving, how much the child is learning, and how happy the child is. The TRF also has open-ended items for reporting illnesses and disabilities, the respondent's concerns about the child, and the best things about the child.

Youth Self-Report

The 2001 edition of the Youth Self-Report (YSR) is designed to obtain 11- to 18-year-olds' reports of their own functioning. The YSR includes 104 specific problem items, 1 open-ended problem item, and 17 competence items. All these items have counterparts on the CBCL/6–18 (Achenbach & Rescorla, 2001). Like the CBCL/6–18, the YSR requests respondents to rate problem items 0, 1, or 2 on the basis of the preceding 6 months. Also like the CBCL/6–18, the YSR has open-ended items for reporting illnesses and disabilities, the youth's concerns, and the best things about the youth. Unlike the CBCL/6–18, the YSR includes 14 socially desirable items (e.g., *I am pretty honest*) that youths rate 0, 1, or 2 according to the same instructions as the problem items.

Relations between Different Editions

In many of the studies cited in this book, data obtained with the CBCL, TRF, and YSR were scored on scales that were published in 1991 (Achenbach, 1991a, 1991b, 1991c). In a few studies, CBCL data were scored on scales that were published in 1983 (Achenbach & Edelbrock, 1983). The 2001 edition of the CBCL/6–18 is a slightly revised version of the CBCL for ages 4–18 (CBCL/4–18) that was the basis for the

1983 and 1991 scales. The CBCL/6–18 has six problem items that differ from the items of the CBCL/4–18.

The 2001 CBCL/6–18 syndromes were derived by using a variety of factor-analytic methods, including exploratory factor analysis (EFA), principal components analysis (PCA), and confirmatory factor analysis (CFA). Although only PCA was used to derive the 1991 CBCL/4–18 syndromes, scores on those syndromes had a mean Pearson correlation (r) of .95 with the 2001 syndromes (correlations between the 1991 and 2001 versions were computed by scoring a large sample of children on both versions and then computing the rs between their scores on the 1991 and 2001 versions; Achenbach & Rescorla, 2001). Scores for Internalizing and Externalizing groupings derived from second-order factor analyses of the 1991 syndromes correlate .98 and .99, respectively, with 2001 Internalizing and Externalizing scores. Total Problems scores from the 1991 CBCL/4–18 correlate 1.00 with Total Problems scores from the 2001 CBCL/6–18.

Like the 2001 CBCL/6–18, the 2001 YSR has six problem items that differ from its 1991 edition. The 2001 TRF has three problem items that differ from its 1991 edition. The mean rs between the 1991 and 2001 scales were .95 for the YSR and .97 for the TRF (Achenbach & Rescorla, 2001). Because the 2001 scales incorporate the few new items and were derived by more comprehensive factor-analytic methodology, we present the 21st-century editions as the most advanced versions of ASEBA scales. When reviewing research findings, we indicate whether they were obtained with the 21st-century or earlier versions of the instruments.

Constructing Empirically Based ASEBA Syndrome Scales

Factor-analytic methodology has been widely used to derive syndromes.We illustrate the construction of syndromes with the procedures that were applied to the CBCL/6–18, TRF, and YSR (Achenbach & Rescorla, 2001). EFA and PCA methodology were used initially to identify syndromes of co-occurring problems that were replicated when different samples and different analytic methods were used. CFA procedures were then used to evaluate and refine the syndromes. (Readers who are not interested in the derivation of the syndrome scales can skim or skip the following sections.)

Factor Analyses of Correlations between Items

To construct the 2001 syndromes, we factor analyzed 4,994 CBCL/6–18 forms. To detect possible gender and age differences in factor structure, we initially performed separate factor analyses for each gender at ages 6–11 and 12–18 years. To ensure that sufficient problems were reported to permit detection of clinically important syndromes, we used only those forms on which the Total Problems scores (sum of 1 and 2 ratings on all problem items) were at, or above, the median of the Total Problems scores obtained for the child's gender and age group in the U.S. National Survey of Children, Youth, and Adults (Achenbach & Rescorla, 2001, provide details of the samples). The children whose forms were included in the factor analyses were assessed in the national survey and in 20 outpatient and inpatient mental health services. The children resided in 40 states of the Unites States, the District of Columbia, Australia, and England. Similar factor analyses were performed on 4,437 TRFs and 2,551 YSRs, for a total of 11,982 forms.

Unidimensional analyses of each factor derived from EFA supported eight factors that were similar in the analyses of each gender/age group on the CBCL/6–18, TRF, and YSR. We identified items that had significant ($p < .01$) loadings of at least .20 on versions of a factor found for the different gender/age groups across the three instruments. (A "factor loading" is like a correlation coefficient that can range from a perfect negative association of –1.00 to a perfect positive association of +1.00. The loading indicates the strength of the association between an item and the syndrome represented by the factor.) The items that met these criteria were then included in tests of correlated eight-factor models for each gender/age group on the CBCL/6–18 and YSR. For the TRF, a combination of a correlated seven-factor model with a hierarchical three-factor model for attention problems was found to be more satisfactory, as explained later.

Multifactor Models in Combined Gender/Age Groups

After the multifactor models were supported in most of the foregoing analyses, we tested the multifactor models with both genders and all ages combined for the CBCL/6–18 and likewise for the TRF and YSR. We evaluated the goodness of fit between the multifactor models and the data by computing the Root Mean Square Error of Approximation (RMSEA; Browne & Cudek, 1993), which has been recommended as the best measure of fit for the types of analyses that were done (Loehlin, 1998; Yu & Muthén, 2002). The RMSEA values were all within the range generally considered to indicate good fit (Yu & Muthén, 2002).

We used the items that loaded significantly on the final versions of the factors to construct eight syndromes for scoring the CBCL/6–18,

TRF, and YSR. The syndromes were given the following names: *Anxious/Depressed, Withdrawn/Depressed* (the 1991 version was called *Withdrawn*), *Somatic Complaints, Social Problems, Thought Problems, Attention Problems, Rule-Breaking Behavior* (the 1991 version was called *Delinquent Behavior*), and *Aggressive Behavior*. A child's score on the CBCL/6–18, TRF, or YSR version of a syndrome is computed by summing the 1 and 2 ratings on the problem items comprising the syndrome. Table 2.2 displays the problem items that comprise each syndrome scale. Chapter 6 reports CFA tests of the syndromes with data from many cultures. Of course, factor analyses of different items could yield different results.

TRF Attention Problems Subscales

Because the items and their mutual associations differ somewhat on the three forms, there are some differences between the items comprising particular syndrome scales scored from the different forms. The biggest difference is between the TRF Attention Problems syndrome and the versions of the Attention Problems syndrome that are scored from the CBCL/6–18 and YSR. Probably owing to the larger pool of attention-related items on the TRF, plus teachers' greater concern about attention problems, the TRF version of the Attention Problems syndrome includes 26 items, whereas the CBCL/6–18 version includes 10 items and the YSR version includes 9 items. Furthermore, factor analyses of the TRF Attention Problems syndrome have supported a hierarchical 3-factor model consisting of a general Attention Problems factor and two specific factors designated as *Inattention* and *Hyperactivity–Impulsivity* (Achenbach & Rescorla, 2001; Dumenci, McConaughy, & Achenbach, 2004).

The general Attention Problems factor can be viewed as representing a construct comprising problems of both inattention and hyperactivity–impulsivity. The TRF Inattention and Hyperactivity–Impulsivity factors can be viewed as representing different phenotypic manifestations of the underlying liabilities encompassed by the general factor. To assess a child in terms of the patterns captured by each of the specific factors, as well as by the general Attention Problems factor, the TRF Attention Problems syndrome is scored in terms of Inattention and Hyperactivity–Impulsivity subscales within the complete Attention Problems syndrome. In Table 2.2 the items of the Inattention subscale are marked with superscript *I*, and the items of the Hyperactivity–Impulsivity subscale are marked with superscript *H*. A child's score for the entire Attention Problems syndrome is the sum of his or her scores

TABLE 2.2. Items Defining the ASEBA School-Age Cross-Informant Syndrome Constructs, plus Items Specific to the CBCL/6–18, YSR, and TRF Syndrome Scales[a]

Anxious/Depressed
14. Cries a lot
29. Fears
30. Fears school
31. Fears doing something bad
32. Must be perfect
33. Feels unloved
35. Feels worthless
45. Nervous, tense
50. Fearful, anxious
52. Feels too guilty
71. Self-conscious
91. Talks or thinks of suicide
112. Worries

Specific to TRF
81. Hurt when criticized[b,d]
106. Anxious to please[b,c]
108. Afraid of making mistakes[b,c]

Withdrawn/Depressed
5. Enjoys little
42. Rather be alone
65. Refuses to talk
69. Secretive
75. Shy, timid
102. Lacks energy
103. Sad
111. Withdrawn

Rule-Breaking Behavior
2. Drinks alcohol[c]
26. Lacks guilt
28. Breaks rules
39. Bad friends
43. Lies, cheats
63. Prefers older kids
67. Runs away[c]
72. Sets fires[c]
73. Sex problems[c,d]
81. Steals at home[c]
82. Steals outside home
90. Swearing
96. Thinks of sex too much
99. Uses tobacco
101. Truant
105. Uses drugs
106. Vandalism[c,d]

Specific to TRF
98. Tardy[b,d]

Somatic Complaints
47. Nightmares[c]
51. Feels dizzy
54. Overtired
56a. Aches, pains
56b. Headaches
56c. Nausea
56d. Eye problems
56e. Skin problems
56f. Stomachaches
56g. Vomiting

Specific to CBCL
49. Constipated[c,d]

Social Problems
11. Too dependent
12. Lonely
25. Doesn't get along
27. Jealous
34. Others out to get him/her
36. Accident-prone
38. Gets teased
48. Not liked
62. Clumsy
64. Prefers younger kids
79. Speech problems

Aggressive Behavior
3. Argues a lot
16. Mean to others
19. Demands attention
20. Destroys own things
21. Destroys others' things
22. Disobedient at home[c]
23. Disobedient at school
37. Gets in fights
57. Attacks people
68. Screams a lot
86. Stubborn, sullen
87. Mood changes
88. Sulks[d]
89. Suspicious
94. Teases a lot
95. Temper
97. Threatens others
104. Loud

Specific to TRF
6. Defiant[b,d]
76. Explosive[b,d]
77. Easily frustrated[b,d]

Thought Problems
9. Can't get mind off thoughts
18. Harms self
40. Hears things
46. Twitching
58. Picks skin
66. Repeats acts
70. Sees things
76. Sleeps less[c]
83. Stores things
84. Strange behavior
85. Strange ideas
100. Trouble sleeping[c]

Specific to CBCL
59. Sex parts in public[c,d]
60. Sex parts too much[c,d]
92. Sleep talks/walks[c,d]

Attention Problems
1. Acts young[I]
4. Fails to finish[I]
8. Can't concentrate[I]
10. Can't sit still[H]
13. Confused[I]
17. Daydreams[I]
41. Impulsive[H]
61. Poor schoolwork[I]
78. Inattentive[I]
80. Stares blankly[d,I]

Specific to TRF
2. Odd noises[b,d,H]
7. Brags[H]
15. Fidgets[b,d,H]
22. Difficulty with directions[b,d,I]
24. Disturbs others[b,d,H]
49. Difficulty learning[b,d,H]
53. Talks out of turn[b,d,H]
60. Apathetic[b,d,I]
67. Disrupts discipline[b,d,H]
72. Messy work[b,d,I]
73. Irresponsible[b,d,I]
74. Shows off[H]
92. Underachieving[b,d,I]
93. Talks too much[H]
100. Fails to carry out tasks[b,d,I]
109. Whining[d,H]

Note. Copyright T. M. Achenbach and L. A. Rescorla. Adapted with permission from Achenbach and Rescorla (2001, p. 88).
[a] Items are designated by the numbers they bear on the CBCL/6–18, YSR, and TRF and summaries of their content.
[b] Not on CBCL.
[c] Not on TRF.
[d] Not on YSR.
[H] TRF Hyperactivity-Impulsivity subscale.
[I] TRF Inattention subscale.

on the Inattention subscale and the Hyperactivity–Impulsivity sub-scale. Consequently, a child can obtain a high score on the Inattention subscale, the Hyperactivity–Impulsivity subscale, both, or neither. In addition, a child's score on the complete Attention Problems syndrome can be deviant if the child obtains at least moderately high scores on both subscales or a high score on one subscale.

Internalizing and Externalizing Groupings

Factor analyses of the correlations between syndromes (i.e., "second-order" factor analyses) have identified an Internalizing group of syndromes that includes the Anxious/Depressed, Withdrawn/Depressed, and Somatic Complaints syndromes. The second-order factor analyses have also identified an Externalizing group of syndromes that includes the Rule-Breaking Behavior and Aggressive Behavior syndromes. Internalizing scores are computed by summing the scores of the three Internalizing syndromes, and Externalizing scores are computed by summing the scores of the two Externalizing syndromes. The Social Problems, Thought Problems, and Attention Problems syndromes are not included in the Internalizing or Externalizing groupings, because they did not load as strongly on either the second-order Internalizing or Externalizing factors as the other syndromes did.

Norming the Scales

To help users evaluate a child's score on ASEBA problem scales in relation to scores obtained by typical children in that child's culture, data from large representative samples of children were used to construct norms. The U.S. norms were constructed from CBCL/6–18, TRF, and YSR scores obtained by a national probability sample (details are provided by Achenbach & Rescorla, 2001). To provide what epidemiologists call a "healthy sample," children who had received mental health, substance abuse, or major special education services in the preceding 12 months were excluded from the normative sample. We assigned standard scores (normalized T scores) to each raw score on each syndrome. The T scores provide a common metric indicating where each child's score stands in relation to the distributions of syndrome scores obtained by the normative sample for that child's age and gender. The syndromes are displayed on profiles for scoring each child in relation to T scores and percentiles derived from the normative sample. Figure 2.2 summarizes the steps by which syndrome scales were constructed for the CBCL/6–18, TRF, and YSR.

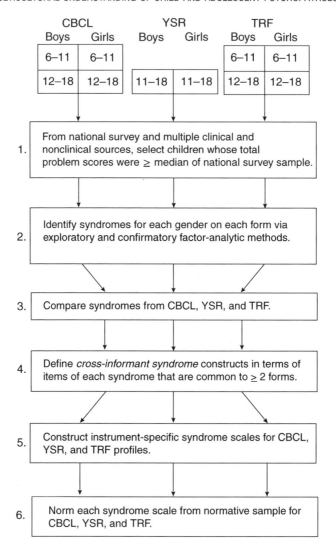

FIGURE 2.2. Summary of steps in constructing the cross-informant syndrome scales for the CBCL/6–18, TRF, and YSR. Copyright T. M. Achenbach and L. A. Rescorla. Adapted with permission from Achenbach and Rescorla (2001, p. 91).

Normal, Borderline, and Clinical Ranges on Scales

The scales for syndromes, Internalizing, Externalizing, and Total Problems provide continuous quantitative measures of various sets of problems. The scales also have cutpoints for distinguishing between the normal range, borderline clinical range, and clinical range, which can be used to identify children who are not likely to need help, those who might need professional help, and those who are most likely to need professional help, respectively.

Constructing DSM-Oriented Scales

An important aim of this book is to integrate different approaches to psychopathology. One way to achieve this integration is by viewing particular data sets from the perspectives of different paradigms. To facilitate applications of diagnostically based constructs to the same data as are used to score empirically based constructs, DSM-oriented scales have been constructed for scoring the CBCL/6–18, TRF, and YSR. The scales were constructed by having an international panel of experts identify CBCL/6–18, TRF, and YSR problem items that they judged to be very consistent with particular DSM-IV diagnostic categories (Achenbach, Dumenci, & Rescorla, 2001, 2003). The experts included 22 psychiatrists and psychologists who had all published on child psychopathology and who came from the following 16 cultures: Australia, Belgium, Canada, China, Germany, Greece, Iceland, Israel, Italy, Jamaica, the Netherlands, Puerto Rico, Spain, Turkey, the United Kingdom, and the United States.

The six scales for which the experts identified substantial numbers of items were designated as follows: *Affective Problems, Anxiety Problems, Somatic Problems, Attention Deficit/Hyperactivity Problems, Oppositional Defiant Problems,* and *Conduct Problems.* The TRF version of the Attention Deficit/Hyperactivity Problems scale also has Inattention and Hyperactivity–Impulsivity subscales consisting of problem items that the experts judged to be very consistent with the DSM-IV Inattentive and Hyperactive–Impulsive types of ADHD, respectively. Table 2.3 displays the problem items that comprise the DSM-oriented scales for the CBCL/6–18, TRF, and YSR.

Like the empirically based syndromes, each DSM-oriented scale is scored by summing the 1 and 2 scores obtained by a child on the items of the scale. The DSM-oriented scales are displayed on profiles in relation to T scores and percentiles based on the same normative samples as the empirically based syndromes. In addition, like the empirically

TABLE 2.3. CBCL/6–18, TRF, and YSR Items[a] Rated by ≥ 64% of Experts as Very Consistent with DSM-IV Categories

		DSM-oriented category			
1. Affective Problems	2. Anxiety Problems	3. Somatic Problems	4. Attention Deficit Hyperactivity Problems	5. Oppositional Defiant Problems	6. Conduct Problems
5. Enjoys little	11. Dependent	56a. Aches	4. Fails to finish[I]	3. Argues	15. Cruel to animals[c]
14. Cries	29. Fears	56b. Headaches	8. Can't concentrate[I]	15. Defiant[b,d]	16. Mean
18. Harms self	30. Fears school	56c. Nausea	10. Can't sit still[H]	22. Disobedient at home[c]	21. Destroys others' things
24. Doesn't eat well[c]	45. Nervous	56d. Eye problems	15. Fidgets[H]	23. Disobedient at school	26. Lacks guilt
35. Feels worthless	50. Fearful	56e. Skin problems	22. Difficulty with directions[b,d,I]	86. Stubborn	28. Breaks rules
52. Feels too guilty	112. Worries	56f. Stomachaches	24. Disturbs others[b,d,H]	95. Temper	37. Fights
54. Overtired		56g. Vomits	41. Impulsive[H]		39. Bad companions
60. Apathetic[b,d]			53. Talks out of turn[b,d,H]		43. Lies, cheats
76. Sleeps less[c]			67. Disrupts class[b,d,H]		57. Attacks
77. Sleeps more[c]			78. Inattentive[I]		67. Runs away[c]
91. Talks suicide			93. Talks much[H]		72. Sets fires[c]
100. Sleep problems[c]			100. Fails to carry out tasks[b,d,I]		73. Behaves irresponsibly
102. Underactive			104. Loud[H]		81. Steals at home[c]
103. Sad					82. Steals outside home
					90. Swears
					97. Threatens
					101. Truant
					106. Vandalism

Note. Copyright T. M. Achenbach and L. A. Rescorla. Adapted with permission from Achenbach, Dumenci, and Rescorla (2001, p. 8).
[a] Items are designated in the table with the numbers they bear on the CBCL/6–18, TRF, and YSR and summaries of their content.
[b] Not on CBCL.
[c] Not on TRF.
[d] Not on YSR.
[H] TRF Hyperactivity–Impulsivity subscale.
[I] TRF Inattention subscale.

based syndromes, the DSM-oriented scales have cutpoints that distinguish between the normal range, borderline clinical range, and clinical range.

Psychometric Properties of ASEBA Empirically Based and DSM-Oriented Scales

Table 2.4 summarizes the psychometric properties of the empirically based syndromes, DSM-oriented scales, Internalizing, Externalizing, and Total Problems scales for the CBCL/6–18, TRF, and YSR. Cronbach's (1951) alpha coefficient measures the internal consistency among the items of each scale. Except for Total Problems, each alpha coefficient shown in Table 2.4 is the mean of the alpha coefficients for scales of a particular type, as scored from one of the three assessment instruments. For example, under the heading *Empirically based syndromes,* the alpha of .83 to the right of *CBCL/6–18* is the mean of the alpha coefficients obtained for the eight empirically based syndromes scored from the CBCL/6–18.

The column to the right of the alpha coefficients displays test–retest reliabilities in terms of *r*s between scale scores obtained at mean intervals of 8–16 days. The *r*s indicate the degree to which children's scores retained the same rank order from the first assessment to the second assessment. Except for the Total Problems score, each *r* is the mean of the *r*s for a set of scales, such as the empirically based syndromes scored from the CBCL/6–18. (All mean *r*s reported in this book were computed via Fisher's *z* transformation, unless otherwise noted.)

Cross-Informant Correlations

The five columns to the right of the test–retest reliability column display mean *r*s between ratings by different combinations of informants, averaged across a particular set of scales scored from the relevant forms. For example, under the heading *Empirically based syndromes*, the CBCL/6–18 row displays mean *r*s between ratings of empirically based syndromes by different respondents, including at least one respondent who completed the CBCL/6–18. Under the heading *Parent × parent*, the mean *r* of .75 is thus the mean of the *r*s between syndrome scales scored from CBCL/6–18 forms completed by children's mothers and fathers.

It should be noted that the cross-informant *r*s are not measures of reliability but of the degree of similarity between ratings by people who may be aware of different aspects of a child's functioning. Cross-

TABLE 2.4. Psychometric Properties of ASEBA Empirically Based and DSM-Oriented Scales

Scales	Alpha[a]	Test–retest reliability[b]	Cross-informant correlations				
			Parent × parent[c]	Teacher × teacher[d]	Parent × teacher[e]	Parent × youth[f]	Teacher × youth[g]
Empirically based syndromes							
CBCL/6–18	.83	.89	.75	NA	.28[h]	.46[h]	NA
TRF	.85	.89	NA	.60	.28[h]	NA	.20[h]
YSR	.79	.79	NA	NA	NA	.46[h]	.20[h]
DSM-oriented scales							
CBCL/6–18	.82	.88	.73	NA	.29[h]	.45	NA
TRF	.84	.85	NA	.58	.29[h]	NA	.21[h]
YSR	.76	.79	NA	NA	NA	.45	.21[h]
Internalizing and Externalizing							
CBCL/6–18	.92	.92	.79	NA	.29[h]	.52[h]	NA
TRF	.93	.88	NA	.71	.29[h]	NA	.23[h]
YSR	.90	.85	NA	NA	NA	.52[h]	.23[h]
Total Problems							
CBCL/6–18	.97	.94	.80	NA	.35[h]	.54[h]	NA
TRF	.97	.95	NA	.55	.35[h]	NA	.21[h]
YSR	.95	.87	NA	NA	NA	.54[h]	.21[h]

Note. Samples included children referred for mental health services and nonreferred children, as detailed by Achenbach and Rescorla (2001). Except for "Total Problems," coefficients are means computed by averaging coefficients for all the relevant scales. Test–retest and cross-informant coefficients are mean rs computed by z transformation. All rs were $p < .05$. Copyright Lawrence Erlbaum Associates. Adapted with permission from Achenbach, Dumenci, and Rescorla (2003, p. 336).

[a]Mean alphas for $N = 1,938–3,210$.
[b]Mean test–retest intervals = 8–16 days; $N = 44$ to 89.
[c]$N = 297$.
[d]$N = 88$.
[e]$N = 1,126$.
[f]$N = 1,038$.
[g]$N = 655$.
[h]Each of these cells duplicates a cell with r for the same combination of raters.

informant differences may occur for many reasons, including the following: (1) differences in how a child behaves in different contexts, such as home versus school (and even in different classes at school); (2) differences in informants' relationships to the child, such as mother versus father and parent versus teacher); (3) differences in what informants notice and remember about a child's behavior; and (4) differences in informants' thresholds for reporting particular problems.

Meta-analyses of cross-informant correlations obtained with many different instruments in many different studies have yielded a mean r of .60 between ratings by people who play similar roles with respect to the children they rate (e.g., pairs of parents, pairs of teachers). The mean r was .28 between people who play different roles with respect to the children they rate (e.g., parents vs. teachers). And the mean r was .22 between children's self-ratings and ratings by adults who know the children, such as parents and teachers (Achenbach, McConaughy, & Howell, 1987). Meta-analyses have shown that cross-informant rs for adult psychopathology are also modest (Achenbach, Krukowski, Dumenci, & Ivanova, 2005).

CONNERS INSTRUMENTS

Parent and teacher rating forms developed by C. Keith Conners have been used in several multicultural studies. Starting with a 39-item version of the Conners Teacher Rating Scale (CTRS-39; Conners, 1969) and a 93-item version of the Conners Parent Rating Scale (CPRS-93; Conners, 1970), there have been many versions, including several "pirate" versions that were not authorized by Conners (Kollins, Epstein, & Conners, 2004, p. 215). Some versions have been very short, with as few as 10 problem items. Prior to publication of the Conners' Rating Scales—Revised (Conners, 1997, 2001), the authorized versions of the Conners forms were scored on diverse scales derived from various factor analyses. However, prior to the factor analytically derived scales of 1997, "a definitive, empirically derived factor structure [had] not been agreed upon" (Conners et al., 1998b, p. 280). Furthermore, as pointed out by Conners et al. (1998b, p. 280), the standardization of the pre-1997 scales was "nonsystematic," and there was no single normative sample.

Since their inception, the Conners forms have been used largely for assessment of attention-deficit/hyperactivity disorder (ADHD), which is their main purpose (Conners, 1997, p. 5). However, the Conners forms are also scored on factorially derived scales for assessing other problems that are considered to be comorbid with ADHD.

Because factor analysis was used as an empirical basis for constructing several of the 1997 scales for scoring the Conners Parent Rating Scale–Revised (CPRS-R) and the Conners Teacher Rating Scale–because Revised (CTRS-R), we summarize these versions of the scales. In reporting multicultural findings for Conners forms, we mention the versions that were used. Because we have found no multicultural studies of other Conners forms, such as the Conners–Wells Adolescent Self-Report Scale (Conners, 2001), we do not address them here. Like ASEBA scales, the Conners scales are scored by summing the ratings for all items comprising the scale. The scores are displayed on profiles in relation to T scores based on normative samples for the child's age and gender. Conners (1997) provides guidelines for evaluating T scores within particular ranges, from "markedly atypical" low scores to "markedly atypical" high scores.

Conners Parent Rating Scale—Revised

One reason for revising the Conners scales was to focus "the revised scales on behaviors that are directly related to ADHD and its associated behaviors"; another reason was to update "the item content to reflect recent knowledge and developments concerning ADHD" (Conners et al., 1998b, p. 258). Starting with a pool of 193 items, Conners et al. (1998b) performed factor analyses of parents' ratings of 2,200 3- to 17-year-old students recruited from approximately 200 schools in the United States and Canada. Based on the student's behavior over the preceding month, the items were rated 0 = Not at all true (Never, Seldom); 1 = Just a little true (Occasionally); 2 = Pretty much true (Often, Quite a bit); or 3 = Very much true (Very often, Very frequently).

The 2,200 CPRS-R forms were randomly divided into derivation and replication samples (N = 1,100 each). The derivation sample was further divided into two random samples of 550 each, which were then subjected to a series of factor analyses. Although the factor analyses provided the basis for syndrome scales, "an item was eliminated from a scale if it lacked conceptual coherence with its factor" (Conners et al., 1998b, p. 259). Based on results for the derivation and replication samples, 57 items were retained for the following scales: A. *Oppositional,* B. *Cognitive Problems/Inattention,* C. *Hyperactivity,* D. *Anxious–Shy,* E. *Perfectionism,* F. *Social Problems,* and G. *Psychosomatic.* The CPRS-R has additional scales comprising items that paraphrase the 18 symptom criteria for the DSM-IV version of ADHD, plus other items, for a total of 80 problem items. Some items are scored on more than one scale, including scales designated as Global Index and ADHD Index. A short form

(CPRS-R:S) includes 27 problem items, which are scored on reduced versions of the Cognitive Problems/Inattention, Oppositional, and Hyperactivity–Impulsivity factor-based scales, plus all 12 items of the ADHD Index.

Conners Teacher Rating Scale—Revised

Conners et al. (1998a) factor analyzed teachers' ratings of 131 items for 1,702 3- to 17-year-old students. Each teacher rated up to 10 students (p. 281). The teachers rated items on 0-1-2-3 response scales like those for the CPRS-R, based on student's behavior over the preceding month.

The 1,702 completed CTRS-R forms were divided into a derivation sample ($N = 1,200$) and a replication sample ($N = 500$). Using procedures like those for the CPRS-R, Conners et al. (1998a) derived syndrome scales via factor analyses and eliminated items that lacked "conceptual coherence" with the factor on which they loaded (Conners et al., 1998a, p. 282), leaving a total of 38 items on the syndrome scales. The following six scales were given the same names as CPRS-R factor-based scales, although there are substantial differences between the items comprising the teacher versus parent versions of the scales: *A. Oppositional, B. Cognitive Problems/Inattention, C. Hyperactivity, D. Anxious–Shy, E. Perfectionism,* and *F. Social Problems.* Because the CTRS-R does not include somatic problems, no equivalent of the CPRS-R Psychosomatic scale was obtained. The CTRS-R also has scales comprising items that paraphrase the 18 DSM-IV symptom criteria for ADHD, plus some other items, for a total of 59 items. A short form (CTRS-R:S) includes 28 items that are scored on reduced versions of the Cognitive Problems/Inattention, Oppositional, and Hyperactivity scales, plus the ADHD Index.

Psychometric Properties of Conners Empirically Based and DSM Scales

Table 2.5 summarizes the psychometric properties of the Conners empirically based scales and its DSM scales for ADHD. The mean alpha coefficients, test–retest reliability rs, and parent × teacher rs were obtained by averaging the coefficients for the relevant scales. The magnitudes of the coefficients are generally comparable to the corresponding coefficients shown in Table 2.4 for the ASEBA scales, except that the somewhat lower test–retest rs for the Conners scales may have resulted from the test–retest intervals of 6–8 weeks versus 8–16 days for the ASEBA scales.

TABLE 2.5. Psychometric Properties of Conners Empirically Based
and DSM Scales

Scales	Alpha[a]	Test–retest reliability[b]	Parent × teacher[c]
Empirically based syndromes			
CPRS-R Scales A to G	.86	.70	.32[d]
CTRS-R Scales A to F	.87	.75	.32[d]
DSM scales for ADHD			
CPRS-R	.91	.75	.43[d]
CTRS-R	.93	.60	.43[d]

Note. Samples for alpha and cross-informant *r*s were from the normative groups recruited from schools, as detailed by Conners (2001). Sources of samples for test–retest *r*s were not specified. Coefficients are means computed by averaging coefficients for all the relevant scales, as reported by Conners (2001). Test–retest and cross-informant coefficients are mean *r*s computed by *z* transformation. All *r*s were *p* < .05.
[a]*N*s were not specified for alphas.
[b]Test–retest intervals = 6–8 weeks; *N* = 49 CPRS-R, 50 CTRS-R.
[c]*N* = 1,024.
[d]Each of these cells duplicates a cell for the same combination of raters.

STRENGTHS AND DIFFICULTIES QUESTIONNAIRE

The Strengths and Difficulties Questionnaire (SDQ) is considered here because some aspects of the empirically based approach have evidently been used in its development, and it has been used in multicultural studies that meet our methodological criteria.

Development of the SDQ

The development of the SDQ appears to have begun when Robert Goodman (1994) used a modified version of a parent rating questionnaire developed by Michael Rutter (1967; Rutter, Tizard, & Whitman, 1970). Goodman added 19 items to the 31 items of the Rutter parent questionnaire. Using parents' ratings of 320 Greater London children with hemiplegia, Goodman subjected the modified Rutter questionnaire to PCA with varimax rotations. Goodman reported that a "rotated solution with just 6 factors was the easiest to interpret and made the greatest clinical sense" (p. 1491). The factors were given the following names: Hyperactivity/Inattention; Prosocial Behavior (comprising many of the prosocial items that Goodman added to the Rutter questionnaire); Conduct Problems/Oppositionality; Somatic/Developmental; Internalization; and Peer Relationships.

Goodman (1997) subsequently reported development of the SDQ to tap five dimensions that he said were suggested by his 1994 factor analysis of the expanded Rutter questionnaire ratings of children with hemiplegia. Goodman now labeled these dimensions as follows: *Conduct Problems; Emotional Symptoms; Hyperactivity; Peer Relationships*; and *Prosocial Behavior* (p. 581). Five items were written for each of these dimensions in a version of the SDQ that could be completed by parents and teachers. No SDQ item was worded identically to any Rutter item, but five items were similarly worded (p. 582). Each SDQ item is rated as *Not True, Somewhat True,* or *Certainly True*. Problem items are scored 0, 1, or 2. Favorably worded items on the problem scales are scored 2, 1, or 0. An example of a favorably worded item on a problem scale is *Generally well behaved, usually does what adults request*; this item is scored on the Conduct Problems scale as *2 = Not True, 1 = Somewhat True,* and *0 = Certainly True*. Items that comprise the Prosocial scale are scored in the opposite direction; high scores indicate high degrees of prosocial characteristics. An example of a Prosocial scale item is *Helpful if someone is hurt, upset or feeling ill*. Parents of 346 children attending either dental clinics or psychiatric clinics in London completed SDQs. Teachers completed SDQs for 185 of the children. Rutter parent questionnaires and Rutter teacher questionnaires were also completed for the children. Four SDQ scales had a mean *r* of .84 with four corresponding scales of the Rutter parent questionnaire and a mean *r* of .90 with corresponding scales of the Rutter teacher questionnaire. (The corresponding Rutter scales were Conduct Problems, Emotional Symptoms, Hyperactivity, and Total Deviance.)

Factor-Analytic Findings

Although Goodman (1997) indicated that the five 5-item scales of the SDQ were not derived directly from empirically based, bottom-up, statistical analyses, he subsequently reported factor analyses of SDQs for the following general population samples of British children: Parent SDQs were analyzed for 9,998 5- to 15-year-olds, teacher SDQs were analyzed for 7,313 5- to 15-year-olds, and self-report SDQs were analyzed for 3,983 11- to 15-year-olds. Goodman (2001) did not specify the measures of association that were analyzed or how the factors were extracted. However, Table 2 in the Goodman (2001) article indicates that the factor loadings were obtained from a varimax rotation of five factors (pp. 1340–1341). According to Goodman's Table 2, all SDQ items rated by parents had their highest loadings on the scale to which Goodman had assigned them. Two SDQ items rated by teachers and two SDQ items rated by youths had loadings on other scales that exceeded or approximated their loadings on the scale to which Goodman had assigned them. The factorial findings displayed in Goodman's Table 2 were thus generally consistent with his previous assignment of items to scales of the SDQ, although the results of a complete bottom-up approach to constructing scales might have been different.

In a study that combined bottom-up EFA analyses with CFA tests of the SDQ scale structure, Dickey and Blumberg (2004) failed to confirm the scale structure in a U.S. national probability sample of 9,574 4- to 17-year-olds. Instead, they found 3 factors, which they designated as "externalizing problems," "internalizing problems," and "positive construal . . . indicating the general extent to which each parent is willing to attribute positive characteristics to the child" (p. 1165). Similar results were obtained in an EFA of SDQ self-ratings by 1,458 Finnish 13- to 17-year-olds (Koskelainen, Sourander, & Vauras, 2001).

Psychometric Properties of the SDQ

Table 2.6 summarizes the psychometric properties of the following SDQ scales: Emotional Symptoms, Conduct Problems, Hyperactivity, Peer Problems, and Total Difficulties (i.e., the sum of the items on the

TABLE 2.6. Psychometric Properties of SDQ Scales

Scales	Alpha[a]	Test–retest reliability[b]	Cross-informant correlations[c] Parent × teacher	Parent × youth	Teacher × youth
Difficulties scales					
Parent SDQ	.66	.64	$.37^d$	$.41^d$	NA
Teacher SDQ	.78	.73	$.37^d$	NA	$.28^d$
Youth SDQ	.59	.56	NA	$.41^d$	$.28^d$
Total Difficulties					
Parent SDQ	.82	.72	$.46^d$	$.48^d$	NA
Teacher SDQ	.87	.80	$.46^d$	NA	$.33^d$
Youth SDQ	.80	.62	NA	$.48^d$	$.33^d$

Note. Samples from the general population of British children (Goodman, 2001). Except for Total Difficulties, coefficients are means computed by averaging the SDQ Emotional Symptoms, Conduct Problems, Hyperactivity–Inattention, and Peer Problems scales. Test–retest and cross-informant coefficients are mean *r*s computed by *z* transformation. All *r*s were *p* < .05.
[a]Alphas for 9,998 Parent SDQs, 7,313 Teacher SDQs, and 3,983 Youth SDQs.
[b]Mean test–retest intervals = 4 to 6 months for 2,091 Parent SDQs, 796 Teacher SDQs, and 781 Youth SDQs.
[c]Cross-informant *r*s for 7,313 Parent × Teacher SDQs, 3,983 Parent × Youth SDQs, and 2,767 Teacher × Youth SDQs.
[d]Each of these cells duplicates a cell for the same combination of raters.

preceding four scales). We computed mean alpha coefficients, test–retest rs, and cross-informant rs for the first four scales by averaging the coefficients for those scales. As shown in Table 2.6, the alphas were smaller than those for the corresponding ASEBA and Conners scales (Tables 2-4 and 2-6, respectively), possibly owing to the smaller number of items on each SDQ scale. The smaller test–retest rs for the SDQ than for the corresponding ASEBA and Conners scales may reflect the longer test–retest interval (4–6 months) for the SDQ. Parent × parent and teacher × teacher rs were not available for the Conners or SDQ scales, but other cross-informant rs were of similar magnitude for all three instruments.

OVERVIEW OF VALIDITY FINDINGS

Validity refers to the accuracy with which instruments assess what they are supposed to assess. The ASEBA and Conners instruments serve many purposes, and their validity can be evaluated in many ways. Because the SDQ is designed primarily as a brief screening instrument, there may be fewer ways to evaluate its validity. One purpose of ASEBA instruments is to identify individuals who may need professional help for behavioral, emotional, or social problems, and/or who need help in strengthening competencies and adaptive functioning. Other purposes include the development of taxonomic groupings of problems and of individuals to advance knowledge of the causes, courses, outcomes, and best treatments for psychopathology. The main purpose of the Conners instruments is to assess ADHD and its related behaviors. Our overview of validity findings is organized in terms of *content validity, criterion-related validity,* and *construct validity.* Most of the validity findings reviewed here are from North America and Europe. Later chapters present diverse findings from many cultures.

VALIDITY OF ASEBA INSTRUMENTS

The most basic kind of validity is *content validity*—that is, the degree to which an instrument's items include what the instrument is intended to assess.

Content Validity of ASEBA Problem Items

Beginning in the 1960s, ASEBA items were developed and refined on the basis of research and practical experience (Achenbach, 1965,

1966; Achenbach & Lewis, 1971). The procedures for selecting items included extensive literature searches, consultation with mental health professionals and special educators, and pilot testing with the kinds of informants for whom the items were intended, such as parents, teachers, and youths. All problem, competence, and adaptive functioning items on the 21st-century editions of the CBCL/6–18, TRF, and YSR were found to be scored significantly ($p < .01$) more favorably for nonreferred than for referred children on one or more of the forms (Achenbach & Rescorla, 2001). (On the problem items, low scores are favorable, because they indicate an absence of problems; on the competence and adaptive functioning items, high scores are favorable, because they indicate good functioning.) These findings support the content validity of the items for measuring characteristics associated with referral for mental health services in the United States. When the items' associations with mental health referral were tested in additional countries, the items have also been found to discriminate significantly between referred and nonreferred children (e.g., Bilenberg, 1999; Montenegro, 1983; Verhulst, 1985; Verhulst & Akkerhuis, 1986; Verhulst, Prince, Vervuurt-Poot, & de Jong, 1989). The content validity of particular ASEBA items with respect to DSM-IV has been supported by international experts' identification of items as being very consistent with particular DSM-IV diagnostic categories (Achenbach et al., 2001).

Criterion-Related Validity of ASEBA Problem Scales

"Criterion-related validity" refers to associations between a particular measure, such as a syndrome scale scored from an ASEBA form, and an external criterion for characteristics that the scale is intended to assess. Separately for each gender, multiple regression analyses of scale scores on referral status, age, ethnicity, and SES have shown that CBCL/6–18, TRF, and YSR scale scores were all associated with referral status much more strongly than with demographic variables (Ns were 3,210 for the CBCL, 3,086 for the TRF, and 1,938 for the YSR). In addition, categorization of children as being in the normal range or combined borderline and clinical ranges was significantly associated with referral status according to odds ratios and chi square tests for every scale (Achenbach & Rescorla, 2001). Significant associations between scale scores and referral for services have also been found in other countries, with appropriate controls for demographic differences (e.g., Bilenberg, 1999; Montenegro, 1983; Verhulst, 1985; Verhulst & Akkerhuis, 1986; Verhulst et al., 1989). Additional validity findings are presented in Chapter 5.

Construct Validity of ASEBA Problem Scales

A "construct" is "an object of thought constituted by the ordering or systematic uniting of experiential elements" (Gove, 1971, p. 489). In other words, constructs are mental abstractions that are derived from data, although they can also be derived from theories. ASEBA scales measure constructs that have been constituted by systematically aggregating scores on the items of ASEBA forms, which tap elements of informants' experience with the children whom they assess.

From a statistical perspective, the constructs measured by ASEBA scales are viewed as *latent variables*. Latent variables are not directly measured by any single score. Instead, a latent variable is inferred from scores on multiple variables that are directly measured. The directly measured variables are called *manifest* (i.e., observed) variables.

As an example, scores on a syndrome scale obtained from ratings by different informants provide multiple ways of measuring a particular latent variable. Because latent variables are collectively measured by multiple manifest variables, the constructs represented by particular latent variables are typically validated on the basis of *nomological* (i.e., lawful) networks of associations between measures of the constructs and measures of other variables, including other constructs (Cronbach & Meehl, 1955). That is, the validity of a construct is supported by findings of systematic associations between measures of the construct and other variables. The more extensive and systematic the networks of findings for a particular construct, the more confidence the construct deserves. Thousands of studies have reported significant associations between ASEBA scales and many other variables (Bérubé & Achenbach, 2006). In the following sections, we summarize findings that support the construct validity of ASEBA scales in relation to other widely used constructs and measures.

Associations with DSM Diagnoses

Numerous studies have reported significant associations between ASEBA scales and DSM diagnoses (e.g., Edelbrock & Costello, 1988; Kasius, Ferdinand, van den Berg, & Verhulst, 1997; Morgan & Cauce, 1999; Weinstein, Noam, Grimes, Stone, & Schwab-Stone, 1990). As an example, in an outpatient clinic sample, empirically based problem scales scored from the CBCL/6–18 had a mean $r = .62$ ($N = 65$) with scores on a checklist of DSM-IV criteria (Hudziak, 1998) and a mean $r = .39$ ($N = 134$) with DSM-IV diagnoses recorded in the children's clinic records (Achenbach & Rescorla, 2001). In the same clinic, DSM-oriented scales scored from the CBCL/6–18 had a mean $r = .71$ ($N = 65$)

with the DSM-IV checklist scores and a mean $r = .46$ ($N = 134$) with the children's DSM-IV clinical diagnoses. (When Pearson r is used to compute a correlation between quantitative scores, such as those of ASEBA scales, and dichotomous categories, such as the presence versus absence of a particular diagnosis, the correlation is knows as a "point-biserial r.") Chapter 5 presents additional findings on associations between ASEBA scales and DSM diagnoses.

Correlations with Conners and BASC Scores

Significant correlations between ASEBA scales and scales scored from various other forms have been reported. As an example, in the same clinic where correlations with DSM diagnoses were obtained, children were rated by parents and teachers on the Conners (1997) CPRS-R and CTRS-R scales, as well as on the CBCL/6–18 and TRF (Achenbach & Rescorla, 2001, p. 130). The mean r was .77 ($N = 53$) between corresponding CPRS-R scales and CBCL/6–18 scales. Between corresponding CTRS-R scales and TRF scales, the mean r was .84 ($N = 46$). In a sample from a different clinic, the mean r was .72 ($N = 82$) between parents' ratings on corresponding scales of the BASC (Reynolds & Kamphaus, 1992) and CBCL/6–18. Between teachers' ratings on corresponding scales of the BASC and TRF, the mean r was also .72 ($N = 51$; Achenbach & Rescorla, 2001, p. 133).

Associations with Genetic Factors

Studies in multiple countries have shown that ASEBA scale scores provide valid phenotypic markers for genetic differences. Although ASEBA scale scores are also influenced by environmental factors, the evidence for the heritability of some ASEBA syndromes means that the syndrome scores can be used to study genetic influences on psychopathology. For example, the Aggressive Behavior syndrome has yielded heritability estimates of .46, .55, .60, .70, and .94 in various studies (Edelbrock, Rende, Plomin, & Thompson, 1995; Eley, Lichtenstein, & Moffitt, 2003; Ghodsian-Carpey & Baker, 1987; Schmitz, Fulker, & Mrazek, 1995; van den Oord, Verhulst, & Boomsma, 1996). The repeated findings of substantial heritability for scores on the Aggressive Behavior syndrome support its construct validity as a measure of genetically influenced aggression.

Unlike the empirically based syndromes, diagnoses of CD do not distinguish between aggressive and unaggressive conduct problems. However, research has shown that the developmental continuity of scores on the CBCL Aggressive Behavior syndrome is influenced largely by genetic factors, whereas the developmental continuity of scores on the Delinquent (now called Rule-Breaking) Behavior syndrome is affected by both genetic and shared environmental factors (Eley et al., 2003). Chapter 5 presents additional findings on associations of ASEBA scale scores with genetic factors.

Associations with Neurophysiological Factors

The genetic findings indicate that the Aggressive Behavior syndrome is significantly influenced by biological factors. Associations with neurophysiological variables have been found in terms of correlations of -.50, -.63, and -.72 between CBCL Aggressive Behavior syndrome scores and measures of serotonergic activity (Birmaher et al., 1990; Hanna, Yuwiler, & Coates, 1995; Stoff, Pollock, Vitiello, Behar, & Bridges, 1987). These findings are consistent with the theory that high levels of aggression are associated with low serotonergic activity (Brown & van Praag, 1991).

Other neurophysiological findings include a correlation of -.81 between CBCL Aggressive Behavior syndrome scores and dopamine-beta-hydroxylase (DBH) levels, and a correlation of .47 between TRF Aggressive Behavior syndrome scores and testosterone (Gabel, Stadler, Bjorn, Shindledecker, & Bowden, 1993; Scerbo & Kolko, 1994). Together with the substantial heritabilities, the neurophysiological correlates found for the Aggressive Behavior syndrome support the construct validity of this syndrome as an index of biological factors. These findings do not mean that the Aggressive Behavior syndrome is not also influenced by environmental factors, as well. For example, genetic factors contribute to differences in the weights of adults. However, adults who consume the fewest calories and exercise the most tend to weigh less than adults who consume the most calories and exercise least, even though genetic factors also affect their weights. The relative influence of genetic and environmental factors on the Aggressive Behavior syndrome may vary with age as well as with other characteristics (Eley et al., 2003).

Developmental Course and Long-Term Outcomes

Another way to test the construct validity of scales is to determine whether their scores predict individual differences over long periods. Several longitudinal studies have found large correlations between initial assessments and scores obtained on the same syndromes years later. For example, parallel studies of representative samples of thousands of American and Dutch children have yielded large correlations between syndrome scores obtained at intervals of 6 years (Achenbach, Howell, McConaughy, & Stanger, 1995a, 1995b, 1995c; Ferdinand,

Verhulst, & Wiznitzer, 1995; Verhulst & van der Ende, 1992b). It has also been found that child and adolescent ASEBA scores predict adult signs of disturbance, such as substance abuse, trouble with the law, suicidal behavior, and referral for mental health services (Achenbach et al., 1998; Ferdinand & Verhulst, 1995). A Dutch longitudinal study that spanned 14 years and included outcomes for ages up to 30 showed that childhood scores on the Anxious/Depressed, Thought Problems, and Delinquent Behavior (Rule-Breaking Behavior) syndrome scales were exceptionally good predictors of adult problems, including DSM diagnoses (Hofstra, van der Ende, & Verhulst, 2000, 2002).

Longitudinal studies have also compared the developmental course of particular ASEBA syndromes. Using CBCL scores for seven birth cohorts of Dutch children assessed five times at 2-year intervals, Stanger, Achenbach, and Verhulst (1997) compared the course of Aggressive Behavior and Delinquent Behavior syndrome scores. Scores for the Aggressive Behavior syndrome tended to decline steadily with age, whereas scores for the Delinquent Behavior syndrome initially declined but then rose from age 10 to 17. Across developmental periods, children's rank orders remained significantly more stable for Aggressive Behavior scores than Delinquent Behavior scores. In addition, the Delinquent Behavior syndrome has yielded lower heritabilities than those cited earlier for the Aggressive Behavior syndrome (Edelbrock et al., 1995; Eley et al., 2003; Schmitz et al., 1995; van den Oord et al., 1996). Coupled with the lower long-term stability of rank orders in Delinquent Behavior scores, these findings suggest that genetic factors affect the Delinquent Behavior scores less than the Aggressive Behavior scores. Additional longitudinal and outcome findings are reported in Chapter 5.

VALIDITY OF CONNERS INSTRUMENTS

As stated by Conners (1997, p. 5), the main use of the Conners scales is for assessment of ADHD, although the scales are also used to assess other kinds of behaviors that are thought to be associated with ADHD.

Content Validity of Conners Problem Items

Because the 1997 CPRS-R and CTRS-R include paraphrased versions of all 18 symptom criteria for DSM-IV ADHD, the content validity of the 1997 forms for assessing DSM-IV ADHD is assumed. Earlier versions of the Conners scales included a variety of items thought to assess ADHD and associated disorders, but the items were not based on specific criteria such as those of the DSM. The many authorized and unauthorized versions of the pre-1997 Conners scales varied too much to afford general conclusions about their content validity.

Criterion-Related Validity of Conners Problem Scales

The main evidence for the criterion-related validity of the Conners problem scales consists of findings that their scores discriminate between children who are diagnosed as having ADHD versus children who do not qualify for this diagnosis. For example, Conners (2001, p. 137) reported scores on the CPRS-R scales for 91 children who had received DSM-IV diagnoses of ADHD, 91 demographically matched children who were randomly selected from the CPRS-R normative sample, and 55 children who were rated as having "emotional problems" by a psychologist or psychiatrist. Analyses of covariance (ANCOVAs) with age as a covariate showed that the ADHD group scored significantly higher than the normative group on all the problem scales except Perfectionism, for which there was no significant difference. The ADHD group also scored significantly higher than the emotional problems group on the Cognitive Problems/Inattention, Hyperactivity, and DSM-IV ADHD scales. The emotional problems group scored significantly higher than the ADHD and normative groups on the Oppositional and Perfectionism scales and significantly higher than the normative group on the Anxious–Shy and Psychosomatic scales.

Conners (2001, pp. 137–138) also reported scores on the CTRS-R for 154 children with DSM-IV diagnoses of ADHD, 154 demographically matched children randomly selected from the CTRS-R normative sample, and 131 children rated by a psychologist or psychiatrist as having emotional problems. ANCOVAs showed that the ADHD group scored significantly higher than the normative group on all scales except Social Problems, for which there was no significant difference. Surprisingly, the ADHD group did not score significantly higher than the emotional problems group on the Hyperactivity scale. The ADHD group did score significantly higher on the other scales, except the Anxious–Shy scale, where the groups did not differ significantly. The normative group scored significantly lower than the emotional problems group on all scales. Multiple studies have shown that pre-1997 Conners scale scores were significantly associated with various criteria for ADHD, as reviewed by Conners (1994, pp. 554–557).

Construct Validity of Conners Problem Scales

Like the factor-based ASEBA scales, the factor-based Conners scales measure constructs (latent variables) that have been formed by systematically aggregating scores on problem items. Because a primary purpose of the Conners scales is to assess ADHD, the findings of significant associations with diagnoses of ADHD constitute evidence for validity in relation to external criteria for measurement of ADHD. To the extent that diagnoses of ADHD are fallible indices of the diagnostic construct of ADHD, the associations of Conners scale scores with diagnoses of ADHD can also be viewed as evidence for construct validity in that both the scale scores and the diagnoses are manifest variables linked by nomological networks of inferred constructs.

Correlations with ASEBA and Children's Depression Inventory Scores

In the section titled "Construct Validity of ASEBA Problem Scales," we reported a mean r of .77 for CPRS-R scales with corresponding CBCL/ 6–18 scales, and a mean r of .84 for CTRS-R scales with corresponding TRF scales. Because the Conners scales focus mainly on ADHD, it is especially important to note that the ASEBA Attention Problems syndrome correlated .77 and .88 in parent and teacher ratings, respectively, with the purest Conners measure of ADHD, the ADHD Index (Achenbach & Rescorla, 2001, p. 130). These large correlations thus support the validity of the Conners and ASEBA scales for measuring a similar construct of Attention Problems.

Although the Conners scales do not focus on depression, Conners (2001, p. 133) reported correlations with scores on scales of the Children's Depression Inventory (CDI; Kovacs, 1992). For scales having the clearest counterparts on the different forms, the correlations of the CDI Negative Mood scale with the Conners Oppositional scale were .56 ($N = 33$) for the CPRS-R and .22 (nonsignificant) for the CTRS-R ($N = 27$). The correlations were .16 and .25 (both nonsignificant) for the CDI Interpersonal Problems scale with the Social Problems scale of the CPRS-R and CTRS-R, respectively. Although the correlation of .56 was statistically significant, significant correlations were also found between other combinations of CDI and Conners scales. The lack of specificity for correlations between the CDI completed by children and the Conners scales completed by adults could reflect the fact that children's self-reports on measures such as the CDI tend not to agree with adults' reports of the children's problems (Achenbach, McConaughy, et al., 1987).

Correlations of pre-1997 Conners scales with other measures completed by the same informants support the construct validity of some of these scales. For example, an early version of the Conners (1973) Parent Questionnaire yielded a mean r of .73 ($N = 60$) with corresponding scales of the 1991 CBCL/4–18 (Achenbach, 1991a, p. 85).

Edelbrock and Rancurello (1985) also reported large correlations between scores on early versions of the Conners Parent Questionnaire and CBCL scales. The 1978 version of the Revised Conners Teacher Rating Scale (Goyette, Conners, & Ulrich, 1978) yielded a mean r of .75 with corresponding scales of the 1991 TRF ($N = 45$; Achenbach, 1991b, p. 70). A mean r of .70 ($N = 135$) has been reported between corresponding scales of the Revised Behavior Problem Checklist (Quay & Peterson, 1987) and the 48-item Revised Conners Parent Rating Scale (Goyette et al., 1978) scored in terms of factors derived by M. Cohen (1988) from data on 135 clinic-referred children.

Associations with Genetic Factors

At least one study has shown that a scale scored from the CPRS-R, the ADHD Index, provides a valid phenotypic marker for genetic differences. In a study of 1,595 7-year-old Dutch twin pairs rated by their mothers on the CPRS-R, some 78% of the variance in the ADHD Index scores was estimated to be accounted for by genetic factors (Hudziak, Derks, Althoff, Rettew, & Boomsma, 2005).

Long-Term Outcomes

Associations have been reported between Conners scale scores and outcomes over significant developmental periods. For example, in a sample of 92 6- to 9-year-old boys, Satin, Winsberg, Monetti, Sverd, and Foss (1985) found that scores on an early version of the Conners Hyperactivity Index identified 90% of the boys who received DSM-III diagnoses of ADHD a year later. In a study of 135 hyperactive boys, Prinz and Loney (1986) found that a 39-item version of the Conners Teacher Questionnaire predicted aggressive behavior over a 3-year period. High initial scores on the Conners Anxiety scale were also found to be associated with poor responses to stimulant medication.

VALIDITY OF THE SDQ

Content Validity of SDQ Problem Items

As it is an outgrowth of the parent and teacher questionnaires developed by Michael Rutter (1967; Rutter et al., 1970), the SDQ's content validity can be evaluated in terms of its correlations with scales of the original Rutter questionnaires. Although Goodman (1997, p. 582) pointed out that no SDQ item is worded identically to any Rutter item, he also indicated that the wording of 5 of the 20 SDQ problem items is similar to Rutter items (p. 582). Considering the overall similarity in purpose, content, format, and rating options, the mean rs of .84 between parents' SDQ and Rutter ratings and .90 between teachers' SDQ and Rutter ratings suggest great similarity between the content of the four corresponding SDQ and Rutter scales.

Criterion-Related Validity of SDQ Problem Scales

As a screen for problems deemed to warrant professional help, Total Difficulties scores on SDQs completed by parents, teachers, and youths have been found to discriminate significantly between 232 children referred to three London mental health clinics and 467 children participating in a pilot study for a national survey of British children (Goodman, 1999). Associations of age, gender, ethnicity, and SES with SDQ scores were evidently not analyzed or controlled. Additional findings are presented in Chapter 5.

Construct Validity of SDQ Problem Scales

Associations with Diagnoses

As described below, several studies have tested associations between the SDQ and clinical diagnoses. Additional details are presented in Chapter 5.

In a study of 7,984 children from a British national survey, SDQ problem scale scores were significantly associated with ICD-10 diagnoses made from the Development and Well-Being Assessment (DAWBA; Goodman, Ford, Simmons, Gatward, & Meltzer, 2000). The DAWBA data were obtained from interviews with parents and youths, plus questionnaires completed by teachers. Clinicians then used the parent, youth, and teacher data to make diagnoses. Goodman et al. concluded that a complex algorithm using data from multiple SDQ informants (parent, teacher, and youth) yielded significantly stronger associations with DAWBA diagnoses (also based on parent, teacher, and youth data) than did data from single informants. No associations or controls for age, gender, ethnicity, or SES were reported.

In a study of 500 of the participants in the same British survey, Goodman (2001) reported that scores above the 90th percentile on each of the SDQ problem scales were significantly associated with at least one category of DSM-IV diagnoses made from the DAWBA. However, associations of age, gender, ethnicity, and SES were neither reported nor controlled.

In a study of children referred to one mental health clinic in London and one in Dhaka, Bangladesh, an algorithm was constructed to use combinations of SDQ problem scale scores and questions about the impact of problems to predict broad categories of ICD-10 clinical diagnoses at a statistically significant level (Goodman, Renfrew, & Mullick, 2000). The diagnostic categories were hyperkinesis, conduct disorder (including oppositional disorder), and emotional disorder (including anxiety, depressive, and obsessive–compulsive disorders).

Correlations with ASEBA Scale Scores

Studies in Finland and Germany have reported significant correlations of SDQ problem scale scores with CBCL and YSR problem scale scores. The Finnish study used a general population sample of 735 7- to 15-year-olds living in two communities (Koskelainen, Sourander, & Kaljonen, 2000). Parent SDQ scores had a mean r of .56 with CBCL scores on scales identified as corresponding to SDQ scales. Self-report scales had a mean r of .62 with corresponding YSR scales.

The German study included 163 4- to 16-year-olds from psychiatric clinics and 110 12- and 13-year-olds from a community sample (Klasen et al., 2000). Correlations between SDQ and CBCL scales were similar for the clinic and community samples, with a mean r of .72. Only the community youths completed the SDQ and YSR, whose corresponding scales had a mean r of .69.

IMPLICATIONS FOR CONSTRUCT VALIDITY

We have presented examples of published findings on the validity of ASEBA, Conners, and SDQ scales as measures of constructs of child psychopathology. In subsequent chapters we provide more detailed evidence relevant to multicultural applications. Validation of constructs related to psychopathology is an ongoing process. Because so much remains to be learned, constructs that can be reliably and validly measured are needed to advance our knowledge of psychopathology. Such constructs can, in turn, foster hypotheses about associations between various aspects of psychopathology, such as etiological, risk, and protective factors, effective treatments, and long-term outcomes. Multicultural data can be especially valuable for deriving constructs that are valid across variations in many potentially relevant influences, such as genes, diets, languages, climates, religions, childrearing practices, schools, and health systems. Furthermore, after constructs have been derived from data in particular cultures, tests of their correlates and utility in multiple cultures can provide especially good ways of refining and extending the nomological networks of associations that support construct validity. The ultimate value of the constructs should be judged according to their contributions to new knowledge. In Chapter 3 we discuss constructs derived from the diagnostically based approach and compare them with constructs from the empirically based approach.

SUMMARY

In this chapter we presented the empirically based, bottom-up, approach to forming taxonomic constructs by deriving syndromes via statistical analyses of problems reported for large samples of children by multiple informants. We also presented ASEBA and Conners instruments, which have generated the most multicultural research on child psychopathology, plus the SDQ, which has brought some aspects of empirically based assessment to bear on multicultural research. Psychometric properties of empirically based syndromes and DSM-oriented scales were presented and found to be similar for the two kinds of scales. Overviews of content, criterion-related, and construct validity findings were presented. Multicultural research presented later in the book extends the evidence for validity.

CHAPTER 3

The Diagnostically Based "Top-Down" Approach to Psychopathology

As outlined in Chapter 1, the diagnostically based approach stems from nosological models of psychopathology whereby children's problems are viewed as symptoms of underlying diseases or disorders. In this chapter we present ways in which the diagnostically based approach has been used to develop assessment procedures for making diagnoses. This approach starts "at the top" with experts' concepts of disorders. These concepts serve as taxonomic constructs for which the experts then formulate definitions in terms of symptoms and other criteria. We begin by outlining the rationale for the top-down approach and the ways in which it has been applied to children's problems before and since the publication of the third edition of the American Psychiatric Association's (1980) *Diagnostic and Statistical Manual of Mental Disorders* (DSM-III). We then present the main assessment procedures that have been developed for making DSM diagnoses of children. Thereafter, we present psychometric and validity findings for the assessment procedures. The chapter closes with comparisons between the empirically based and diagnostically based approaches to psychopathology.

RATIONALE FOR THE DIAGNOSTIC APPROACH

The top-down approach to psychopathology is modeled largely on nosologies of physical diseases. Most physical diseases are defined in terms of tissue pathology, the presence of pathogenic agents, and/or deviant physical parameters, such as high blood pressure. However, in the absence of known physical causes or correlates, psychopathology is defined mainly in terms of deviant behavioral, emotional, social, and cognitive characteristics.

In the 19th century progress in medical research helped to bring the study and treatment of psychopathology out of the realm of demonology and into the realm of medicine. An influential 19th-century medical view contended that psychopathology results from brain diseases (Griesinger, 1845/1867). When Emil Kraepelin (1883) developed the psychiatric nosology that continues to shape diagnostic concepts, he assumed that different symptom patterns of psychopathology could ultimately be traced to different brain diseases. This assumption was strongly reinforced in 1897 by Krafft-Ebing's confirmation of syphilis as the cause of general paresis, a pattern of mental and motor symptoms that had been described with increasing precision over the preceding 100 years. According to Kraepelinian nosology, the task of assessment is to identify symptoms from which particular diseases can be diagnosed. This perspective has engendered a top-down approach whereby experts who are assumed to know what disorders exist collaborate in formulating diagnostic categories. The experts draw on their clinical and research experience to select symptoms and other criteria for determining which disorder(s) an individual has. As explained by Robert Spitzer and Dennis Cantwell (1980), the formulation of diagnostic categories for DSM childhood disorders started

> with a clinical concept for which there is some degree of face validity. Face validity is the extent to which the description of a particular category seems on the face of it to describe accurately the characteristic features of persons with a particular disorder. It is the result of clinicians agreeing on the identification of a particular syndrome or pattern of clinical features as a mental disorder. Initial criteria were generally developed by asking the clinicians to describe what they consider to be the most characteristic features of the disorder. (p. 369)

Figure 3.1 illustrates the top-down strategy of starting with categories of disorders and then specifying symptoms and other criteria for each disorder.

DSM Versions of the Diagnostic Approach

Although applications of the diagnostic approach to adult psychopathology emerged in the 19th century, diagnostic concepts of children's disorders remained quite undifferentiated throughout much of

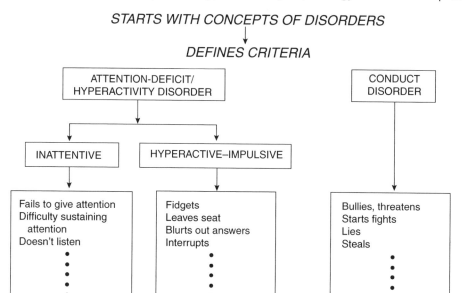

FIGURE 3.1. The "top-down" approach to assessment and taxonomy of psychopathology. Copyright T. M. Achenbach. Reprinted by permission.

the 20th century. Formulations of childhood disorders in the DSM emerged in two phases, as outlined in the following sections.

Phase 1: Childhood Disorders in DSM-I and DSM-II

DSM-I and DSM-II (American Psychiatric Association, 1952, 1968) specified most diagnostic categories in terms of general descriptions and inferences. The DSM-I categories for child and adolescent disorders were specified as follows:

> *Schizophrenic reaction, childhood type*—"those schizophrenic reactions occurring before puberty. The clinical picture may differ from schizophrenic reactions occurring in other age periods because of the immaturity and plasticity of the patient at the time of the reaction" (American Psychiatric Association, 1952, p. 28).
>
> *Adjustment reaction of childhood*—"the transient symptomatic reactions of children to some immediate situation or internal emotional conflict" (American Psychiatric Association, 1952, p. 41).

Subcategories of adjustment reactions were provided for cases where particular kinds of symptoms predominated; these included *habit disturbance, conduct disturbance,* and *neurotic traits.* An additional category was provided for *adjustment reaction of adolescence,* specified as "those transient reactions of the adolescent which are the expression of his emancipatory strivings and vacillations with reference to impulses and emotional tendencies" (American Psychiatric Association, 1952, p. 42). However, adult diagnoses could also be applied to children and adolescents.

DSM-II (American Psychiatric Association, 1968) retained the categories for adjustment reactions and childhood schizophrenia (now omitting the term *reaction*) but added the following behavior disorders of childhood and adolescence: *hyperkinetic reaction, withdrawing reaction, overanxious reaction, runaway reaction, unsocialized aggressive reaction,* and *group delinquent reaction.* The distinction between the unsocialized aggressive reaction and group delinquent reaction was based on early statistical studies of case records by Jenkins and his colleagues (Hewitt & Jenkins, 1946; Jenkins & Glickman, 1946). However, the DSM-II categories were specified in terms of general descriptions and inferences, like those of the DSM-I categories, rather than in terms of the specific problem clusters identified by Jenkins and colleagues.

Phase 2: Childhood Disorders in DSM-III and Its Successors

DSM-III (American Psychiatric Association, 1980) departed significantly from DSM-I and DSM-II by providing explicit criteria and decision rules for each diagnostic category. For example, attention deficit disorder with hyperactivity (ADHD) was defined in terms of five symptoms of inattention, six symptoms of impulsivity, and five symptoms of hyperactivity. The decision rule for diagnosing ADHD was that a child had to manifest at least three symptoms of inattention, three symptoms of impulsivity, and two symptoms of hyperactivity, with onset before age 7 and a duration of at least 6 months. Exclusionary criteria specified that the symptoms were not due to schizophrenia, affective disorder, or severe or profound mental retardation (American Psychiatric Association, 1980, pp. 43–44). Although the criteria used in DSM-III and its successors have been said to provide "operational definitions" (e.g., Rapoport & Ismond, 1996), the DSM has not specified assessment operations for determining whether its criteria are met, other than the use of IQ tests for determining whether individuals meet the criterion of IQ ≤ 70 for diagnoses of mental retardation (American Psychiatric Association, 1980, 1987, 1994, 2000).

In addition to providing explicit criteria and decision rules, DSM-III also provided five axes for evaluating people's functioning. The first three axes constituted the "official diagnostic assessment" (American Psychiatric Association, 1980, p. 23); *Axis I* consisted of clinical syndromes plus conditions that are not attributable to a mental disorder but that are a focus of attention or treatment; *Axis II* consisted of personality disorders and developmental disorders; and *Axis III* consisted of physical disorders and conditions. *Axis IV* provided ratings of psychosocial stressors, and *Axis V* provided ratings of the highest level of adaptive functioning in the past year. DSM-III provided many more diagnostic categories for "disorders first evident in infancy, childhood, or adolescence" than had been provided by DSM-I or DSM-II.

Many of the DSM-III categories and criteria were subsequently revised in DSM-III-R and DSM-IV. Table 3.1 lists DSM-IV diagnoses for common behavioral and emotional problems of children and adolescents. The composition and names of the five axes also changed somewhat; the DSM-IV versions follow:

Axis I.   Clinical disorders and other conditions that may be a focus of clinical attention
Axis II. Personality disorders and mental retardation
Axis III. General medical conditions
Axis IV. Psychosocial and environmental problems
Axis V.   Global assessment of functioning

TABLE 3.1. DSM-IV Diagnoses for Behavioral and Emotional Problems of Childhood and Adolescence Most Relevant to Multicultural Research

Adjustment disorders	Depressive disorders
These can be specified with depressed mood, anxiety, disturbance of conduct, and mixtures of these problems.	Dysthymic disorder Major depressive disorder (MDD)
	Disruptive disorders
Anxiety disorders	Attention-deficit/hyperactivity disorder (ADHD)
Generalized anxiety disorder (GAD) Obsessive–compulsive disorder (OCD) Posttraumatic stress disorder (PTSD) Separation anxiety disorder (SAD) Social phobia Specific phobia	Conduct disorder (CD) Oppositional defiant disorder (ODD)
	Eating disorders
	Anorexia nervosa Bulimia nervosa

Note. DSM-IV diagnoses from American Psychiatric Association (1994, 2000). Other DSM-IV child and adolescent diagnostic categories include pervasive developmental disorders, feeding disorders of infancy or early childhood, tic disorders, and elimination disorders.

The ICD

The ICD is published by the World Health Organization (WHO) to provide a standard classification system for diseases, including diagnostic categories for child psychopathology. Initially proposed by a WHO seminar (Rutter, Shaffer, & Shepherd, 1975), a multiaxial approach to diagnoses of childhood disorders was included in the ninth revision of the ICD (ICD-9; World Health Organization, 1978), prior to the DSM-III multiaxial system.

Although the DSM provides crosswalks between its diagnostic categories and codes for the ICD diagnostic categories, the DSM and ICD categories for childhood disorders differ in many ways. A fundamental difference is that the DSM provides explicit criteria for each category whereas the ICD lacks such explicit criteria, although the tenth revision of the ICD includes explicit diagnostic criteria for research purposes, separate from the clinical diagnostic criteria (ICD-10; World Health Organization, 1993). The DSM and ICD also differ in the names that they assign to diagnostic categories and in the ways in which particular categories are combined or separated. For example, DSM-IV specifies one set of criteria for all conduct disorders, although it allows for specification as childhood-onset type versus adolescent-onset type according to whether at least one criterial symptom was evident prior to age 10. ICD-10, by contrast, distinguishes among the following types of conduct disorders: conduct disorder confined to the family context; unsocialized conduct disorder; socialized conduct disorder; and oppositional defiant disorder (which DSM-IV defines as a disorder separate from conduct disorder).

DIAGNOSTICALLY BASED ASSESSMENT INSTRUMENTS

In the empirically based, bottom-up approach, assessment instruments provide data from which taxonomic constructs are derived. In the diagnostically based approach to child psychopathology, by contrast, "the diagnostic categories were developed before the tools that could measure their defining features (primarily symptoms)" (McClellan & Werry, 2000, p. 19). In this chapter we highlight interviews and rating forms that have been developed to assess children in terms of the criteria for diagnostic categories. Table 3.2 outlines the steps that are typically followed in developing interviews for diagnosing childhood disorders. Later chapters present data obtained with diagnostically based instruments that have been used in multiple cultures.

TABLE 3.2. Developing Interviews for Diagnosing Childhood Disorders

1. Formulate questions to ascertain the presence of each criterial symptom and other criterial features for each diagnosis.
2. Construct versions of interviews appropriate for children and parents.
3. Provide instructions and training for interviewers.
4. Pilot test and revise instruments based on responses by children and parents.
5. Use instruments to assess large clinical and epidemiological samples.
6. Tabulate prevalence rates of diagnoses obtained with child and parent interviews.
7. Test reliability and other psychometric properties.
8. Test validity in relation to external criteria.

It is important to note that the diagnostically based instruments are intended to operationalize diagnostic criteria via standardized assessment procedures—an essential step for doing research on diagnoses, including multicultural research. However, diagnoses are used for many important purposes, and they have correlates that do not depend on standardized interviews. For example, clinicians often make diagnoses, decide on treatments, and obtain reimbursements for clinical services on the basis of information that is not obtained with standardized diagnostic interviews. Similarly, researchers often use information from sources other than standardized interviews to study correlates of diagnoses, such as the results of genetic analyses, neuroimaging, evaluations of treatment, and long-term outcome assessments (e.g., Devito et al., 2005; Todd et al., 2005). Thus, standardized interviews are by no means the only basis for making diagnoses. Nevertheless, to maintain comparability of data across different cultures, our reviews of diagnostically based findings give priority to studies in which diagnoses were explicitly operationalized. Standardized interviews such as those described in the following sections have been the main methods for operationalizing diagnoses in studies that afford multicultural comparisons.

Respondent-Based Interviews

One method for determining whether children meet criteria for diagnoses is to ask respondents structured questions about whether the children display each of the criterial features for each diagnosis. Applications of this method to childhood disorders are modeled largely on the Diagnostic Interview Schedule (DIS; Robins, Helzer, Croughan, & Ratcliff, 1981), which was developed for epidemiological studies of adults. To make such studies cost effective, the DIS was designed to be administered by "lay interviewers," that is, interviewers who are not trained clinicians. Unlike trained clinicians, lay interviewers are not expected to tailor their questions to characteristics of the interviewees, nor to probe beneath the surface of interviewees' responses, nor to synthesize information into diagnoses. Instead, lay interviewers are trained to ask standardized questions and to follow strict rules for recording the answers. Algorithms are then used to determine whether interviewees' report enough features of a disorder to meet the diagnostic criteria for the disorder. Interviews that use responses to structured questions as the basis for making diagnoses are called *respondent-based*, because the diagnostic decisions are directly determined by the respondents' answers to the interview questions.

Diagnostic Interview Schedule for Children

The most direct application of the DIS's respondent-based methodology to children is the Diagnostic Interview Schedule for Children (DISC), which was commissioned by the U.S. National Institute of Mental Health (NIMII) in 1980 to make DSM-III diagnoses of children in epidemiological samples (Costello, Edelbrock, Kalas, Kessler, & Klaric, 1982). Like the DIS, the DISC is administered by lay interviewers who ask structured questions about the criterial features of each diagnostic category. Algorithms are then applied to the respondents' answers to determine whether they meet criteria for disorders defined by the DSM. Thus, if a child affirms enough criterial features of a disorder, he or she is diagnosed as having the disorder.

It soon became clear that the diagnoses obtained with the version of the DISC (DISC-C) administered to children did not agree well with other information about the children. Consequently, a parallel version of the DISC, called the DISC-P, was developed for administration to parents (Costello et al., 1982).

The DISC has undergone numerous revisions to incorporate changes in diagnostic categories and criteria from DSM-III to DSM-III-R and DSM-IV. Changes have also been made in administration procedures, the wording of questions, and the scoring criteria. It was found that young children could not provide meaningful answers to many of the DISC questions. The intended age range for the self-report DISC was therefore narrowed to 9–17 years, and it became known as the DISC-Y (*Y* = youth; Shaffer, Fisher, Lucas, Dulcan, & Schwab-Stone, 2000). The DISC-P is designed to obtain parents' reports for ages 6–17 years.

The version of the DISC for DSM-IV diagnoses (DISC-IV) includes nearly 3,000 questions, 358 of which are "stem" questions to be asked of every respondent (Shaffer et al., 2000). Some 1,300 "contingent" questions can be asked when stem questions or previous contingent questions are answered affirmatively. An additional 732 questions ask about age of onset, impairment, and previous treatment. And nearly 700 other questions are included in an optional module for assessing lifetime symptoms. Shaffer et al. (2000) reported that administration time averages about 70 minutes per informant in community samples and about 90–120 minutes for "known patients" (p. 33). Because it is often impractical to administer the entire DISC, modules for a limited number of diagnoses are usually administered, typically with the aid of a computer program.

Diagnostic Interview for Children and Adolescents

In addition to the DISC, other interviews have been designed to derive diagnoses from respondents' answers. Like the DISC, the Diagnostic Interview for Children and Adolescents (DICA) was originally modeled on the DIS as a structured, respondent-based interview for administration by lay interviewers (Herjanic & Reich, 1982). However, later editions of the DICA are more semistructured, in that they permit interviewers to probe and ask additional questions (Reich, 2000). Because interviewers are taught how to deviate from the structured questions, the DICA may require more training than the DISC. Like the DISC, the DICA has separate versions for children and their parents. Reich (2000) reported that the DICA typically takes about 1–2 hours to administer and 50–55 minutes to edit.

Interviewer-Based Interviews

In contrast to the respondent-based diagnoses made from the DISC, interviewer-based diagnoses require interviewers to judge information obtained from respondents before deciding whether to record symptoms as present.

Child and Adolescent Psychiatric Assessment

The Child and Adolescent Psychiatric Assessment (CAPA) was explicitly developed to make interviewer-based diagnoses (Angold & Costello, 2000). The CAPA is described as providing "a structure for the *mind of the interviewer.* The interview serves as a guide in determining whether a symptom is present; the interviewer makes that decision on the basis of information collected from the patient or respondent. . . . The interviewer is expected to question until he or she can decide whether a symptom meeting each definition is present" (Angold & Costello, 2000, p. 39). An extensive glossary provides definitions of the symptoms that are criteria for diagnoses. Although previous clinical experience is not deemed essential, extensive training and certification by a qualified CAPA trainer are required. The CAPA is designed to make diagnoses of 9- to 17-year-olds based on separate child and parent interviews. Angold and Costello (2000) reported that CAPA interviews in community samples averaged about 66 minutes for parents and 59 minutes for children. Interviewers then need about 15 minutes to code responses, and supervisors need 30 minutes to check the responses.

Schedule for Affective Disorders and Schizophrenia for School-Age Children

Prior to the emergence of the explicit distinction between respondent-based and interviewer-based diagnostic interviews, the Schedule for Affective Disorders and Schizophrenia for School-Age Children (K-SADS) was developed as a downward extension of the Adult SADS (Endicott & Spitzer, 1978; Puig-Antich & Chambers, 1978). Both the K-SADS (*K* stands for *kiddie*) and the Adult SADS must be administered by trained clinicians. Within a semistructured format, "suggested verbal probes assist the examiner in clarifying both the presence and severity of symptoms. The examiner can ask as many questions as necessary to achieve this goal. With this system, the interviewer makes a clinical judgment based purely on clarification of the patient's subjective reports" (Ambrosini, 2000, p. 50). The target age range is 6–18 years. A version of the K-SADS is administered first to the child's parent. The parent is asked to rate the severity of the child's symptoms when the symptoms were at their worst during a particular period and then during the previous week or during the current episode of a disorder. The same clinician then administers the K-SADS to the child. Thereafter, the clinician rates the severity of symptoms on the basis of all available information. If there are major discrepancies between reports by the child and parent, they are interviewed together to clarify their views. The clinician, rather than a diagnostic algorithm, ultimately decides the diagnoses. Ambrosini (2000) reported that administration of the K-SADS averages about 1.25–1.50 hours.

Combining Respondent-Based and Interviewer-Based Approaches

Respondent-based interviews that enable lay interviewers to obtain diagnoses directly from respondents' answers to structured questions are less costly to administer than interviews requiring highly trained interviewers to make clinical judgments of respondents' answers. Questions, response options, and diagnostic algorithms that are standardized also minimize variations in respondent-based assessment procedures from one interviewer to another and from one interviewee to another. On the other hand, diagnoses based on more flexible questioning and clinical judgment may reduce misunderstandings by interviewees and inaccuracies in determining whether interviewees' reports indicate problems that are severe enough to meet diagnostic criteria. However, interviews that involve flexible questioning and clinical judgment require higher levels of training and vary more across interviewers and interviewees.

Development and Well-Being Assessment

To combine the economy and standardization of respondent-based interviews with the flexibility of clinical judgment, the Development and Well-Being Assessment (DAWBA) includes a structured interview administered to parents of 5- to 16-year-olds by lay interviewers (Goodman, Ford, Richards, Gatward, & Meltzer, 2000). The questions in the structured interview are said to be "closely related" to DSM-IV and ICD-10 criteria (Ford, Goodman, & Meltzer, 2003, p. 1204). When the structured questions identify definite symptoms, interviewers can use open-ended questions and prompts to elicit descriptions of problems in the interviewees' own words, which are then transcribed verbatim by the interviewers. In community samples the 36 pages of DAWBA questions take about 50 minutes to administer if "skip" rules are followed for omitting questions whenever screening questions yield negative replies (Goodman, Ford, Richards, et al., 2000, p. 647). A similar DAWBA interview is used to obtain 11- to 16-year-olds' reports of their own problems. DAWBA questionnaires are sent to teachers to obtain their reports of conduct, emotional, and hyperactivity symptoms and their inferences about whether the symptoms cause impairment.

A computer program prints summaries of the information obtained from the informants, plus algorithm-generated diagnoses. These are given to clinicians, who make the final diagnostic decisions. The input to the clinicians is limited to data obtained from the DAWBA interviews and teacher questionnaires, but the clinicians decide how to use these data in making diagnostic decisions. Among their decisions, clinicians must "decide which informant to believe when presented with conflicting information" (Goodman, Ford, Richards, et al., 2000, p. 648). Because the DAWBA clinicians do not conduct interviews, Goodman et al. refer to the DAWBA as "investigator-based" (p. 653) rather than "interviewer-based." Having clinicians mentally combine the data is intended to mimic the typical clinical process for making diagnoses. However, much remains to be learned about how best to combine data from multiple sources, including interviews and questionnaires completed by parents, teachers, youths, and others.

DSM-Based Rating Forms

In addition to the interviews for making DSM diagnoses, forms have been developed for rating DSM criterial symptoms. Some of the DSM-based rating forms focus on a particular diagnostic category. For example, the ADHD Rating Scale–IV consists of the DSM-IV symptom criteria for the inattentive and hyperactive–impulsive types of ADHD (DuPaul, Power, Anastopoulous, & Reid, 1998). Parent and teacher versions are available on which each symptom is rated as *0 = Never or rarely; 1 = Sometimes; 2 = Often;* or *3 = Very often.* The symptom scores are then summed to yield scale scores for Inattention, Hyperactivity–Impulsivity, and Total ADHD. Factor analyses have supported both a single-factor model and a two-factor Inattention and Hyperactivity–Impulsivity model. However, DuPaul et al. (1998) reported a correlation of .94 between the two factors, which suggested that they measure a single construct.

Other rating forms have been developed to assess a broader range of DSM diagnostic categories. For example, Gadow and Sprafkin (1998) developed the Adolescent Symptom Inventory–4 (ASI-4) to obtain parent and teacher ratings of symptoms specified for several DSM-IV diagnostic categories. The symptoms are rated 0, 1, 2, or 3 according to gradations like those of the ADHD Rating Scale–IV (DuPaul et al., 1998). The Youth Inventory–4 (YI-4; Gadow & Sprafkin, 1999) is a parallel self-rating form that includes many of the same DSM symptoms as the ASI-4.

PSYCHOMETRIC PROPERTIES
OF DIAGNOSTICALLY BASED INSTRUMENTS

Psychometric concepts may not seem applicable to diagnoses. However, procedures for making diagnoses need to be evaluated for reliability and for agreement between sources of data, just as procedures for assessing other constructs do. In Chapter 2 we summarized findings for internal consistency (coefficient alpha), test–retest reliability, and cross-informant agreement for empirically based scales. Because procedures for making diagnoses embody preexisting diagnostic criteria, measures of internal consistency among items for assessing the diagnostic criteria are not typically reported. However, statistics for test–retest reliability and cross-informant agreement have been reported for some of the DSM instruments. Although we later report multicultural findings obtained with the DAWBA, the authors of the DAWBA have argued against computing test–retest reliability on the grounds that interviewees tend to report fewer problems at a second interview than at an initial interview (Goodman, Ford, Richards, et al., 2000, p. 654). Called "test–retest attenuation," the tendency to report fewer problems at second interviews is addressed in later chapters.

Psychometric Properties of the DISC

Table 3.3 summarizes test–retest reliability findings from a massive study that was funded by the NIMH to improve epidemiological research on childhood disorders defined in terms of DSM criteria (Schwab-Stone et al., 1996). Called the Methods for Epidemiology of Child and Adolescent Mental Disorders (MECA) Study, it applied a version of the DISC (the DISC-2.3) to community samples in Atlanta, Georgia; New Haven, Connecticut; Westchester County, New York; and San Juan, Puerto Rico. Because the DISC is designed to make yes/no diagnoses according to the DSM's fixed decision rules, the kappa statistic is typically used to measure test–retest reliability in terms of percent-

TABLE 3.3. Psychometric Properties of DISC Interviews

| DSM-III-R diagnoses | Test–retest reliability[a] | | Cross-informant agreement |
	Parent	Youth	Parent × youth[b]
ADHD	.60	.10	.09
ODD	.68	.18	.14
CD	.56	.64	.10
Overanxious	.60	.28	.15[c]
Separation anxiety	.45	.27	—
Social phobia	.45	.33	—
Major depression	.55	.37	.11[d]
Dysthymia	.30	.43	—
Mean kappa	.52	.33	.12

Note. Statistics in table are kappa coefficients. Youths were 9–18 years old.
[a]$N = 247$ (Schwab-Stone et al., 1996) for computer-assisted DISC interviews administered in the MECA study at intervals of 1–15 days. Addition of impairment criteria reduced the mean test–retest kappa to .48 for parent interviews and .24 for youth interviews.
[b]$N = 1,283$ (Jensen et al., 1999) for mean kappas obtained in the MECA study by averaging results with and without impairment criteria for ages 9–11 and 12–18.
[c]Includes any anxiety disorder.
[d]Includes major depression and dysthymia.

ages of agreement between Time 1 and Time 2 diagnoses that are corrected for chance agreement. The kappas in the first two columns of
Table 3.3 indicate the agreement between yes/no diagnoses obtained
from two administrations of the DISC by trained lay interviewers to
parents and to their 9- to 18-year-old children at intervals of 1–15 days.
As Table 3.3 shows, the mean test–retest kappa was .52 for parent interviews and .33 for child interviews.

In a Puerto Rican study where child psychiatrists administered
DISC interviews separately to 91 parents and their children at a mean
interval of 19 days, the mean test–retest kappa was .44 for the psychiatrists' DSM-III diagnoses based on a combination of parent and child
data (Canino et al., 1987). A subsequent Puerto Rican study yielded a
mean kappa of .42 over test–retest intervals averaging 12 days for the
Spanish language DISC-IV, administered by trained lay interviewers to
parents of a clinical sample of 146 children (Bravo et al., 2001).

In a Quebec study where trained lay interviewers administered the
DISC-2.25 twice to 260 parents (mean interval = 13.8 days) and twice to
145 adolescents (mean interval = 12.8 days), the mean test–retest kappa
for DSM-III-R diagnoses was .51 for parents and .52 for adolescents
(Breton, Bergeron, Valla, Berthiaume, & St. Georges, 1998). In a multiethnic U.S. clinical sample of 101 adolescents, a mean test–retest kappa
of .47 was obtained for DSM-III-R diagnoses made from the DISC-2.1
administered by trained lay interviewers over 7- to 14-day intervals
(Roberts, Solovitz, Chen, & Casat, 1996).

The kappas in the righthand column of Table 3.3 indicate the
agreement between diagnoses based on data from separate DISC interviews administered to parents and to their children (Jensen et al.,
1999). The mean cross-informant kappa was .12. Consistent with this
low kappa, several studies that did not specify cross-informant kappas
have reported finding very little overlap between diagnoses made from
the parent and child DISC (e.g., Breton, Bergeron, Valla, Berthiaume,
& Gaudet, 1999; Shaffer et al., 1996; Verhulst et al., 1997).

According to the inventor of kappa (Cohen, 1960, p. 43), this statistic is usually about the same size as the phi coefficient, which is the
Pearson r computed for 2×2 tables. Because binary data (e.g., yes vs.
no responses) typically yield smaller correlations than would be found
if the same variables were scored in terms of more than two values,
kappa and phi may be smaller than if the diagnostic data were scored
continuously (e.g., the numbers of symptoms reported). However, the
smaller coefficients are not mere methodological artifacts. Instead,
they reflect the actual levels of agreement obtained when diagnoses
are made categorically, as is the case with the DSM and with the assessment procedures that make yes/no diagnoses.

Psychometric Properties of DSM-Based Rating Forms

According to the *Manual for the ADHD Rating Scale-IV* (DuPaul et al., 1998), a mean of .91 was obtained for the alpha coefficients (internal consistency) of parent and teacher ratings of Inattention, Hyperactivity–Impulsivity, and total score. The mean test–retest r was .86. The mean cross-informant r between parent and teacher ratings was .42.

For the YI-4, Gadow et al. (2002) reported a mean alpha of .78. The mean test–retest r was .67. The mean cross-informant r between youth and parent ratings was .30. The higher test–retest and cross-informant correlations for DSM rating forms than interviews may be partly due to the continuous scoring of the rating forms versus the yes/no "scoring" of the interviews.

OVERVIEW OF VALIDITY FINDINGS

The main purpose of the diagnostic interviews reviewed in this chapter is to make DSM diagnoses. Consequently, the main criterion for judging the validity of the interviews is the degree to which they agree with DSM diagnoses made by other means. Because DSM diagnostic categories and criteria have been formulated according to clinicians' concepts of disorders, clinical diagnoses provide the most compelling external validity criteria for DSM diagnostic interviews.

Agreement between DISC Diagnoses and Clinical Diagnoses of Children

To test the validity of the DISC-2.3 in relation to clinical diagnoses, Jensen and Weisz (2002) compared DSM-III-R diagnoses made by clinicians with diagnoses generated independently from DISC-2.3 interviews with parents of 245 7- to 17-year-olds referred to five outpatient clinics. The interviewers had received the standard DISC training program operated by the DISC development team at Columbia University. In addition to the DISC-P, Jensen and Weisz used children's reports obtained with the DISC-C for diagnostic categories for which children's reports were particularly important, including depressive disorders and CD. For the 10 diagnostic categories that yielded diagnoses for at least 20 children, the kappas between the DISC and the clinical diagnoses ranged from –.03 to +.27, with a mean of +.12. The only kappas that were statistically significant were .14 for ADHD and .27 for CD.

In another study, DSM-IV diagnoses made by multidisciplinary teams of clinicians for 240 6- to 18-year-olds were compared with diagnoses made from the DSM-IV version of the DISC (DISC-IV) administered independently to parents and to 11- to 18-year-old youths (Lewczyk, Garland, Hurlburt, Gearity, & Hough, 2003). Diagnoses were made from the DISC if either the parent's or youth's responses to the DISC met criteria for a DSM-IV disorder and at least moderate impairment was reported to result from a disorder that met DSM-IV criteria. To maximize chances for detecting agreement, specific diagnoses were aggregated into the following four categories: Any ADHD disorder, any disruptive behavior disorder, any mood disorder, and any anxiety disorder. For these four broad categories, kappas between DISC diagnoses and diagnoses made by teams of clinicians ranged from –.04 to +.22, with a mean of +.09, which approximated the mean kappa of +.12 in the Jensen and Weisz (2002) study. Only the kappas of .22 for ADHD and .11 for any mood disorder were statistically significant.

Both the Jensen and Weisz (2002) and Lewcyk et al. (2003) articles reported tests of possible methodological explanations for the low kappas between clinical diagnoses and those obtained from the DISC. Based on their tests of possible methodological artifacts and their extensive reviews of other studies, the authors concluded that their findings accurately reflected typical levels of agreement between the DISC and diagnoses made independently by clinicians. Meta-analyses of multiple studies have yielded a mean kappa of .15 between diagnoses of children derived from standardized diagnostic interviews and diagnoses derived from clinical evaluations (Rettew, Doyle, Achenbach, Dumenci, & Ivanova, 2006).

Agreement between DIS Diagnoses and Clinical Diagnoses of Adults

The DISC was originally based on the DIS, which was designed to make diagnoses of adult disorders in epidemiological studies. Because the DIS preceded the DISC and because adult diagnostic categories have much longer histories than child diagnostic categories, validity findings for the DIS might be viewed as setting a standard to which the DISC should aspire.

How high a standard does the DIS set? In a study designed to test the agreement of DIS diagnoses of depression with clinicians' diagnoses, 349 adults were diagnosed according to the DIS administered in home interviews. The same 349 adults were later clinically assessed by psychiatrists who administered the Schedules for Clinical Assessment in Neuropsychiatry (SCAN; Wing et al., 1990), an extensive semi-structured clinical interview (Eaton, Neufeld, Chen, & Cai, 2000). The clinical assessment also included personality and neuropsychological tests, as well as assessment of risk factors. After assessing a participant and reviewing the DIS results, the psychiatrist dictated a two- to three-page summary of findings, including explanations for possible disagreements with the DIS. Diagnoses were ultimately made on the basis of conferences with other psychiatrists.

Eaton et al. reported a kappa of .20 between DIS diagnoses and clinical diagnoses of major depressive disorder, which was the main focus of the study. This kappa of .20 was somewhat better than the kappas of .12 and .09 found in the Jensen and Weisz (2002) and Lewczyk et al. (2003) studies of childhood diagnoses. However, the psychiatrists in the Eaton et al. study of adults reviewed the DIS results, and neither their diagnoses nor the DIS diagnoses required cross-informant comparisons. Despite these potential advantages, agreement between DIS diagnoses and the psychiatrists' diagnoses of adults were not materially better than agreement between the DISC diagnoses and clinical diagnoses of children. On the other hand, Eaton et al. (2000) reported that the number of different symptom groups (e.g., dysphoria, anhedonia) identified by the DIS had a Pearson r of .49 with the number of different symptom groups identified in the psychiatrists' clinical assessment of each participant. Considering that the magnitudes of kappas are similar to those of phi coefficients (Pearson rs for binary data), the Pearson r of .49 versus the kappa of .20 suggests that better agreement might be obtained when interview data are quantified than when they are categorized into yes/no diagnostic decisions. In addition to the Eaton Study, meta-analyses of multiple studies have yielded only moderate agreement between diagnoses of adults derived from clinical evaluations and diagnoses made from standardized diagnostic interviews, as indicated by a mean kappa of .29 (Rettew et al., 2006).

Agreement between DAWBA Diagnoses and Clinical Diagnoses

In the only published study that we found that reported agreement between DAWBA diagnoses and diagnoses based on clinical assessments, a child psychiatrist reviewed case notes recorded in the psychiatric clinic records of 39 children who were independently assessed with the parent DAWBA (Goodman, Ford, Richards, et al., 2000). Sixteen of the 20 11- to 15-year-olds in the sample were interviewed with the youth version of the DAWBA, and teachers completed DAWBA questionnaires for 17 of the total sample of 39.

Based on the case notes, the child psychiatrist judged diagnoses as absent, possible, or definite for the three broad categories of emotional disorders, conduct–oppositional disorders, and ADHD–hyperkinetic disorders. A disorder was judged present if the psychiatrist felt that it corresponded to either ICD-10 or DSM-IV criteria. The psychiatrist was blind to the DAWBA diagnoses. Computed separately for each of the three broad diagnostic categories for all 39 children, Kendall *tau b* rank-order correlations between DAWBA yes/no diagnoses and the psychiatrist's judgments of absent, possible, and definite were .52 for emotional disorders, .47 for conduct–oppositional disorders, and .70 for ADHD–hyperkinetic disorders, with a mean of .56. The *tau b* coefficients are larger than the mean kappa coefficients of .12 and .09 obtained for agreement between yes/no clinical diagnoses and DISC diagnoses in the Jensen and Weisz (2002) and Lewczyk et al. (2003) studies and the mean meta-analytic kappa of .15 (Rettew et al., 2006). The larger coefficients for the DAWBA could reflect the quasi-quantitative nature of the psychiatrist's judgments as absent–possible–definite, the properties of the *tau b* coefficient, the aggregation of diagnoses into three very broad categories, and/or the crediting of agreement for diagnoses that corresponded to either ICD-10 or DSM-IV criteria.

Agreement between DSM-Based Rating Scales and Clinical Diagnoses

DSM-based rating scales are scored quantitatively, by summing ratings for the symptom items, but are intended to assess DSM diagnoses. Cutpoints can be used to categorize scale scores as indicating a diagnosis versus no diagnosis. However, reports of agreement between scale scores and diagnoses have preserved the quantitative scale scores by using point-biserial correlations between the quantitative scale scores and yes/no diagnoses. The manual for the ADHD Rating Scale-IV reports correlations that averaged .31 between various combinations of DSM ADHD diagnoses and scores from the ADHD Rating Scale-IV completed by parents and teachers (DuPaul et al., 1998). (Although the correlations were computed using logistic regressions in which each scale score was the only predictor of yes/no diagnoses, the correlations are equivalent to point-biserial rs.) For DSM scales scored from the YI-4, Gadow et al. (2002) reported that the highest point-biserial rs with diagnoses found in clinic case records averaged .25 for the following diagnostic categories: ADHD, ODD, CD, depressive disorders, and anxiety disorders.

Like DISC diagnoses, scores obtained from rating scales comprised of DSM criterial items are thus weakly associated with DSM clinical diagnoses. Nevertheless, DuPaul et al. (1998) reported that teachers' ratings on the CTRS (Conners, 1989) Hyperactivity scale correlated .73 and .79, respectively, with the teachers' ratings on the Inattention and Hyperactivity–Impulsivity scales of the ADHD Rating Scale-IV. Similarly, Gadow et al. (2002) reported many rs in the .60s and .70s between youths' self-ratings on the YI-4 and their self-ratings on non-DSM scales of the CDI (Kovacs, 1992), the Multidimensional Anxiety Scales for Children (MASC; March, 1997), and the YSR (Achenbach, 1991c). These findings indicate that the DSM-based rating scales are significantly associated with other kinds of rating scales completed by the same informants, even if their associations with clinical diagnoses are minimal.

In summary, the findings indicate that diagnostic conclusions obtained from interviews and rating scales based on DSM criteria do not agree well with clinical diagnoses. The reasons for the low agreement may include factors such as the following: the difficulty of making reliable and valid judgments of the absence versus presence of each criterial feature required for each DSM diagnosis; the difficulty of making reliable and valid decisions about whether all the necessary criteria are met for each DSM diagnostic category; high rates of comorbidity that may make it hard to decide which DSM categories should have priority in classifying each child's disorders; and the difficulties of reconciling discrepancies between reports from different sources into yes/no judgments of DSM diagnoses. We now turn to comparisons between important characteristics of the empirically based and diagnostically based approaches.

COMPARISONS BETWEEN THE EMPIRICALLY BASED APPROACH AND THE DSM VERSION OF THE DIAGNOSTICALLY BASED APPROACH

The empirically and diagnostically based approaches to child psychopathology have many points of contact; both seek to improve assessment, understanding, prevention, and treatment of similar problems; both provide explicit statements of the problems to be assessed. And there are statistically significant associations between a variety of empirically based syndromes and DSM diagnoses (e.g., Achenbach & Rescorla, 2001; Conners, 2001; Kasius et al., 1997; Morgan & Cauce, 1999; Weinstein et al., 1990). The empirically based and diagnostically based approaches also face similar challenges; for example, determining which characteristics can discriminate best between children who do, versus do not, need professional help and between children who need different kinds of help. The challenges also include perfecting procedures for assessing characteristics relevant to psychopathology and for combining data from multiple sources in order to optimize decisions about how to help each child.

Despite these similarities, the two approaches differ in a variety of ways. As summarized in Table 3.4, the differences include the quantitative scoring of problems in the empirically based approach versus the yes/no judgments of problems in the DSM approach; the derivation of

TABLE 3.4. Similarities and Differences between the Empirically Based Approach and the DSM Version of the Diagnostically Based Approach to Child Psychopathology

Similarities between approaches

1. Both seek to improve assessment, understanding, prevention, and treatment of similar problems.
2. Both provide explicit statements of problems to be assessed.
3. Some empirically based syndromes and DSM categories comprise similar problems.
4. Statistically significant agreement has been found between some syndrome scores and diagnoses.
5. Both face similar challenges with respect to determining criterial characteristics, perfecting assessment procedures, and combining multisource data.

Differences between approaches

Empirically based	DSM
1. Problems are scored quantitatively.	1. Problems are judged as absent versus present.
2. "Bottom-up" approach: Syndromes are derived from problem scores.	2. "Top-down" approach: Categories and criteria are chosen by committees of experts.
3. Clinical cutpoints and norms are based on data for each gender, age, and source of data.	3. Clinical cutpoints are the same for both genders, different ages, and different sources of data.
4. Clinicians use parallel standardized forms and scoring profiles for data from multiple sources.	4. Clinicians choose sources of data, data to obtain, and assessment procedures.
5. Provides cross-informant comparisons of scores and profiles.	5. Does not specify procedures for comparing data from different sources.
6. End products are multi-informant item and syndrome scores displayed on norm-referenced profiles.	6. End products are diagnoses that are judged as absent versus present.

syndromes from problem scores versus the choice of categories and criteria by committees of experts; and the use of distributions of scores obtained by children of each gender and different ages from different sources of data to construct norms and to select clinical cutpoints versus experts' formulations of fixed rules for diagnostic decisions that are the same for both genders, different ages, and different sources of data.

Other differences concern methods for obtaining and using data: Practitioners using the empirically based approach obtain data from multiple informants on parallel standardized forms, which are scored on parallel profiles. The practitioners then compare data from multiple informants by using multi-informant item and syndrome scores that indicate problem levels according to reports by each informant. The end products are multi-informant item and syndrome scores displayed on norm-referenced profiles. By contrast, each practitioner using the DSM version of the diagnostically based approach chooses the sources of data, the data to obtain, and the assessment procedures. Each practitioner also decides whether to obtain data from multiple informants and how to reconcile contradictory data from different informants. The end products are diagnoses that must be categorized as absent versus present.

Throughout the book, we draw on findings from both the empirically based and diagnostically based approaches as we work toward new ways to understand, assess, prevent, and treat child psychopathology in multiple cultures.

SUMMARY

In this chapter we presented the diagnostically based "top-down" approach to psychopathology. This approach starts "at the top" with experts' concepts of disorders. These concepts serve as taxonomic constructs for which the experts then formulate definitions in terms of symptoms and other criteria. Although the diagnostic approach to adult psychopathology emerged in the 19th century, explicitly defined diagnostic categories for childhood disorders were added to the DSM only in 1980 (American Psychiatric Association, 1980). Explicit categories for childhood disorders were also added to the International Classification of Diseases during the same period (ICD-9, ICD-10; World Health Organization, 1978, 1992, 1993).

Other than specifying IQ tests for diagnosing mental retardation, the DSM and ICD do not specify assessment operations for determining whether diagnostic criteria are met for childhood disorders. Efforts have been made to operationalize DSM criteria for childhood disorders by means of structured diagnostic interviews that ask parents and children whether criterial symptoms have been present during particular periods. The "respondent-based" DISC and DICA base diagnoses mainly on respondents' endorsements of symptoms. However, the CAPA and K-SADS are more "interviewer based" in that interviewers probe and evaluate respondents' answers before deciding whether diagnostic criteria are met. The DAWBA is intended to combine respondent-based and interviewer-based methods by using lay interviewers to obtain informants' responses but then using clinicians to make diagnostic judgments from computer printouts of the responses. Rating scales have also been developed to obtain parent, teacher, and self-ratings of symptoms specified by the DSM.

Because current versions of diagnoses must be judged as absent versus present, test–retest reliability and cross-informant agreement for diagnostic interviews have been measured with kappa coefficients. The kappa coefficients for diagnoses have been smaller than the Pearson rs found for test–retest reliability and cross-informant agreement for empirically based syndrome scales and quantitative DSM-oriented scales. Because binary data tend to yield smaller correlations than data scored continuously, the reliability and cross-informant coefficients for DSM diagnoses may be limited by the yes/no decisions required by categorical diagnoses. When symptom ratings on DSM-based scales are scored on continuous scales, the Pearson rs for reliability and cross-informant agreement are larger than the kappas between categorical diagnoses.

The main validity criteria for DSM interviews and rating forms are DSM diagnoses made by practitioners on the basis of diverse kinds of data obtained for clinical cases. When practitioners making clinical diagnoses were blind to the DISC results, the mean kappas between the clinical diagnoses and DISC diagnoses were .09 and .12 in two exceptionally thorough studies. In meta-analyses of agreement between child diagnoses made from various standardized interviews and clinical evaluations, the mean kappa was .15. For adult diagnoses, the mean meta-analytic kappa was .29. Point-biserial correlations between DSM clinical diagnoses and scores on the DSM-based ADHD Rating Scale-IV and the YI-4 have averaged .31 and .25, respectively.

Comparisons between the empirically based approach and the DSM version of the diagnostically based approach indicate many points of contact and some similar challenges, as well as a variety of differences. In the following chapters, we draw on findings from both approaches as we seek to advance understanding of child psychopathology across cultures.

CHAPTER 4

Multicultural Findings on Scores Obtained with Empirically Based Assessment Instruments

In this chapter we review multicultural research using empirically based assessment instruments. Most studies have used the CBCL, TRF, or YSR, the three school-age instruments of the ASEBA. Our review of ASEBA multicultural research compares cultures with respect to mean scores on scales, syndromes, and items. We also review gender and age effects across multiple cultures. Next we review findings from research using other empirically based instruments, such as the CTRS and CPRS (Conners, 1997) and the SDQ (Goodman, 2001). In selecting studies for review we gave priority to those that met the following criteria:

1. They were published or accepted for publication in peer-reviewed journals.
2. Their findings were based on standardized procedures used in two or more cultures.
3. They employed samples that were reasonably representative of important populations, rather than "convenience" samples.
4. Samples had a minimum of 300 participants per culture, recommended as the minimum sample size by Nunnally and Bernstein (1994, p. 228).
5. They reported appropriate and well-documented statistical analyses.

ASEBA MULTICULTURAL RESEARCH

Multicultural research using ASEBA instruments started in the 1980s. Many of the first studies provided bicultural comparisons with findings from the United States. For instance, Weisz et al. (1987) compared Thai and U.S. samples. Verhulst and Achenbach (1995) subsequently published an integrative review of the early bicultural ASEBA studies. Crijnen, Achenbach, and Verhulst (1997) then pioneered a new approach to multicultural research when they compared 12 cultures on CBCL Total Problems, Externalizing, and Internalizing scores. Later studies compared CBCL syndrome scores in the same 12 cultures (Crijnen, Achenbach, & Verhulst, 1999) and YSR scores in 7 cultures (Verhulst et al., 2003). Subsequent multicultural comparisons included CBCLs from 31 cultures (Rescorla et al., 2006a), TRFs from 21 cultures (Rescorla et al., in press), and YSRs from 24 cultures (Rescorla et al., 2006b).

Because of the very high statistical power afforded by the studies reviewed, we omit any findings with $p > .001$ and concentrate on findings with effect sizes (ESs) $\geq 1\%$. We interpret the magnitude of ESs using J. Cohen's (1988) criteria for ANOVAs, whereby an ES of 1–5.9% is *small*, an ES of 5.9–13.8% is *medium*, and an ES > 13.8% is *large*. All analyses of CBCL, TRF, and YSR data were conducted using raw scores, as recommended by Achenbach and Rescorla (2001). Unless otherwise noted, all analyses summarized in this chapter were analyses of variance (ANOVAs), analyses of covariance (ANCOVAs), multivariate analyses of variance (MANOVAs), or multivariate analyses of covariance (MANCOVAs).

CBCL STUDIES

At the time of the Verhulst and Achenbach (1995) review, bicultural comparisons of CBCL data from large general population samples had been published for nine cultures. We summarize findings from these bicultural studies and from the Crijnen et al. (1997, 1999) CBCL multicultural comparisons. We then review findings from the CBCL multicultural comparisons for 31 cultures, reported by Rescorla et al. (2006a).

Bicultural Comparisons of the CBCL Scores

In the Verhulst and Achenbach (1995) review, scores from Australia, China, France, Greece, Jamaica, the Netherlands, Puerto Rico, and Thailand were compared to scores from one of two U.S. samples

(Achenbach, 1991a; Achenbach & Edelbrock, 1981), whereas scores from Belgium were compared to Dutch scores. Total Problems scores ranged from 20.0 for the Achenbach and Edelbrock (1981) U.S. sample to 35.4 for the Greek sample (MacDonald, Tsiantis, Achenbach, Motto-Stefanidi, & Richardson, 1995), out of a possible range of 0–236. About half of the bicultural comparisons for Total Problems scores yielded significant differences between pairs of cultures, with ESs ranging from 1% for Thailand versus the United States to 11% for Sydney, Australia versus the United States. All significant gender, age, and SES effects for Total Problems were < 1%. Gender differences for Internalizing and Externalizing were reported in two of the bicultural studies reviewed. In the Jamaica–U.S. comparison (Lambert, Lyubansky, & Achenbach, 1998), as well as in the Puerto Rico–U.S. comparison (Achenbach, Bird, et al., 1990), girls scored higher on Internalizing problems, whereas boys scored higher on Externalizing problems. In the Thailand–U.S. comparisons (Weisz et al., 1987; Weisz, Suwanlert, et al., 1993), Thai children had higher scores than U.S. children on Overcontrolled problems (a composite the authors computed that is analogous to Internalizing), but did not differ significantly from U.S. children on Undercontrolled problems (a composite analogous to Externalizing).

Crijnen's Multicultural Comparisons of CBCL Scores

Crijnen et al. (1997) compared CBCL data from 12 cultures (Australia, Belgium, China, Germany, Greece, Israel, Jamaica, the Netherlands, Puerto Rico, Sweden, Thailand, and the United States) in a single set of analyses (N = 13,697). Bicultural data from several of these cultures were presented previously in the Verhulst and Achenbach (1995) review. Response rates were all ≥ 80%, and sample sizes ranged from 466 for Greece to 2,863 for Germany. For Total Problems scores, Crijnen et al. (1997) found that cultural differences accounted for 11% of the variance for ages 6–11 in 12 cultures and for 8% of the variance for ages 6–17 in 9 cultures. The mean Total Problems score for ages 6–11 across 12 cultures was 22.4 (the "omnicultural" mean), whereas the omnicultural mean for ages 6–17 across 9 cultures was 20.3. Most cultures scored within 4 points of the omnicultural mean for both the 6–11 and 6–17 age analyses. Further analyses for ages 6–11 indicated that the ES for culture was 9% for Internalizing and 7% for Externalizing. Gender and age effects were significant but < 1%, and no interactions with culture were significant. In other words, the gender and age effects were similar in all cultures. Girls scored higher than boys on Internalizing, whereas boys scored higher than girls on Externalizing.

Internalizing scores increased with age, whereas Externalizing scores decreased.

In the Crijnen et al. (1997) 12-culture analysis, the mean Total Problems score of 35.2 for Puerto Rico was the highest, whereas the mean score of 13.3 for Sweden was the lowest. Crijnen et al. (1997) suggested that these differences in problem scores may have been due in part to differences in sampling procedures. The Puerto Rican sample was obtained by randomly sampling households on the entire island, with a 92% response rate, which was the highest of any culture. The Swedish sample, by contrast, was obtained by sampling from schools in a relatively affluent area of Sweden, the response rate was lower (84%), and special schools for children with problems were excluded. These selection factors meant that more children who would have obtained high problem scores may have been omitted in Sweden than in Puerto Rico.

In a second study Crijnen et al. (1999) compared scores for children ages 6–17 from nine cultures on the eight CBCL syndromes ($N = 11,887$). Culture ESs ranged from 1% on the Delinquent Behavior syndrome (now designated as Rule-Breaking Behavior; Achenbach & Rescorla, 2001) to 9% on Withdrawn (now designated as Withdrawn/Depressed). Girls had significantly higher scores than boys on Somatic Complaints and Anxious/Depressed (ESs < 1%).

To measure similarities in mean item scores across cultures, Crijnen et al. (1997) computed rs between the mean score obtained on each item by all children in one culture and the mean score obtained on each item in another culture. The mean of the rs between all pairs of cultures was .78, indicating substantial similarity, on average. In other words, the 12 cultures were quite similar in terms of which CBCL items had high versus low mean scores. The largest mean r of any one culture with all other cultures was .84 for the United States, while the smallest mean r was .68 for China.

Rescorla's Multicultural Comparisons of CBCL Scores

Using the procedures pioneered by Crijnen et al. (1997, 1999), Rescorla et al. (2006a) compared CBCL problem scores from general population samples in 31 cultures ($N = 55,508$). Ns ranged from 513 (Ethiopia) to 4,858 (China). ESs for culture ranged from 3% to 14% across the 17 CBCL scales.

CBCL Total Problems Scores

Mean CBCL Total Problems scores for ages 6-16 in the 31 cultures ranged from 13.1 for Japan to 34.7 for Puerto Rico. An omnicultural mean of 22.5 (*SD* = 5.6) was obtained by averaging the Total Problems scores of the 31 cultures. This omnicultural mean was quite close to Crijnen et al.'s (1997) CBCL omnicultural mean of 20.3 for ages 6–17 in 9 cultures. Nineteen of the 31 cultures in the Rescorla et al. (2006a) study scored within one *SD* of the omnicultural mean, six scored below this range and six scored above this range.

Figure 4.1 shows the distributions of CBCL Total Problems scores for the 6 "low" scoring cultures, the 19 "medium" scoring cultures, and the 6 "high" scoring cultures. Each point on the *X* axis represents an interval of three Total Problems scores (e.g., T1 = Total Problems scores of 0, 1, and 2). The three groups of cultures have highly overlapping distributions, with similar shapes over much of the range. The main difference between the low-, medium-, and high-scoring cultures is in the percentage of children who obtained very low Total Problems scores. For example, 15% of the low-scoring samples, 7% of the medium-scoring samples, and 3% of the high-scoring samples obtained Total Problems scores of 0, 1, or 2 (i.e., T1). In contrast, 5% of the low-scoring, 6% of the medium-scoring, and 7% of the high-scoring samples obtained Total Problems scores around the omnicultural mean (i.e., T22 = 21, 22, or 23). This convergence of the three samples is even more marked at T61: 0.3%, 0.7%, and 1.4% obtained Total Problems scores of 60, 61, and 62. The convergence of the low, medium, and

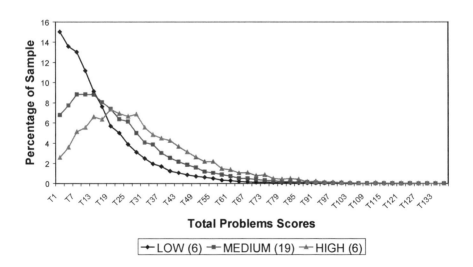

FIGURE 4.1. CBCL Total Problems score distributions for low-, medium-, and high-scoring cultures. Copyright T. M. Achenbach and L. A. Rescorla. Reprinted by permission.

high scoring samples at higher scores is important, because a major purpose of the CBCL is to identify children with high scores who may be in need of help.

CBCL Internalizing and Externalizing Scores

Girls obtained higher CBCL Internalizing scores than boys, with the differences being significant in more cultures at ages 12–16 than at ages 6–11. As Figure 4.2 shows, Internalizing scores increased significantly more with age for girls than for boys. Boys obtained higher CBCL Externalizing scores than girls (ES < 1%), with the differences being significant in more cultures at ages 6–11 than at ages 12–16. Externalizing scores decreased with age for boys but not for girls.

CBCL Syndrome Scores

The smallest ES of culture on the CBCL syndrome scores was 4% for Rule-Breaking Behavior, an Externalizing syndrome. The largest ES for culture was 9% on Anxious/Depressed, an Internalizing syndrome. Girls generally had higher scores on Somatic Complaints and Anxious/Depressed, whereas boys generally had higher scores on Attention Problems, Rule-Breaking Behavior, and Aggressive Behavior. For

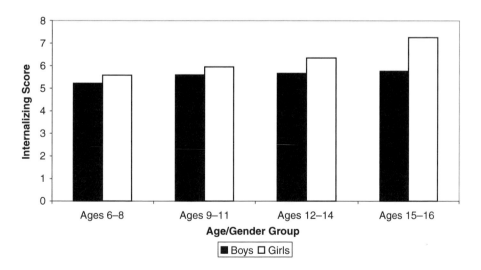

FIGURE 4.2. CBCL Internalizing scores by gender and age for 24 cultures (N = 47,987).

Internalizing syndromes, gender differences were more consistent across cultures at ages 12–16 than at ages 6–11. Conversely, for Externalizing syndromes, gender differences were more consistent across cultures at ages 6–11 than at ages 12–16. For example, boys scored significantly higher than girls on Aggressive Behavior in fewer cultures at ages 12–16 (5 cultures) than at ages 6–11 (21 cultures). As Figure 4.3 shows, Aggressive Behavior scores decreased significantly more with age for boys than for girls.

CBCL DSM-Oriented Scale Scores

The smallest ES of culture on the CBCL DSM-oriented scales was 3% on Conduct Problems, while the largest was 8% for Anxiety Problems. The range of ESs was comparable to the ESs for the empirically based syndromes. For both sets of scales, ESs for culture were smaller for Externalizing kinds of problems than for Internalizing kinds of problems. Girls scored higher than boys on Affective Problems, Anxiety Problems, and Somatic Problems, and lower than boys on Attention Deficit Hyperactivity Problems, Oppositional Defiant Problems, and Conduct Problems. The DSM-oriented scales displayed the same pattern of changing gender differences with age as the empirically based syndromes.

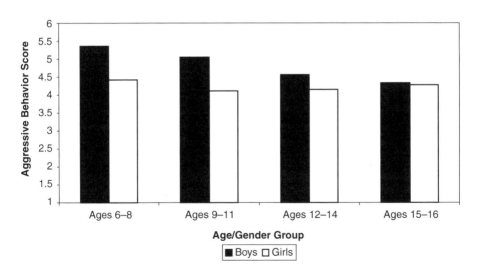

FIGURE 4.3. CBCL Aggressive Behavior scores by gender and age for 24 cultures ($N = 47,987$).

CBCL Mean Item Scores

Rescorla et al. (2006a) reported *r*s between mean CBCL item scores obtained in each of the 31 cultures. The mean *r* across all pairwise comparisons was .74, very close to the .78 found by Crijnen et al. (1997) for CBCL item scores. Among the 10 items with the highest mean scores were problems of attention, self-control, noncompliance, shyness, perfectionism, and jealousy. Sex problems, suicide attempts, sees things that aren't there, using alcohol or drugs, running away from home, vandalism, stealing, and daytime enuresis were among the 10 items with the lowest mean scores.

Multicultural Module

CBCL problem scores from many cultures have made it possible to create scoring software that enables users to display a child's CBCL scale scores in relation to three sets of norms. One set of norms reflects scores for the six cultures whose mean Total Problems scores were more than one standard deviation *below* the omnicultural mean. A second set of norms reflects scores for the six cultures whose mean Total Problems scores were more than one standard deviation *above* the omnicultural mean. To create norms for the low-scoring cultures, for example, Achenbach and Rescorla (in press) averaged the distributions of scores on that scale from the six low-scoring cultures to produce a single distribution. The sample sizes differed among the cultures, but each culture was given equal weight by averaging that culture's distribution of scores together with the distributions obtained in the other five low-scoring cultures. The distribution for the six low-scoring cultures was then used as the basis for the percentiles and standard scores (*T* scores) for each scale. The same procedure was used to derive percentiles and standard scores for the six high-scoring cultures. To represent the cultures whose mean Total Problems scores were between one standard deviation below and one standard deviation above the omnicultural mean (i.e., the medium-scoring cultures), Achenbach and Rescorla used percentiles and *T* scores based on the 2001 U.S. norms. The U.S. norms were used because the mean U.S. Total Problems score was at about the middle of the medium-scoring group and because so many publications and practical applications have been based on the U.S. percentiles and *T* scores.

The software containing the three sets of norms is called the Multicultural Module for Ages 6–18. When data from a CBCL are entered into the module, the user can elect to have the scale scores displayed in relation to percentiles and *T* scores for the low, medium, or high norms. In addition, TRF and YSR data can be entered into the module and can then be displayed in relation to percentiles and T scores for the low-, medium-, and high-scoring samples described in the following sections.

The availability of low, medium, and high norms for the CBCL, TRF, and YSR makes it possible to display parent, teacher, and self-ratings for a child in relation to different sets of norms. For example, consider a girl whose family has emigrated from a culture in the low-scoring group to a culture in the medium-scoring group. The girl's parents complete the CBCL in a language that they know. An evaluator can then use the module to display the girl's CBCL scale scores in relation to the low norms characteristic of her home culture and also to display her scale scores in relation to the medium norms characteristic of the host culture. By viewing the girl's CBCL scale scores in relation to norms for both the home and the host cultures, the evaluator can see whether the girl's problem scores exceed the normal range in relation to either or both sets of norms. If the girl attends school in the host culture, her teachers can be asked to complete the TRF. The module can then be used to display scores in relation to TRF norms for the girl's home culture and the host culture. If the girl is at least 11 years old, she can complete the YSR. The module can then be used to display her YSR scale scores in relation to norms for her home culture and the host culture. The evaluator can thus see whether problems reported by parents, teachers, or youths deviate from various combinations of potentially relevant norms. The normed scores computed by the module can also be used for research on problem scores in relation to the distributions of scores from various cultures. Information about the module can be obtained at www.ASEBA.org.

TRF STUDIES

Verhulst and Achenbach (1995) reviewed findings from five bicultural comparisons of the TRF. After briefly summarizing findings from these five bicultural comparisons and two subsequent ones, we review findings from the Rescorla et al. (in press) TRF study comparing 21 cultures.

Bicultural Comparisons of TRF Scores

The Verhulst and Achenbach (1995) review included bicultural comparisons between teachers' ratings for general population samples of students in the United States versus demographically similar students in Jamaica, the Netherlands, Puerto Rico, Thailand, and China. Mean TRF Total Problems scores ranged from 17.6 (the Netherlands) to 39.0 (rural China), out of a possible range of 0–236. The largest culture ES for Total Problems was 5%. Significant effects for culture were also reported for some TRF problem items, syndromes, and for the Internalizing and Externalizing scales (with ESs for culture ranging from < 1 to 9%). Teachers scored boys significantly higher than girls on Total Problems in all cultural groups. Significant SES effects were reported on TRF scores in the Netherlands, Puerto Rico, Jamaica, and the United States, with children from lower SES families obtaining higher problem scores in all comparisons.

Since the Verhulst and Achenbach (1995) review, TRF data have also been reported for Greece (Roussos et al., 1999) and Portugal (Fonseca et al., 1995). Although direct comparisons with U.S. data were not reported in either study, mean Total Problems scores were quite similar to those from the 1991 U.S. normative sample current at the time of the reports (Achenbach, 1991b).

Two bicultural studies have reported correlations between mean TRF item scores obtained in pairs of cultures. An r of .78 was obtained between TRF item scores in the U.S. mainland and Puerto Rican samples (Achenbach et al., 1990). An r of .72 was obtained between Chinese and American TRF item scores in urban areas, whereas an r of .44 was obtained for TRF item scores in rural areas of the two cultures (Weine, Phillips, & Achenbach, 1995).

Rescorla's Multicultural Comparisons of TRF Scores

Using procedures similar to those employed by Rescorla et al. (2006a), Rescorla et al. (in press) tested the effects of culture, gender, and age on TRF scores for students ages 6–15 in 21 cultures ($N = 30,957$). ESs for culture ranged from 3 to 13% across all TRF scales.

TRF Total Problems Scores

Fifteen of the 21 cultures scored within one standard deviation of the TRF omnicultural mean of 21.6, which was very close to the omnicultural mean of 22.5 found for 31 cultures on the CBCL (Rescorla, 2006a). Three cultures scored more than one standard deviation below the overall mean, whereas three other cultures scored more than one standard deviation above this mean. Mean TRF Total Problems scores ranged from 8.4 for Japan to 31.6 for Puerto Rico.

TRF Internalizing and Externalizing Scores

Girls' Internalizing scores on the TRF were significantly higher than boys' scores in fewer cultures than on the CBCL. Internalizing scores increased with age for both genders, but more so for girls than for boys.

The gender ES for Externalizing was larger for the TRF (2%) than for the CBCL (< 1%). As Figure 4.4 shows, boys obtained higher Externalizing scores than girls in all cultures, significantly so in all cultures except Iran and Jamaica. There was no consistent association between age and Externalizing scores across cultures.

TRF Syndrome Scores

On the TRF syndromes, ESs for culture ranged from 3% for Thought Problems to 13% for Anxious/Depressed. Gender ESs were largest for Attention Problems, Rule-Breaking Behavior, and Aggressive Behavior, with boys obtaining higher scores than girls in nearly all cultures. These gender differences were larger than those found for the CBCL. Across cultures, girls did not obtain consistently higher scores than boys on any TRF syndrome, unlike the pattern found for the CBCL. Age trends varied across syndromes and cultures.

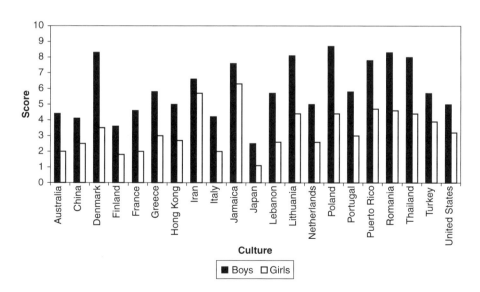

FIGURE 4.4. TRF Externalizing scores by gender for 21 cultures ($N = 30,957$).

TRF DSM-Oriented Scale Scores

On the TRF DSM-oriented scales, ESs for culture were smallest for Somatic Problems, Oppositional Defiant Problems, and Conduct Problems (all 3%) and largest for Anxiety Problems (8%). Boys scored
higher than girls on Oppositional Defiant Problems, Attention Deficit
Hyperactivity Problems, and Conduct Problems in most cultures. Figure 4.5 depicts the striking gender differences for TRF DSM-oriented
Attention Deficit Hyperactivity Problems. Girls scored significantly
higher than boys on Affective Problems and Somatic Problems, but in
fewer than half the cultures. The only DSM-oriented scale with a consistent age pattern across cultures was Affective Problems, on which
scores generally increased with age.

Mean TRF Item Scores

The mean bicultural r of .74 for TRF mean item scores, identical to the
mean bicultural r obtained for the CBCL, indicates similar rank order-
ings of item scores for teachers' ratings in very diverse cultures. Five of
the 10 TRF items with the highest mean scores across cultures were
from the Attention Problems syndrome (e.g., failing to concentrate, to
finish tasks, and to work up to potential). The other five items were
from the Internalizing grouping (e.g., being afraid of making mistakes,

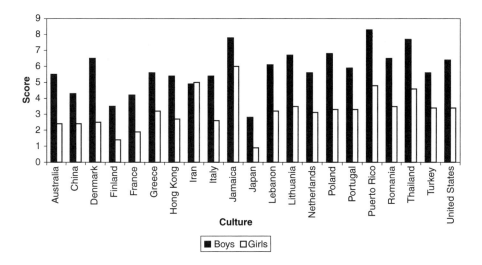

FIGURE 4.5. TRF DSM-oriented Attention Deficit/Hyperactivity Problems
scores by gender in 21 cultures (N = 30,957).

being shy, feeling hurt when criticized). Hearing or seeing things that aren't there, somatic complaints, suicidal thoughts and attempts, stealing, using alcohol or drugs, and strange ideas were among the 10 TRF items with the lowest mean scores.

YSR STUDIES

Verhulst and Achenbach (1995) summarized two bicultural YSR studies. A third bicultural study was published shortly thereafter (Lambert et al., 1998). We briefly review findings from these three bicultural studies and then summarize multicultural comparisons of YSR scores from seven cultures (Verhulst et al., 2003). Thereafter, we present findings from the Rescorla et al. (in press) comparison of YSR scores from 24 cultures.

Bicultural Comparisons of YSR Scores

Verhulst and Achenbach (1995) reviewed bicultural comparisons of YSR scores from the United States with YSR scores from the Netherlands and Puerto Rico. Whereas CBCL and TRF scores were similar for the United States and the Netherlands, Dutch YSR scores were significantly lower than U.S. YSR scores on Total Problems (ES = 13%). In both cultures, YSR scores were higher than CBCL and TRF scores. Girls obtained significantly higher scores than boys on the YSR Internalizing scale but lower scores than boys on the YSR Externalizing scale. Older youths scored higher than younger youths on Internalizing, Withdrawn, and Delinquent Behavior. Verhulst and Achenbach (1995) also reported that Puerto Rican YSR Total Problems scores were significantly lower than mainland U.S. YSR scores (ES = 4%), whereas Puerto Rican CBCL and TRF Total Problems scores were significantly higher than those in the mainland sample. CBCL, TRF, and YSR Total Problems scores were quite similar to each other in Puerto Rico, whereas CBCL and TRF scores were much lower than YSR scores in the mainland sample. Girls obtained significantly higher YSR Total Problems scores than boys in both cultures. In addition, low-SES youths reported significantly more problems than upper YSR youths in both cultures.

Lambert et al. (1998) reported that YSR Total Problems scores were similar in Jamaica and the United States. YSR scores were higher than CBCL and TRF scores in both cultures. Boys scored significantly higher than girls on Externalizing and lower on Internalizing in both cultures, and lower SES was associated with higher Internalizing and Externalizing scores on the YSR in both cultures.

Verhulst's Multicultural Comparisons of YSR Scores

Verhulst et al. (2003) compared YSR scores for 7,137 youths from seven cultures (Australia, Hong Kong, Israel, Jamaica, the Netherlands, Turkey, and the United States). Response rates were all ≥ 78%. The culture ES for Total Problems scores was 5% and the YSR omnicultural mean was 37.6. The highest mean Total Problems score was in Hong Kong, whereas the lowest was in Israel. For all five cultures having parent as well as youth ratings, YSR Total Problems scores were much higher than CBCL Total Problems scores. Girls obtained significantly higher YSR Total Problems scores than boys (ES < 1%). Boys obtained significantly higher Externalizing scores but lower Internalizing scores than girls. Culture ESs for YSR syndromes ranged from 3% (Aggressive Behavior) to 8% (Thought Problems). The mean of the bicultural correlations between YSR item scores was .75. The United States had the largest mean r (.83) with all other cultures, whereas Turkey had the smallest (.69). The largest bicultural correlation was between Australia and the United States (.92).

Rescorla's Multicultural Comparisons of YSR Scores

Using procedures similar to those employed by Rescorla et al. (2006a, in press), Rescorla et al. (2006b) tested the effects of culture, gender, and age on YSR scores in 24 cultures (N = 27,206). Data from five of the cultures were included in the Verhulst et al. (2003) study. The 14 YSR items that tap positive qualities (e.g., *6. I like animals*; *59. I can be pretty friendly*; and *98. I like to help others)* were analyzed separately as a Positive Qualities scale. ESs for culture ranged from 3 to 9% across the 17 YSR problem scales, which is the same as the range for the CBCL.

YSR Total Problems Scores

Contrary to the pattern found on the CBCL and the TRF but consistent with Verhulst et al.'s (2003) YSR findings, girls obtained significantly higher YSR Total Problems scores than boys. Youths ages 14 to 16 reported significantly more problems than youths ages 11–13, also consistent with Verhulst et al.'s findings.

The omnicultural mean for the YSR Total Problems score was 35.3 (SD = 6.0), slightly lower than the mean of 37.6 reported by Verhulst et al. (2003) for seven cultures. Four cultures scored more than one standard deviation below the omnicultural mean, three cultures scored more than one standard deviation above the omnicultural mean, and 17 cultures scored within one standard deviation of the omnicultural mean.

For 19 cultures, CBCL and YSR data were available for many of the same participants. CBCL and YSR means for adolescents ages 11–16 in each culture were computed using the same 98 problem items common to both forms. The CBCL Total Problems mean was 20.5, which was 13.5 points lower than the YSR omnicultural mean of 34.0. Thus, adolescents across these 19 cultures clearly reported many more problems than their parents reported about them.

YSR Internalizing and Externalizing Scores

Girls obtained significantly higher Internalizing scores than boys in most cultures, as shown in Figure 4.6. This gender difference for Internalizing scores was found in more countries for the YSR than for the CBCL. Youths ages 14–16 obtained significantly higher Internalizing scores than youths ages 11–13.

As was true on the CBCL and TRF and in the Verhulst et al. (2003) study of the YSR, boys obtained significantly higher Externalizing

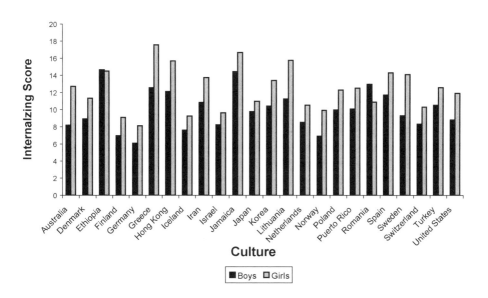

FIGURE 4.6. YSR Internalizing scores by gender in 24 cultures ($N = 27,206$).

scores than girls. Youths ages 14–16 obtained significantly higher Externalizing scores than youths ages 11–13.

YSR Syndrome Scores

Culture ESs for YSR syndrome scores ranged from 5% for Withdrawn/ Depressed, Somatic Complaints, and Aggressive Behavior to 9% for Attention Problems. Girls obtained significantly higher scores than boys on Anxious/Depressed, Withdrawn/Depressed, and Somatic Complaints, whereas boys obtained significantly higher scores than girls on Rule-Breaking Behavior and Aggressive Behavior. Consistent with the Verhulst et al. (2003) findings, boys and girls did not differ on YSR Attention Problems. This is notable because parents and teachers in most cultures rated boys higher than girls on Attention Problems (Rescorla et al., 2006a, in press). In many cultures, youths ages 14–16 obtained higher scores than youths ages 11–13 on Withdrawn/Depressed, Attention-Problems, Rule-Breaking Behavior, and Aggressive Behavior.

YSR DSM-Oriented Scale Scores

On the YSR DSM-oriented scales, ESs for cultures ranged from 3% for Conduct Problems to 8% for Attention Deficit Hyperactivity Problems. Girls scored higher than boys in more than half the cultures on Affective Problems, Anxiety Problems, and Somatic Problems. Conversely, boys scored higher than girls on Conduct Problems in more than half the cultures. For all DSM-oriented scales except Somatic Problems, scores were significantly higher for ages 14–16 than for ages 11–13. As shown in Figure 4.7, girls obtained slightly higher scores than boys on the DSM-oriented Affective Problems scale at ages 11–13 but much higher scores than boys at ages 14–16.

YSR Positive Qualities Scale Scores

As Figure 4.8 shows, most cultures had mean Positive Qualities scores in the range of 19–21. Standard deviations for Positive Qualities scores were quite small within each culture, which resulted in a very large culture ES of 27%. Although youths in many diverse cultures were similar in rating their positive qualities, youths in Ethiopia, Korea, Hong Kong, and Japan rated themselves less positively. Rescorla et al. (2006b) suggested that this may reflect cultural differences in how appropriate it is considered to praise oneself or to "boast" about positive qualities. Girls scored significantly higher on the Positive Qualities scale than

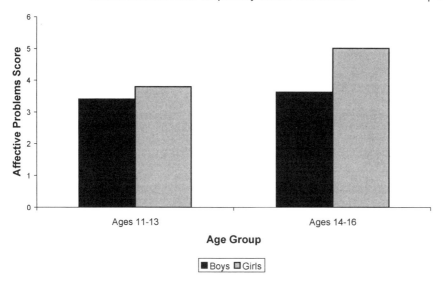

FIGURE 4.7. YSR DSM-Oriented Affective Problems scores by gender and age for 24 cultures (*N* = 27,206). Copyright T. M. Achenbach and L. A. Rescorla. Reprinted by permission.

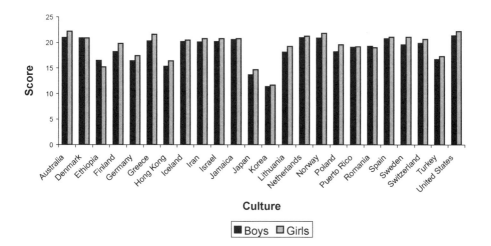

FIGURE 4.8. YSR Positive Qualities scores by gender in 24 cultures (*N* = 27,206).

boys, and youths ages 14–16 scored significantly higher than youths ages 11–13. As would be expected, mean scores on the 14-item Positive Qualities scale were much higher than scores on any of the YSR syndrome or DSM-oriented scales.

Mean YSR Item Scores

When bicultural rs between the 98 mean problem item scores obtained on the YSR in each culture were computed, the mean bicultural r was .69. The mean r across cultures was slightly lower for the YSR (.69) than for the CBCL or the TRF (both .74). The 10 YSR problem items with the highest mean scores included shyness; mood swings; perfectionism; problems concentrating; daydreaming; and being stubborn, secretive, and argumentative. Conversely, the 10 items with the lowest mean scores included stealing; deliberate self-injury; suicidal ideation; hearing and seeing things that are not there; running away from home; setting fires; destroying things belonging to others; being afraid of school; and vomiting without known medical cause.

CONNERS RATING SCALES

The Conners scales for parents and teachers have been used in a few multicultural studies that met our methodological criteria for inclusion. We summarize this research next.

Conners Parent Rating Scale

Al-Awad and Sonuga-Barke (2002) reported scores from a 48-item Arabic version of the 1978 CPRS (Goyette et al., 1978) administered to parents of 300 6- to 10-year-olds in Khartoum and Medani, the two main cities of Sudan. The sample was stratified to include equal numbers of boys and girls from upper, middle, and lower-SES families. Response rates were not reported. Single-sample t tests were used to compare the Sudanese CPRS scale scores with the mean scale scores previously published for a Canadian sample (Trites, Blouin, & Laprade, 1982). For both genders, the Sudanese scores were significantly ($p <$ .001) lower than the Canadian scores on four of the five CPRS scales.

In another study, Rosenberg and Jani (1995) obtained parents' ratings on a 48-item version of the CPRS (Conners, 1990) for 863 children living around Bombay, India. For upper-SES children (N = 132), parents completed the English language CPRS. For lower-SES children (N = 731), parents completed a Gujarati translation. The authors did not provide information about sampling procedures, response rates, administration procedures, or the age range of the children, although the mean age was about 8.5 years. No direct statistical comparisons of the Indian scores with scores from other countries were reported, but Rosenberg and Jani did report that the mean T scores on the five scales scored from the CPRS were within one standard deviation of the mean T scores reported by Conners (1990) for American children.

Conners Teacher Rating Scale

Two studies have reported multicultural comparisons of scores on the CTRS. Al-Awad and Sonuga-Barke (2002) compared mean CTRS scores (39-item version) obtained by 300 Sudanese students with the mean CTRS scores previously published by Trites et al. (1982) for a Canadian sample. Like their findings for the CPRS, Al-Awad and Sonuga-Barke found that Sudanese students tended to obtain lower scores than the Canadian sample, with the differences being significant ($p < .001$) on four of the six CTRS scales for both genders.

Using an early version of the 39-item CTRS (Conners, 1973), Luk, Leung, and Lee (1988) obtained teachers' ratings for 914 randomly selected 6- to 12-year-olds attending schools in Hong Kong. A table comparing the mean Hong Kong scores on four CTRS scales with scores from New Zealand (Werry & Hawthorne, 1976), England (Taylor & Sandberg, 1984), and a town in the United States (Werry, Sprague, & Cohen, 1975) showed that the New Zealand sample had the highest scores in most comparisons, and the American sample had the lowest. However, statistical comparisons were precluded by the many differences among the studies.

Several studies have reported prevalence rates for scores above certain cutpoints on 10-item versions of the CTRS (called the Abbreviated Conners Teacher Rating Scale or "ATRS"; summarized by O'Leary, Vivian, & Nisi, 1985). However, many of the studies were unpublished or lacked detailed reports in peer-reviewed journals. We know of no published statistical comparisons for the same CTRS item sets scored for students selected randomly from different cultural groups.

Using a very early version of the 39-item CTRS (Conners, 1969), O'Leary et al. (1985) had 23 teachers in 14 Italian schools complete the CTRS on all students in their classes (total $N = 344$). Based only on the 10 items that are on the ATRS, O'Leary et al. found that the cutpoint used in most studies classified 19.9% of Italian boys but only 2.6% of Italian girls as hyperactive. On both the ATRS and the Hyperactivity factor derived from the 39-item CTRS, boys obtained much higher scores than girls. O'Leary et al. concluded that the large gender differences should be taken into account in establishing cutpoints.

STRENGTHS AND DIFFICULTIES QUESTIONNAIRE

Since Goodman (1997) published the SDQ, it has been translated into many languages and has been used for research in numerous cultures other than the United Kingdom, where it was developed. Many studies report SDQ results in a single culture. In addition, SDQ studies in several cultures have been summarized in two reviews, one of which reported some statistical comparisons. Only a few studies met our methodological criteria of $N \geq 300$ per culture from representative samples, similar standardized procedures employed in at least two cultures, and statistical comparisons of results across cultures. Nonetheless, to illustrate ways in which the SDQ has been used in diverse cultures, we include some studies that failed to meet our methodological criteria.

SDQ Findings from Single-Culture Studies

SDQ findings from large general population samples have been published for the United Kingdom, Finland, Sweden, Norway, Germany, the Netherlands, and the United States. Most of these studies examined effects of gender and age on SDQ scores, and several examined informant differences.

SDQ Findings in the United Kingdom

Goodman (1997) reported the first findings for the SDQ. Samples were from mental health clinics ($N = 188$) and dental clinics ($N = 158$). Although no means or standard deviations were provided for the SDQ, an appendix suggested "provisional" normal, borderline, and abnormal score bands. The 90th percentile cutpoint for Total Difficulties, which demarcated the abnormal range, was a score of 17 for parent reports and a score of 16 for teacher reports. It was unclear whether these cutpoints were derived from the mental health and/or dental clinic samples or from some other samples, but it was stated that the cutpoints were not adjusted for age and gender.

As we summarized in Chapter 2, Goodman, Ford, Simmons, et al. (2000) reported SDQ findings for 7,984 5- to 15-year-olds in the British Child Mental Health Survey. Ratings on the SDQ (scored *not true*, *somewhat true*, or *certainly true*) were obtained from parents and teachers, as well from 11- to 15-year-olds. Goodman, Ford, Simmons, et al. (2000) did not report statistical comparisons of scores by age or gender, nor did they provide means or standard deviations for SDQ scores.

Goodman, Meltzer, and Bailey (1998) reported data from a pilot study using the self-report version of the SDQ with 11- to 16-year-olds (N = 83 in a community sample and 116 in a mental health clinic). Mean Total Difficulties score was 11.4 in the community sample and 18.6 in the clinic sample, but no statistical tests for group, gender, or age were reported, nor were scores on SDQ subscales provided. An appendix provided provisional score ranges for normal, borderline, and abnormal status, unadjusted for age and gender, but did not specify the sample on which these ranges were based. A score of 20 demarcated the 90th percentile for Total Difficulties.

SDQ Findings in Finland

A comparison of the SDQ and the CBCL was conducted in a school-based sample in two areas of southwest Finland (N = 735; Koskelainen et al., 2000). SDQs were obtained from 96% of the parents, from 99% of the adolescents for whom parents gave consent, and from 90% of the primary school teachers. Total Difficulties means and standard deviations for parent and self-reports on the SDQ were provided for boys and girls in grades 1, 3, 5, 7, and 9. Total Difficulties scores based on teacher reports for children in grades 1, 3, and 5 were also reported. Self-report scores were significantly higher than parent report scores, and scores for younger children were significantly higher than those for older children. Gender differences were significant only for teacher reports, with boys rated as having more problems. For the primary school sample, teacher ratings were higher than parent ratings for Total Difficulties. There were also significant gender × informant interactions, with teachers rating boys higher on Hyperactivity and Conduct Problems and rating girls higher on Prosocial. The correlations between SDQ Total Difficulties and CBCL Total Problems was .75; for the SDQ and TRF, the correlation was .71.

Koskelainen et al. (2001) reported self-report SDQ findings for 1,458 Finnish 13- to 17-year-olds in seventh- and ninth-grade classes in two cities (89% of those sampled). Girls had significantly higher scores than boys on Total Difficulties, Prosocial, Hyperactivity, and Emotional Symptoms but significantly lower scores than boys on Conduct Problems and Peer Problems. Older adolescents had significantly higher scores than younger adolescents on Emotional Symptoms. The 90th percentile cutpoint for deviance on Total Difficulties was a score of 18, lower than the cutpoint of 20 in the United Kingdom. No statistical comparisons were made between scores obtained for this Finnish sample and those obtained for Goodman et al.'s (1998) U.K. sample, although the means for Total Difficulties were very similar (11.2 in Finland vs. 11.4 in the United Kingdom).

SDQ Findings in Sweden

Smedje, Broman, Hetta, and von Knorring (1999) reported parent ratings on the SDQ for 760 Swedish 6- to 8-year-olds and 140 Swedish 10-year-olds recruited through local health clinics for a study on sleep behaviors (73% completion rate). Boys scored significantly higher than girls on Total Difficulties and Hyperactivity and significantly lower than girls on Emotional Symptoms and Prosocial. The 90th percentile cutpoint for Total Difficulties was 14. No statistical comparisons with SDQ data from other cultures were reported, but Smedje et al. stated that their cutpoint was lower than the cutpoint of 17 reported by Goodman (1997).

SDQ Findings in the Netherlands

Van Widenfelt, Goedhart, Treffers, and Goodman (2003) presented self-report SDQ findings for 970 11- to 16-year-old Dutch adolescents. Parent and teacher SDQ data were also collected for some participants, but only 63% of parents and 36% of the schools approached agreed to participate. Relative to children whose parents completed the SDQ, children whose parents refused to complete the SDQ had significantly higher Total Difficulties scores, according to self-reports, and significantly higher Conduct Problems and lower Prosocial scores, according to teacher reports. Boys scored significantly higher than girls on Total Difficulties in both parent and teacher reports but not in self-reports. In parent reports, Total Difficulties scores were higher for younger children than for older children. For all three informants, boys had significantly higher scores than girls on Conduct Problems and significantly lower scores than girls on Prosocial. Teachers and parents rated boys higher than girls on Hyperactivity. Self-reports yielded higher scores for girls than for boys on Emotional Symptoms.

Van Widenfelt used J. Cohen's (1988) measure of effect size, d, to compare Dutch SDQ scores with British SDQ scores reported on the SDQ website. Significantly lower scores were found for Dutch than for British children on Total Difficulties and on three subscales for parent reports. On the other hand, the two significant differences for teacher reports and the three significant differences for self-reports were inconsistent in direction. Van Widenfelt also reported correlations of .74 and .70 between SDQ Total Difficulties and Total Problems on the CBCL and YSR, respectively.

SDQ Findings in Germany

Klasen et al. (2000) reported SDQ, CBCL, and YSR data for a Bavarian community sample of 12- to 13-year-olds participating in a birth cohort study (N = 110), as well as for a clinical sample (N = 163). Mean Total Difficulties scores were significantly lower in the community sample (6.6 for boys and 5.1 for girls) than in the clinical sample (17.4 for boys and 14.9 for girls). No tests of gender differences were reported. The r between SDQ Total Difficulties and CBCL Total Problems was .78; between the SDQ and YSR, the r was .77.

Woerner, Becker, and Rothenberger (2004) reported normative data for the SDQ based on forms completed by 930 German parents whose 6- to 16-year-old children were participating in a nationwide study of weight problems and eating habits. Boys obtained significantly higher scores than girls on Total Difficulties, Conduct Problems, Hyperactivity, and Peer Problems. Age had a significant but small negative correlation of –.09 with Hyperactivity scores, indicating slightly higher scores among younger children. The 90% cutpoint for deviance on Total Difficulties was a score of 16. No statistical comparisons of these German SDQ scores with those from other cultures were provided, but Woerner et al. stated that only "small deviations" were found between the German and British results.

SDQ Findings in Norway

Rønning, Handegaard, Surander, and Mørch (2004) obtained self-report SDQs from 4,167 11- to 16-year-olds in 66 schools in Norway, with a completion rate of 80%. Girls had significantly higher scores than boys on Emotional Symptoms and Prosocial and lower scores than boys on Hyperactivity, Conduct Problems, and Peer Problems. Emotional Problems scores tended to increase with age for girls, whereas Prosocial scores generally decreased with age for boys. The 90th percentile cutpoint for Total Difficulties was 18. No statistical comparisons were reported between these Norwegian scores and those obtained from other cultures. Rønning et al. did state that their mean scores and cutpoints were "generally somewhat lower" than those reported by Goodman (1997).

SDQ Findings in the United States

Bourdon, Goodman, Rae, Simpson, and Koretz (2005) reported SDQ data for a U.S. sample of 10,367 4- to 17-year-olds rated by their parents as part of the 2001 National Health Interview Survey (NHIS). Mean Total Difficulties scores obtained from ratings by U.S. parents were slightly lower than those obtained from U.K. parent ratings (7.1 vs. 8.4), but no statistical test of this difference was reported, nor were the U.S. scores compared to SDQ scores from any other cultures. Cut-points for "high," "medium," and "low" difficulties judgments, based on weighted cumulative frequency distributions, were slightly lower in the United States than in the United Kingdom. For example, Bourdon et al. (2005) reported that the cutpoint for "high" difficulties was 16 in the United States (91st percentile).

Comparison of SDQ Findings across Cultures

Obel et al. (2004) published a narrative comparison of SDQ findings in five Nordic countries (Sweden, Norway, Iceland, Denmark, and Finland). The authors stated that because the samples varied widely in their representativeness, age and gender distributions, and informants, no statistical comparisons were attempted. However, descriptive tables allowed visual comparisons of results across cultures for some age groups. For example, parent reports on the SDQ for 7-year-olds were available for five samples (one in Denmark and two each in Norway and Sweden). Mean Total Difficulties scores ranged from a low of 5.7 in one Norwegian sample to a high of 7.2 in one Swedish sample. Similarly, in four samples of 15-year-olds who completed the SDQ, the mean Total Difficulties scores ranged from 9.8 in a Norwegian sample to 11.4 in a Finnish sample.

Marzocchi et al. (2004) published a summary of SDQ studies in five Southern European countries (France, Italy, Spain, Portugal, and Croatia). For several of the studies, no results were reported because the projects were still in progress. The only statistical comparisons were for teacher SDQs for community samples of 7- to 8-year-olds in Italy, Spain, and Portugal. Consistent gender differences were found in all three countries, with boys obtaining higher scores than girls on Hyperactivity and Conduct Problems and lower scores than girls on Prosocial. ANOVAs indicated significant differences between cultures on the Hyperactivity and Prosocial scales for both boys and girls. Portuguese children obtained higher scores than children in the other two cultures on Hyperactivity, whereas Italian children obtained lower scores than children in the other two cultures on Prosocial.

SUMMARY

In this chapter, we presented findings from multicultural comparisons of scores on the CBCL, the TRF, and the YSR, three empirically based assessment instruments for school-age children from the ASEBA family of instruments. We also reviewed findings for the CPRS, the CTRS, and the SDQ. Major conclusions from our review include the following:

1. In multicultural comparisons of CBCL, TRF, and YSR scores from 31, 21, and 24 cultures, respectively, most ESs for culture were < 10% for all three instruments. On all three instruments, the mean Total Problems scores for most cultures were within one standard deviation of the omnicultural mean. However, ESs for culture were larger than ESs for gender or age, and culture often interacted significantly with these factors. Although variance within cultures was much larger than variance between cultures for all three instruments, cultural differences were certainly present.

2. Gender differences were found for many ASEBA scales. With considerable consistency across instruments, girls scored higher than boys on Internalizing problems but lower than boys on Externalizing problems. Teachers' reports yielded larger gender differences than parents' reports on scales where boys typically score higher. On the CBCL, gender differences on scales assessing Internalizing problems became more consistent across cultures with age. Conversely, gender differences on CBCL scales assessing Externalizing problems became less consistent across cultures with age. Gender differences on the YSR generally mirrored those found on the CBCL, with a few notable exceptions. There were no significant gender differences on the YSR Attention Problems or DSM-oriented Attention Deficit Hyperactivity Problems scales, whereas boys were rated significantly higher on both the CBCL and TRF versions of these scales.

3. Age effects varied across the three instruments as well as across scales and cultures. On the CBCL, Internalizing scores generally increased with age, Externalizing scores generally decreased, and scores for syndromes and DSM-oriented scales showed less consistency across ages. For the TRF, Internalizing scores generally increased with age, but Externalizing scores did not typically decrease. Age trends varied across syndromes and cultures, but scores on the DSM-oriented Affective Problems, Somatic Problems, and Conduct Problems scales typically increased with age. On the YSR, youths ages 14–16 typically reported more problems than youths ages 11–13 on most scales.

4. Mean bicultural rs of .74 for the CBCL, .74 for the TRF, and .69 for the YSR indicated substantial consistency in mean item score rankings across very different cultures in parent, teacher, and self-reports.

5. To date, very few studies comparing scores between two or more cultures have been published for the Conners scales. Findings that have been reported for these instruments suggest some significant cultural differences in scores.

6. SDQ studies have proliferated in many cultures since the instrument was published in 1997. Although very few statistical comparisons across cultures have been published to date, many studies in single cultures have compared their findings informally to U.K. findings. Findings from SDQ studies include the following: self-report problem scores have typically been higher than parent and teacher report scores; boys have typically obtained higher scores than girls on Hyperactivity, Conduct Problems, and Total Difficulties; girls have typically obtained higher scores than boys on Prosocial and sometimes obtained higher scores than boys on Emotional Symptoms; and 90th percentile cutpoints in most cultures have been slightly lower than the cutpoints published by Goodman (1997; Goodman et al., 1998), which were presumably based on U.K. samples.

CHAPTER 5

Multicultural Findings on Correlates of Empirically Based Scale Scores

In Chapter 4 we summarized studies comparing scores on empirically based scales in general population samples from many cultures. We also summarized findings about effects of age and gender reported in all the studies reviewed. Therefore, we do not include age and gender among the correlates of scores in this chapter. Instead, we present findings on other correlates of empirically based scales. We begin by reviewing associations between scores on empirically based instruments and measures of SES and parental marital status. We then review associations of scores on empirically based instruments with psychiatric diagnoses and referral for mental health services. Next we review longitudinal findings on scores derived from empirically based instruments, followed by findings on genetic correlates of empirically based scores. Thereafter we review findings regarding empirically based scores for immigrant children. Because so much research has examined correlates of the CBCL, TRF, and YSR, most of the studies report findings from these instruments. However, insofar as we could find relevant studies, we also review findings reported for the CTRS and CPRS (Conners, 1997) as well as the SDQ (Goodman, 2001).

As much as possible, we summarize results using measures that are easily interpretable. As stated in Chapter 4, we use the term *effect size* (ES) to refer to percent of variance accounted for, such as indexed by η^2 (eta square), which can be interpreted using J. Cohen's (1988) criteria for the magnitude of effects. Pearson correlations (rs) between variables can also be interpreted using Cohen's (1988) criteria (*small* = .10–.29, *medium* = .30–.49, *large* ≥ .50). Cohen's (1988) *d* represents the mean difference between two groups in standard deviation units. Benchmarks for interpreting *d* as an ES are *small* = .20–.49, *medium* = .50–.79, and *large* ≥ .80. Odds ratios (ORs) indicate how much more likely an outcome is in the presence, than in the absence, of a particular risk factor. ORs are very influenced by how common the risk factor and the outcome are in the sample (i.e., the base rates). We also report findings in terms of two widely used measures of screening efficiency: *sensitivity* (percent of "cases" correctly identified as deviant by an assessment instrument) and *specificity* (percent of "noncases" correctly identified as nondeviant by the instrument). Like ORs, sensitivity and specificity are influenced by base rates. Sensitivity and specificity are typically inversely related because lowering the cutpoint for defining deviance both increases the chance of correctly identifying all true cases and of incorrectly identifying noncases as deviant.

CRITERIA FOR STUDIES OF CORRELATES

Our criteria for studies of correlates of empirically based scale scores are similar to those specified in Chapter 4 for studies of the effects of age, gender, and culture. That is, we gave priority to studies published in peer-reviewed journals that used standardized assessment procedures with large general population samples ($N \geq 300$ per culture) and that reported results of statistical analyses.

ASSOCIATIONS BETWEEN SCORES
ON EMPIRICALLY BASED SCALES AND SES

Table 5.1 summarizes studies from 15 cultures that tested associations between scores on empirically based scales and measures of SES in large general population samples. Most studies used the CBCL, but some also included the TRF and YSR, and two studies used the SDQ. Correlates of competence scores as well as problem scores were reported in some studies. Measures of SES varied across studies, but most used the occupation and/or education of the child's parents and grouped participants into low-, medium-, and high-SES groups. Some studies also used measures of family income. Although the studies varied in statistical details, they were consistent in reporting higher problem scores for children from lower-SES families than from higher-SES families.

TABLE 5.1. Studies Reporting Effects of SES and Parental Marital Status on Empirically Based Assessment Scores

Culture	Reference	N	Ages	SES measures	SES effects	Marital status effects
Australia	Sawyer et al. (1990)	528	10–11, 14–15	School SES	CBCL (TP): L > H, 12–14% prevalence of "cases" (low SES), 7–9% (middle SES), 5–7% (high SES)	
	Sawyer et al. (2001)	4,083	4–17	Education, income, jobs	High CBCL TP score more common in low-SES families	Higher CBCL TP scores in single/blended families
Belgium	Hellinckx et al. (1994)	2,222	6–12	Occupation scale	CBCL (TP, I, E, 6 syndromes, 31 items): L > H, ESs < 1–2% Competence: L < H, ESs 2–5%	
China	Liu, Kurita, Guo, et al. (1999)	2,940	6–11	Education	CBCL (TP): L > H, OR = 2.0	CBCL TP deviance: OR =15.9 for divorce
	Liu, Kurita, Sun, and Wang (1999)	1,695	6–11	Education	CBCL (TP): L > H, OR = 1.4–1.5	
	Liu et al. (2000)	174	6–15			CBCL TP deviance: OR = 18.4 for divorce
Denmark	Bilenberg (1999)	779	4–16	Occupation	CBCL and TRF (TP): L > H	
Germany	Woerner et al. (2004)	930	6–16	Occupation, education, income	SDQ: L > H, r = .15 (TD), .21 (H/I), and .09 (PP)	
Greece	Roussos et al. (1999)	1,213	6–11	Education, occupation	CBCL and TRF (TP) L > H Competence: L < H	
Iceland	Hannesdottir and Einarsdottir (1995	943	4–16	Occupation	CBCL (TP): L > H	

(continued)

TABLE 5.1. (continued)

Culture	Reference	N	Ages	SES measures	SES effects	Marital status effects
Italy	Frigerio et al. (2004)	1,423	6–16	Occupation	CBCL and TRF (TP, E, SP, AP, DB): L > H	
Jamaica	Lambert et al. (1994)	1,306	6–11	Occupation	CBCL (18 items): L > H, ESs < 1–4%	
	Lambert et al. (1998)	730	12–16	Occupation	CBCL (I, E, 8 syndromes): L > H (no ESs reported)	
Lithuania	Zukauskiene et al. (2003)	1,296	7–14	Education	CBCL (TP, I, E): L > H	Lower CBCL scores in intact families
Netherlands	Achenbach, Verhulst, Baron, et al. (1987)	3,333	4–16	Occupation	CBCL (TP, 36 items): L > H, ESs < 1% Competence: L < H, ESs < 1–3%	
	Achenbach, Verhulst, Edelbrock, et al. (1987)	1,348	6–11	Occupation	TRF: L > H, < 1–3%	
	Kalff, Kroes, Vles, Bosma, et al. (2001) Kalff, Kroes, Vles, Hendrickson, et al. (2001)	734	5–7	Occupation, education	CBCL (TP, E): L > H	Higher CBCL TP scores in divorced, single-parent families
Puerto Rico	Achenbach, Bird, et al. (1990)	1,448	4–16	Occupation, education	CBCL (TP): L > H	
Russia	Hellinckx et al. (2000)	2,002	12–16	Income and estimated financial status	CBCL (TP, I, E, A/D, SC, DB): L > H, ESs < 1%	
				Own room	L > H, 6–8%	

Norway	Novik (1999)	1,170	6–16	Occupation	CBCL (TP, I, E): L > H, ES = 3% Competence: ES = 8%
Sweden	Larsson & Frisk (1999)	1,308	6–16	Occupation	CBCL (TP, E, DB): L > H, ESs < 1–5% Competence: ES = 4%
United States	Achenbach et al. (2003a)	3 × 670	7–16	Occupation	CBCL (TP, E, 6 syndromes, 3 DSM scales): L > H, ESs = 1% Competence: ESs = 3–6%
	Achenbach et al. (2002)	3 × 696	7–16	Occupation	TRF (TP, E, 8 syndromes, 5 DSM scales): L > H, ESs < 1–2% Competence: 4–7%
	Achenbach and Rescorla (2001)	3,210 and 3,086	6–18	Occupation	CBCL and TRF (TP, E, some syndromes): L > H, ESs = 1–2% CBCL Competence: 3–4% YSR Competence: 2–4%
	Achenbach, Howell, et al. (1991)	2,726	4–16		ACQ Total: Larger % > 90th %ile in divorced or single-parent families
	National Institute of Child Health and Human Development Early Child Care Research Network (2005)	803	8.5	Income	CBCL and TRF: L > H Higher CBCL and TRF scores if mother never married
	Bourdon et al. (2005)	10,367	4–17	Income	SDQ: OR = 2.5 SDQ: ORs = 2.4–2.7

Note. TP, Total Problems; I, Internalizing; E, Externalizing; A/D, Anxious/Depressed; SC, Somatic Complaints; SP, Social Problems; AP, Attention Problems; DB, Delinquent Behavior; L, Lower SES; H, Higher SES; OR, Odds Ratio; ES, Effect Size; TD, SDQ Total Difficulties; H/I, SDQ Hyperactivity/Inattention; PP, SDQ Peer Problems.

SES Effects on ASEBA Problem Scores in the United States

To provide a benchmark for findings from cultures other than the United States, we first summarize findings on associations between CBCL, TRF, and YSR scores and SES in general population samples in the United States (Achenbach et al., 2002, 2003a). For the CBCL, participants were nonreferred children ages 7–16 from three general population samples (N = 670 each), whose parents provided CBCL information during home interviews conducted in 1976, 1989, and 1999 (Achenbach et al., 2003a). The three samples were matched exactly on gender and as closely as possible on age, ethnicity, and SES. Significant but small ESs (1%) for SES were found for Total Problems, Externalizing, six syndromes, and three DSM-oriented scales, with higher problem scores for children from lower-SES families than from higher-SES families.

A parallel study reported TRF data for three demographically matched cohorts of children in the United States who were assessed in 1981, 1989, and 1999 and matched on demographic factors (N = 696 in each cohort; Achenbach et al., 2002). Significant SES effects were found for Total Problems, Externalizing, six syndromes, and five DSM-oriented scales. The largest ESs (2%) were for Attention Problems, Rule-Breaking Behavior, and the DSM-oriented Attention Deficit Hyperactivity Problems scale.

Comparable ESs for SES were reported in the 2001 manual for the CBCL and the TRF (Achenbach & Rescorla, 2001). In those analyses, children from the 2001 national normative sample were compared with referred children matched on age, gender, SES, and ethnicity. The ESs for SES on the CBCL were 1–2% for Total Problems, Externalizing, Aggressive Behavior, Rule-Breaking Behavior, and the DSM-oriented Conduct Problems scale. On the TRF, ESs were also 1–2% for Total Problems, Externalizing, and several syndromes and DSM- oriented scales. No SES effects were significant for YSR scores.

SES Effects on ASEBA Problem Scores in Nine European Cultures

When Achenbach, Verhulst, Baron, and Akkerhuis (1987) tested SES effects on CBCL problem scores for 2,033 Dutch children and 1,300 American children, SES (based on parental occupation) was a significant covariate for Total Problems, as well as for 34 problem items (all ESs ≤ 1%). In a parallel study of TRF scores for 748 Dutch children and 600 American children (Achenbach, Verhulst, Baron, and Althaus,

1987), SES was a significant covariate for Total Problems and for 36 problem items. All ESs were ≤ 1%, except for TRF item *49. Difficulty learning,* which had an ES of 3%. In a study comparing 1,120 Belgian children with 1,122 Dutch children (Hellinckx, Grietens, & Verhulst, 1994), SES was a significant covariate for CBCL Total Problems, Internalizing, Externalizing, six syndromes, and 31 items. SES had its largest ES on Attention Problems (2%).

In a Norwegian sample of 2,600 children, Novik (1999) reported a 3% ES for SES on CBCL Total Problems. For a sample of 943 Icelandic 4- to 16-year-olds, Hannesdottir and Einarsdottir (1995) reported that children from the highest SES level had significantly lower CBCL Total Problems scores (mean = 12.9) than children from the other five SES levels (mean scores = 17.1–20.6). In a sample of 1,308 Swedish 6- to 16-year-olds, children from lower-SES families had significantly higher CBCL Total Problems, Externalizing, and Delinquent Behavior scores than children from higher-SES families (Larsson & Frisk, 1999). In Lithuania (*N* = 1,296), 7- to 14-year-olds from lower-SES families had significantly higher scores on Total Problems, Internalizing, and Externalizing than children from higher-SES families (Zukauskiene, Ignataviciene, & Daukantaite, 2003). In Italy (*N* = 1,423), significant SES effects were reported for CBCL Total Problems, Externalizing, Social Problems, Attention Problems, and Delinquent Behavior (Frigerio et al., 2004). Bilenberg (1999) reported significant effects for SES on CBCL and TRF Total Problems scores for a Danish sample (*N* = 779), and Roussos et al. (1999) reported that Greek children from lower-SES families had higher problem scores than children from higher-SES families on both the CBCL and TRF (*N* = 1,213).

For a Russian sample of 2,002 adolescents ages 12–16, Hellinckx, Grietens, and De Munter (2000) reported that both income and the family's estimate of its financial position had ESs < 1% on CBCL Total Problems, Internalizing, Externalizing, and three syndromes. Interestingly, much larger ESs were found for the higher problem scores obtained by adolescents who did not have their own room versus those who did. These ESs included 8% for Total Problems, 6% for Internalizing, and 6% for Externalizing. It is possible that having one's own room was a proxy for SES effects, but lack of a private room may also have contributed to problems.

SES Effects on ASEBA Problem Scores in Two Caribbean Cultures

When 360 Jamaican children ages 6–11 were compared with 946 American children (Lambert, Knight, Taylor, & Achebach, 1994), SES was a significant covariate for 18 CBCL problems items but not for Total Problems scores. The largest ES (4%) was for item *61. Poor school work.* SES was also a significant covariate for all CBCL syndromes and for Internalizing and Externalizing scores in a sample of 365 Jamaican adolescents ages 12–16, who were compared with an age- and gender-matched sample of American adolescents (Lambert et al., 1998), but ESs were not reported. When comparing Puerto Rican with U.S. mainland children, Achenbach, Bird, et al. (1990) reported that SES was a significant covariate for Total Problems scores on all three ASEBA school-age instruments.

SES Effects on ASEBA Problem Scores in China

In a Chinese sample of 2,940 children ages 6–11, Liu, Kurita, Guo, et al. (1999) obtained an OR of 1.8 that indicated significantly higher CBCL Total Problems scores for children whose parents had low educational attainment. However, income and type of occupation were not significantly associated with CBCL scores. In a different Chinese sample, Liu, Kurita, Sun, and Wang (1999) reported an OR of 1.5 between CBCL Total Problems and father's education and of 1.4 with mother's education.

SES Effects on ASEBA Problem Scores in Australia

Associations between SES and ASEBA problem scores have been found for two Australian samples. In a South Australia sample, Sawyer, Sarris, Baghurst, Cornish, and Kalucy (1990) reported that the mean prevalence of deviant "cases" on the CBCL was 13% in a low-SES school, 8% in a middle-SES school, and 6% in a high-SES school. Additionally, in a national sample of 4,509 children, Sawyer et al. (2001) reported that children with high CBCL scores were more likely than children with low CBCL scores to come from families with lower incomes, more unemployment, and lower levels of education.

SES Effects on Competence Scores

In all the studies we found that reported effects of SES on competence scores, higher SES was consistently associated with higher competence scores. Furthermore, ESs for competence scores were typically larger than those for problem scores. As Table 5.1 shows, ESs for SES were 6% for CBCL Total Competence and 3–4% for the Activities, Social, and School scales in the 1976, 1989, and 1999 demographically matched samples analyzed by Achenbach et al. (2003a). In the 1981,

1989, and 1999 TRF samples, ESs were 7% for Academic Performance and 4% for Total Adaptive scores. Findings for the 2001 U.S. normative sample included SES ESs of 4% for CBCL Total Competence and 3% for Activities, Social, and School; 4% for YSR Total Competence and Activities and 2% for YSR Social scale scores; and 6% for TRF Academic Performance and 3% for TRF Total Adaptive scores. As shown in Table 5.1, significant associations between SES and CBCL competence scores were also found in the Netherlands, Belgium, Norway, Greece, and Sweden. ESs for Total Competence ranged from 3% in the Netherlands to 8% in Norway. ESs for the Activities, Social, and School scales ranged from < 1 to 5%.

ASSOCIATIONS BETWEEN SDQ SCORES AND SES

Woerner et al. (2004) tested associations between SDQ scores and SES for a general population sample of 930 children ages 6–16 in Germany, collected as part of a nationwide study of weight problems and eating habits. SES was based on a composite of parental education, occupation, and income. Significant correlations between SES and Hyperactivity/Inattention Problems ($r = .21$), Peer Problems ($r = .09$), and Total Difficulties ($r = .15$) were reported. Children from lower-SES families had higher scores for all three scales.

Bourdon et al. (2005) reported associations between the SDQ and family income in a sample of 10,367 children in the United States. The OR for a high SDQ Total Difficulties score was 2.5 for families below, versus above, the poverty line.

Summary of SES Effects

Significant SES effects on ASEBA problem scores have been reported in at least 15 cultures, including 10 in Europe, 2 in the Caribbean, and 1 in Asia, plus Australia and the United States. Studies varied in which ASEBA forms and scales were analyzed and which statistical results were reported. Nonetheless, findings consistently indicated that across very diverse cultures, lower SES was associated with higher problem scores. ESs on Total Problems, Internalizing, Externalizing, many syndromes, and numerous problem items were generally 1–5%. In two bicultural analyses—the United States and the Netherlands reported by Achenbach, Verhulst, Baron, et al. (1987), and the United States and Jamaica reported by Lambert et al. (1994)—the largest SES ESs were for items dealing with schoolwork and learning problems. In Russia, an adolescent who did not have his or her own room, which is a proxy variable for SES but may have its own consequences as well, had a larger ES on problem scores than more conventional SES measures such as family income (Hellinckx et al., 2000). In the few studies that have assessed SES effects on ASEBA competence scores, larger ESs have been reported than for problem scores. SES effects on the SDQ have been reported in Germany (Woerner et al., 2004) and the United States (Bourdon et al., 2005). In both cases, lower SES was associated with higher SDQ scores.

ASSOCIATIONS BETWEEN SCORES
ON EMPIRICALLY BASED SCALES AND MARITAL STATUS

A few studies have reported associations between parental marital status and problem scores on empirically based instruments. In some studies, such as the Sawyer et al. (2001) study in Australia, an association between higher CBCL problems scores and single parent/blended families was reported, but statistical details were lacking. Similarly, for Lithuanian children, Zukauskiene et al. (2003) reported that children living in intact families had lower CBCL problem scores than children in single-parent families; again, statistical details were not provided.

Achenbach, Howell, Quay, and Conners (1991) reported effects of marital status on problem scores on the Achenbach, Conners, Quay (ACQ) Behavior Checklist, which contained 115 CBCL items as well as items from the Conners (1978) Parent Questionnaire and the Quay–Peterson (1982) Revised Behavior Problem Checklist. In a sample of 2,734 American children, the proportion of children with high ACQ Total Problems scores was significantly greater in divorced, separated, and single-parent families than in intact and widowed families. Additionally, the proportion of children who had much higher Externalizing than Internalizing scores was significantly greater in divorced, separated, and single-parent families than in intact and widowed families.

In a Chinese sample of children ages 6–12, the OR between having separated/divorced parents and having an elevated problem score on the CBCL was 15.9 (Liu, Kurita, Guo, et al., 1999). This family factor was the strongest predictor of behavioral problems among all the variables tested in the Chinese study. Drawing from their general population sample of 4,862 children, Liu et al. (2000) compared 58 Chinese children whose parents were divorced with 116 children of non-divorced parents matched on age, gender, and school class. To control for the lower family incomes in the divorced families, the authors covaried income in all analyses. Results indicated that children in divorced families had consistently higher CBCL problem scores than children in intact families, even after controlling for differences in income. The OR for scoring > 90th percentile on CBCL Total Problems in divorced versus intact families was 18.4. The OR for scoring > 98th percentile on TRF Attention Problems was 13.4 for children in divorced versus intact families. It is unfortunate that ASEBA studies in other cultures have not reported ORs between marital status and problem scores. It is possible that ORs between marital status and problem scores would be lower in cultures where the base rates for divorced and single-parent families are higher than they are in China.

Bourdon et al. (2005) reported an OR of 2.7 between high SDQ Total Difficulties scores and being from single-parent versus intact families in their U.S. national sample. They also reported an OR of 2.4 between high SDQ scores and being from reconstituted versus intact families.

Multilevel Modeling of SES and Marital Status

Research on a general population sample of 734 5- to 7-year-olds in the Dutch city of Maastricht examined the effects of family type, parental education and occupation, immigrant status, and neighborhood SES level on CBCL scores using multilevel modeling (Kalff, Kroes, Vles, Bosma, et al., 2001; Kalff, Kroes, Vles, Hendricksen, et al., 2001). As would be expected, the most deprived neighborhoods had higher concentrations of divorced/single-parent families and parents with low education and occupation levels. Parental education and occupation, marital status, and neighborhood SES were all significant predictors of CBCL Total Problems scores. Multilevel regression analyses indicated that neighborhood SES had an independent effect on CBCL Total Problems scores over and above family-level SES factors. That is, children from low-SES and divorced/single-parent families had higher risks of behavioral and emotional problems if they lived in low-SES rather than higher-SES neighborhoods. The authors speculated that this effect may result from low social cohesion in disadvantaged neighborhoods.

Research reported by the National Institute of Child Health and Human Development (NICHD) Early Child Care Research Network (2005) also used multilevel modeling to test effects of SES and marital status on CBCL and TRF problem scores. Data from birth to age 8.5 years were analyzed for 803 children, comprising all members of a longitudinal sample of 1,364 for whom complete parental income data were available. Based on a ratio of family income to the poverty threshold, families were identified as (1) never poor from the time the children were 6 months old through third grade; (2) poor when the children were 6–36 months old; (3) poor when the children were 54 months old through third grade; or (4) poor during both the early and later periods from age 6 months through third grade. From age 2 to 8.5 years, children whose families were never poor had lower CBCL and TRF Internalizing and Externalizing scores than children whose families were poor across the whole period. Children whose families were poor only during the later period tended to have higher problem scores than children whose families were poor only during the earlier period. Low maternal education, mother living without a partner, and maternal depressive symptoms were found to be significant mediators of the group differences in problem scores. These mediators accounted for much of the association between poverty and problem scores.

Summary of Marital Status Effects on Problem Scores

It is surprising that so few findings have been published regarding associations between parents' marital status and children's problem scores, because information about marital status is relatively easy to collect. The few published studies have consistently reported that children from intact families have lower problem scores than children from divorced, single-parent, and reconstituted families. Furthermore, as the Kalff et al. (Kalff, Kroes, Vles, Bosma, et al., 2001; Kalff, Kroes, Vles, Hendrickson, et al., 2001) and NICHD Early Child Care Research Network (2005) studies indicate, children in divorced and single-parent families are more likely to be poor and to live in poor neighborhoods. The adults in these families tend to have lower educational and occupational levels than adults in intact families. All these factors are associated with higher problem scores for children.

ASSOCIATIONS BETWEEN SCORES ON EMPIRICALLY BASED SCALES AND DIAGNOSES

Table 5.2 summarizes associations between scores on empirically based scales and psychiatric diagnoses obtained from structured diagnostic interviews. Some of the studies employed *two-stage sampling* procedures. In two-stage sampling, a low-cost assessment procedure such as the CBCL is administered in Stage 1 to screen all individuals in a sample. The low-cost assessment procedure is used to identify individuals who are likely to be *cases* (i.e., *screen-positive* individuals who have high problem scores and are therefore likely to meet criteria for diagnoses) versus individuals who are likely to be *noncases* (i.e., *screen-negative* individuals who have low problem scores and are thus unlikely to meet criteria for diagnoses). In Stage 2 the screen-positive individuals identified as potential cases in Stage 1, plus a small proportion of screen-negative individuals who were identified as potential noncases, are assessed with diagnostic interviews in order to make diagnoses.

CBCL, TRF, and YSR Findings from the Netherlands

An early study using a two-stage design was reported by Verhulst, Berden, and Sanders-Woudstra (1985) for 8- and 11-year-olds from their South Holland general population sample. Out of 334 children, 78 screen-positives were identified (scores > 85th percentile on either the CBCL or the TRF constituted the cutpoint for deviance). From the screen-negatives (scores ≤ 85th percentile, i.e., not deviant), 75 children were randomly selected as controls. Based on separate parent and child clinical interviews for 57 of the screen-positive and 59 of the screen-negative children, ratings of moderate to severe disturbance were used to define psychiatric "caseness." Sensitivity and specificity were calculated using caseness as the outcome, with scores > 85th percentile on either the CBCL or the TRF as the cutpoint for deviance. Sensitivity and specificity values were 77 and 70%, respectively, for 8-year-olds and 70 and 63%, respectively, for 11-year-olds. When caseness was defined as a psychiatric rating in the severe range, sensitivity increased but specificity decreased.

Verhulst et al. (1997) used the CBCL, TRF, and YSR to screen a national general population sample of Dutch 13- to 18-year-olds. This procedure identified 200 screen-positive adolescents, whose mean scores across the CBCL, TRF, and YSR were above the 75th percentile, and 112 screen-negative adolescents, whose mean scores were below the 75th percentile. DISC-P and/or DISC-C interviews were conducted with 87% of these 312 adolescents and their parents in order to obtain DSM-III-R diagnoses. After administering the DISC-P and the DISC-C, interviewers completed the Children's Global Assessment Scale (CGAS) for each adolescent. Sensitivity and specificity of the combined CBCL/TRF/YSR cutpoint were generally good, but they varied across the 20 different permutations of DISC-P, DISC-C, and CGAS results used to define caseness in the study. For example, when ≥ 1 diagnosis based on the DISC-P alone was used to define caseness, sensitivity and specificity were 51 and 82%, respectively. However, when either the DISC-P *or* the DISC-C plus a CGAS score < 61 were used to define psychiatric caseness, sensitivity and specificity were 90 and 80%, respec-

TABLE 5.2. Studies Reporting Associations between Empirically Based Scores and Diagnoses and/or Referral Status

Culture	Reference	N	Ages	Design	Diagnoses	Referral status
Australia	Graetz et al. (2001)	3,597	6–17	Community sample	Higher CBCL scores associated with ADHD diagnoses, based on DISC-P	
Denmark	Bilenberg (1999)	779	4–16	Community versus clinic samples		Clinic scores higher on CBCL, TRF, and YSR
Finland	Helstelä et al. (2001)	598	15–16	Community sample		Higher CBCL and YSR scores if parents reported referral or maladjustment
	Helstelä & Sourander (2001) Sourander et al. (2004)	2,316	18	Community sample		Higher YSR scores if self-reports of maladjustment YASR: OR = 9.0 (TP), 5.1 (I), 8.1 (E) for mental health services
	Koskelainen et al. (2000)	735	7–15	Community sample		SDQ: ORs = 10.0 (P), 3.2 (T), and 4.4 (S) predicting parent report of having difficulties
	Sourander et al. (2005)	2,347	18	Military recruits	YASR: ORs = 22.8 (TP), 15.9 (I), 9.7 (E), and 2.7–16.5 (syndromes) for ICD-10 diagnoses	YASR: ORs = 7.93 (TP), 8 (I), 4.1 (E), and 2.2–8.7 (syndromes) for self-reported problems
France	Fombonne (1992)	2,090	6–11	Community versus clinic samples		D = 1.0 for group difference on CBCL TP

Germany	Schmeck et al. (2001)	4,116	4–18	Community versus clinic samples		ROC-AUC = 92% for CBCL TP
	Klasen et al. (2000)	110 163	4–16	Community versus clinic samples		SDQ (P): AUC = 91% for TD; CBCL: AUC = 87% for TP
	Becker, Woerner, et al. (2004)	543	5–17	Clinic sample	SDQ (P/T) AUCs: TD = .77/.75, ES = .69/.65, CP = .81/.82, H/I = .77/.79 BCL/TRF AUCs: TP = .78/.76, I = .73/.67, E = .84/.83, AP = .70/.72	
	Becker, Hagenberg, et al. (2004)	214	11–17	Clinic sample	SDQ (S) AUCs: TD = .84, ES = .69, CP = .77, H/I = .68 YSR AUCs: TP = .81, I = .70, E = .74, AP = .62	
Hawaii	Loo and Rapport (1998)	812	6–18	Community versus clinic samples		ES = 25% for CBCL TP
Netherlands	Kasius et al. (1997)	231	6–16	Clinic cases	SENS = 59%, SPEC = 73% for TP/any diagnosis	
	Verhulst et al. (1997)	200+ 112–	6–18	Two-stage screening	SENS = 90%, SPEC = 80% for ≥ 1 diagnosis on DISC-P or C plus CGAS < 61	
	Verhulst, Berden, et al. (1985)	78+ 75–	8, 11	Two-stage screening	SENS = 70–77%, SPEC = 63–70% for caseness = psychiatric ratings of moderate to severe	

(continued)

TABLE 5.2. (continued)

Culture	Reference	N	Ages	Design	Diagnoses	Referral status
Puerto Rico	Bird et al. (1991)	317+ 69–	4–16	Two-stage screening	SENS = 61%, SPEC = 87% for > 1 diagnosis on DISC-P and C	
Switzerland	Steinhausen et al. (1997)	577+ 128–	6–17	Two-stage screening	CBCL syndrome scores elevated for relevant diagnoses based on DISC-P	
United Kingdom	Goodman et al. (2001)	10,438	5–15	Community sample	OR = 15 (P), 14 (T), 7 (S) between SDQ and any diagnosis from DAWBA	
	Goodman, Ford, Simmons, et al. (2000)	7,894	11–15		Community sample	SENS/SPEC = 63/95% for any diagnosis from DAWBA
	Goodman (1997)	188/146 158/39	4–16	Psychiatric versus dental clinic		AUC = 87% (P) and 85% (T) for predicting clinic group
	Goodman (1999)	699	5–15	Community versus clinic samples		SDQ kappas = .68 (P), .56 (T), and .40 (S) for predicting clinic group

	Author	N	Age range	Sample	Findings
	Goodman, Renfrew, & Mullick (2000)	190	11–16	Psychiatric clinic samples in London and Dhaka	SENS = 81–90% and SPEC = 47–84% for conduct disorder; emotional disorder, and hyperactivity disorder diagnoses from records
	Goodman et al. (2003)	83 116	11–16	Community and clinic samples	SDQ (S) AUC = 82% for TD
United States	Achenbach and Rescorla (2001)	3,210 3,086 1,938	6–18 6–18 11–18	Matched community versus clinic samples Matched community versus clinic samples	CBCL (TP): ES = 36%, OR = 14 TRF (TP): ES = 26%, OR = 9 YSR (TP): ES = 15%, OR = 5
	Conners et al. (1998)	182 320	3–17 3–17	Matched community versus clinic samples Matched community versus clinic samples	CPRS-R: SENS = 92%, SPEC = 95% for ADHD diagnoses CTRS-R: SENS = 92%, SPEC = 95% for ADHD diagnoses
	Bourdon et al. (2005)	10,367	4–17	Community sample	SDQ OR = 12 for mental health referral and OR = 21 for special ed referral

Note. TP, Total Problems; I, Internalizing; E, Externalizing; SENS, sensitivity; SPEC, specificity; ROC, receiver operating characteristic; AUC, area under the curve; P, parent report; T, teacher report; S, self-report; TD, SDQ Total Difficulties; ES, SDQ Emotional symptoms; CP, SDQ Conduct Problems; H/I, SDQ Hyperactivity/Inattention Problems.

tively. When 1 diagnosis on both the DISC-P *and* the DISC-C plus a CGAS score < 61 were required to define caseness, sensitivity and specificity were 100 and 76%, respectively.

Kasius et al. (1997) reported associations between DSM-III-R diagnoses made from the DISC and scores on the CBCL for a sample of 231 children referred for outpatient mental health services. Sensitivity and specificity for predicting at least one DSM diagnosis from a CBCL Total Problems T score > 63 were 59 and 73%, respectively. The relatively low sensitivity was probably due to a difference in base rates for the two assessment procedures. Specifically, 63% of the sample met criteria for ≥ 1 DSM-III-R diagnosis, whereas only 47% of the sample scored in the clinical range ($T > 63$) on CBCL Total Problems.

Kasius et al. (1997) used logistic regression to test associations between scores on each CBCL syndrome and 10 specific DSM diagnoses, plus four broad groupings of diagnoses (anxiety, mood, disruptive, and psychotic). Many significant ORs were reported between CBCL syndromes and relevant diagnoses, after effects of other syndromes were partialed out (e.g., Anxious/Depressed and any mood disorder = 27.3; Anxious/Depressed and any anxiety disorder = 23.2; Attention Problems and ADHD = 14.8; Aggressive Behavior and ODD = 37.9). Often, more than one CBCL syndrome was significantly associated with a given diagnosis. Additionally, many CBCL syndromes had high ORs with several diagnoses. Kasius et al. (1997) suggest that this multiplicity of associations between syndromes and diagnoses was probably due to the high level of comorbidity manifested by the children (i.e., 64% of the 146 children with one diagnosis had at least one additional diagnosis).

CBCL and TRF Findings from Puerto Rico

A two-stage sampling design was used in Puerto Rico to test associations between CBCL and TRF scores and DSM-III diagnoses. Diagnoses were based on psychiatrists' conclusions from information integrated from DISC interviews with both children and parents, as well as information from teachers (Bird, Gould, Rubio-Stipec, Staghezza, & Canino, 1991). The DISC was used to assess 386 children, 317 of whom were screen-positive on either the CBCL or the TRF and 69 of whom were screen-negative. Cutpoints on the CBCL and TRF were not specified, but sensitivity and specificity values for the CBCL and TRF were reported for various definitions of psychiatric caseness. When ≥ 1 DSM diagnosis was used as the criterion for caseness, sensitivity and specificity for the CBCL were 61 and 87%, respectively. When TRF information was also used, sensitivity increased (71%) but specificity decreased (82%). The CBCL and the TRF were comparable in screening value for ages 6–11, whereas the CBCL provided better screening than either the TRF or the YSR for ages 12–16.

CBCL Findings from Switzerland

Steinhausen, Winkler Metzke, Meier, and Kannenberg (1997) conducted a two-stage study of 1,964 6- to 17-year-old residents of the canton of Zurich. Screening was done with the CBCL, although cutpoints were not reported. Of 577 screen-positives and 128 randomly selected screen-negatives, 399 parents (57%) were seen for DISC interviews. Steinhausen et al. (1997) presented profiles of CBCL syndrome scores for four diagnostic groups. Children with no diagnosis had mean scores in the normal range on all CBCL syndromes. Children diagnosed with only anxiety disorders had somewhat elevated scores on the Withdrawn, Somatic Complaints, and Anxious/Depressed syndromes and normal range scores on all other syndromes. Children diagnosed with ADHD had elevated scores on the CBCL Social Problems, Attention Problems, Delinquent Behavior, and Aggressive Behavior syndromes. Finally, children with comorbid anxiety and ADHD diagnoses had elevated scores on all syndromes.

CBCL Findings from Australia

Graetz, Sawyer, Hazell, Arney, and Baghurst (2001) reported associations between CBCL scores and ADHD diagnoses made from DISC-IV interviews in an Australian national general population sample of 3,597 6- to 17-year-olds. Children diagnosed with any of the three ADHD types had much higher scores on all CBCL syndromes and scales than children with no ADHD diagnosis. For example, the 3,298 children in the non-ADHD group had a mean Total Problems score of 16.1, whereas the 67 children with ADHD combined type had a mean Total Problems score of 62.1. The 133 inattentive type children and the 68 hyperactive–impulsive type children had mean Total Problems scores of 39.6 and 43.8, respectively.

YASR Findings from Finland

Sourander et al. (2005) reported associations between Young Adult Self-Report (YASR; Achenbach, 1997), an upward extension of the YSR, scores and psychiatric diagnoses in a sample of 2,347 Finnish 18-

year-olds being called up for military service. Based on a medical examination at call-up, 4.7% of the sample obtained an ICD-10 psychiatric diagnosis. The OR was 22.8 for having a psychiatric diagnosis, given a YASR Total Problems score ≥ 90th percentile versus a score < 90th percentile. ORs for a psychiatric diagnosis based on scores ≥ 90th percentile on Internalizing and Externalizing were 15.9 and 9.7, respectively. For YASR syndromes, ORs ranged from 2.7 for Attention Problems to 16.5 for Somatic Complaints. The Intrusive syndrome was not significantly associated with psychiatric diagnosis. It is notable that, despite these substantial ORs, only 21% of those scoring > 90th percentile on YASR Total Problems obtained a psychiatric diagnosis.

CPRS-R and CTRS-R Findings from the United States

Two studies have reported associations between diagnoses of ADHD and scores on the CPRS-R and the CTRS-R, although only one of these studies met our minimum N of 300. For parent reports, 91 3- to 17-year-olds from an outpatient ADHD clinic who had been diagnosed with ADHD using standard clinic procedures based on DSM-IV criteria (not including the CPRS-R) were matched on age, sex, and ethnicity with 91 children who did not have ADHD diagnoses. The children who did have ADHD diagnoses were drawn from the school-based community sample used to standardize the CPRS-R (Conners et al., 1998a). Sensitivity and specificity were 92 and 95%, respectively, for differentiating between children in the ADHD versus the non-ADHD groups based on scores on the CPRS-R, with 93% correctly classified. In a parallel study, 160 children from an ADHD clinic who had been diagnosed with DSM-IV ADHD using standard clinic procedures were compared with 160 children matched on age, sex, and ethnicity without ADHD diagnoses from the standardization sample (Conners et al., 1998b). For the CTRS-R, sensitivity and specificity were 78 and 91%, respectively, in relation to ADHD diagnoses, with 85% correctly classified. Unfortunately, neither study reported which specific CPRS-R scales and cut-points yielded these results.

SDQ Findings from the United Kingdom

Goodman (2001) reported associations between the SDQ and DSM-IV diagnoses made with the DAWBA for 10,438 British 5- to 15-year-olds in a community sample. Children were classified on each SDQ scale as deviant (> 90th percentile) or nondeviant (≤ 90th percentile), based on ratings by parents, teachers, or the children themselves. ORs between deviance on SDQ Total Difficulties and any DSM diagnosis were 15.2 for parent reports, 13.5 for teacher reports, and 6.6 for self-reports. ORs were also reported between SDQ subscales and diagnoses relevant to those scales. For parent reports, ORs ranged from 11.7 (between Emotional Symptoms and any anxiety or depression diagnosis) to 32.3 (between Hyperactivity and any ADHD diagnosis). For teacher reports, ORs ranged from 5.3 (between Emotional Symptoms and any anxiety or depression diagnosis) and 33.4 (between Conduct Problems and ODD or CD diagnoses). For self-reports, ORs ranged from 5.0 (between Hyperactivity Problems and any ADHD diagnosis) to 9.7 (between Emotional Symptoms and any anxiety or depression diagnosis).

Goodman, Ford, Simmons, Gatward, and Meltzer (2000) tested associations between SDQ scores and ICD-10 diagnoses in a sample of 7,984 11- to 15-year-olds taking part in the British Child Mental Health Survey. A computer scoring algorithm, which was not explained, combined SDQ scores from parent, teacher, and self ratings, plus scores on the SDQ impact questions, to yield predictions of diagnoses of conduct–oppositional disorder, anxiety–depressive disorder, or hyperactivity–inattention disorder as being *unlikely, possible,* or *probable.* Results indicated that 2% of those for whom a diagnosis was predicted to be *unlikely* received a diagnosis, whereas 47% of those for whom a diagnosis was predicted to be *probable* received a diagnosis. Using a prediction of *probable* to identify screen-positives, sensitivity and specificity for any diagnosis were 63 and 95%, respectively. Prediction was reportedly stronger when the child received a "severe" rather than a "mild" rating for the diagnosis. Additional analyses indicated that sensitivity was lower when only one informant was used than when two or three informants were used. Adding self-reports to parent and teacher reports improved sensitivity for anxiety and depressive diagnoses but not for the other diagnoses.

SDQ Findings from the United Kingdom and Bangladesh

Goodman, Renfrew, et al. (2000) reported associations between the SDQ and ICD-10 diagnoses based on reviews of case records for clinic samples in the United Kingdom (N = 101) and in Dhaka, Bangladesh (N = 89). Although this study did not meet our criterion of $N \geq 300$, we include it because it compared findings in two cultures. The SDQ computer scoring algorithm used by Goodman, Ford, Simmons, et al. (2000) generated predictions of a conduct disorder, an emotional disorder, or a hyperactivity disorder as *probable* (screen positive) versus *possible* or *unlikely* (screen negative). For a definite conduct disorder diagnosis given a *probable* prediction, sensitivity/specificity were 90/ 47% in London and 86/82% in Dhaka. For an emotional disorder diagnosis, sensitivity/specificity were 81/80% in London and 86/84% in Dhaka. For a hyperactivity disorder diagnosis, sensitivity/specificity were 89/78% in London and 89/81% in Dhaka.

SDQ Findings from Germany

Becker, Woerner, Hasselhorn, Banaschewski, and Rothenberger (2004) tested associations between the parent and teacher SDQ, the CBCL, the TRF, and clinic diagnoses in a sample of 543 5- to 17-year-olds attending a mental health clinic in Göttingen, Germany. Clinic diagnoses were grouped into three categories: emotional disorders, oppositional/conduct disorders, and hyperactivity/attention deficit disorders. Becker, Woerner, et al. (2004) reported findings for the *area under the curve* (AUC), which derives from *receiver operating characteristic analysis* (ROC). ROC analysis provides a bivariate graph of *sensitivity* on the Y axis against *1 minus specificity* on the X axis for various cutpoints on a distribution of scores. Larger AUCs indicate better prediction. Most AUCs were similar for the SDQ and the CBCL/TRF. For example, AUCs were .77 for parent report and .75 for teacher report for SDQ Total Difficulties, whereas AUCs were .78 and .76 for CBCL/TRF Total Problems. For predicting emotional disorders, CBCL Internalizing had a significantly higher AUC than SDQ Emotional Symptoms (.73 vs. .69). On the other hand, for predicting hyperactivity/attention deficit disorders, parent and teacher SDQ Hyperactivity scores had higher AUCs (.77 and .79) than CBCL and TRF Attention Problems scores (.70 and .72).

Becker, Hagenberg, Roessner, Woerner, and Rothenberger (2004) compared the self-report SDQ, the YSR, and clinical diagnoses in 214 11- to 17-year-olds attending the same mental health clinic in Göttingen, Germany used by Becker, Woerner, et al. (2004). The same three broad diagnostic groupings used by Becker, Woerner, et al. (2004) were applied: emotional disorders, oppositional/conduct disorders, and hyperactivity/attention deficit disorders. There were no significant differences in AUCs between the self-report SDQ and the YSR. For example, AUCs were .84 for SDQ Total Difficulties and .81 for YSR Total Problems. For parent reports in the same samples, the AUCs for the SDQ and the CBCL were similar for predicting emotional disorders or conduct disorders. For predicting hyperactivity/attention deficit disorders, the SDQ AUC of .76 was significantly higher than the CBCL AUC of .71. Adding self-ratings to either parent or teacher ratings improved prediction for all three diagnostic groupings. However, self-ratings did not significantly improve prediction after parent and teacher ratings had been taken into account.

Summary of Associations between Diagnoses and Scores on Empirically Based Instruments

Associations between scores on ASEBA scales and DSM diagnoses have been reported for at least five cultures. The studies varied in methodology, the measures of association used, and the strength of the associations reported. Even within a single study, sensitivity and specificity values varied widely as a result of differences in criteria for psychiatric caseness (e.g., Verhulst et al., 1997). Despite this heterogeneity, research has generally indicated significant and moderately strong associations between ASEBA scores and diagnoses. Relative base rates had a major influence on associations. That is, when more stringent diagnostic criteria were employed, fewer children were classified as cases, and the sensitivity of ASEBA scales generally increased. Additionally, because comorbidity was often high, particularly in clinical samples such as the one studied by Kasius et al. (1997), ASEBA syndromes typically predicted more than one diagnosis, and the same diagnosis typically had significant associations with several syndromes.

Strong associations between the Conners scales and a diagnosis of ADHD have been reported in the United States (Conners et al., 1998a, 1998b). Significant associations between SDQ scores and ICD or DSM diagnoses have been reported in two cultures (Goodman, Ford, Simmons, et al., 2000; Goodman, Renfrew, et al., 2000). Although details of how cutpoints on the SDQ were determined have not been consistently provided in these studies, ORs and sensitivities/ specificities have generally been high and comparable to those reported for the ASEBA scales. AUCs for the SDQ and the CBCL were generally similar in predicting three broad groupings of diagnoses in a German clinical sample (Becker, Hagenberg, et al., 2004a; Becker, Woerner, et al., 2004b).

ASSOCIATIONS BETWEEN SCORES ON EMPIRICALLY BASED SCALES AND REFERRAL STATUS

Several studies have reported associations between CBCL, YSR, and/ or TRF scores and referral for mental health or special education services. Several other studies have examined associations between SDQ scores and referral status. We summarize both sets of studies here and in the last column of Table 5.2.

Associations of ASEBA Scores with Referral Status in Six Cultures

Achenbach and Rescorla (2001) compared large demographically matched samples of referred and nonreferred children on scores from the CBCL (N = 3,210), TRF (N = 3,086), and YSR (N = 1,938). On all competence and adaptive functioning scales and on all problem scales, referral status ESs were highly significant and large. For example, as shown in Figure 5.1, the ESs were 36 and 28% for Total Competence on the CBCL and YSR and 29% for Total Adaptive Functioning on the TRF. Referral status ESs for Total Problems scores were 36% on the CBCL, 15% on the YSR, and 26% on the TRF. CBCL Total Problems scores across age and gender groups ranged from 22.8 to 25.2 for nonreferred children and from 58.5 to 68.2 for demographically matched referred children. ORs for being in the referred group, given deviant ($T \geq 60$) versus nondeviant ($T < 60$) scores on Total Problems, were 14, 5, and 9 for the CBCL, YSR, and TRF, respectively.

Bilenberg (1999) reported a mean CBCL Total Problems score of 17.7 for a general population sample of 779 Danish 4- to 16-year-olds, compared to a mean Total Problems score of 57.7 for 146 children attending mental health clinics. Bilenberg (1999) also reported similarly large differences between general population and referred sam-

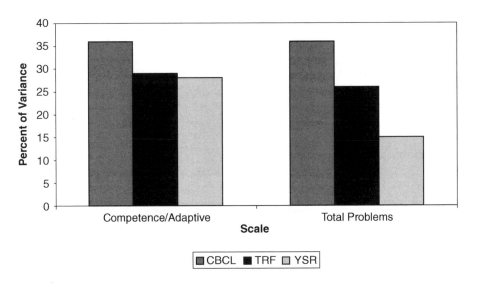

FIGURE 5.1. Effect sizes for referral status for the CBCL, TRF, and YSR in the United States. Data from Achenbach and Rescorla (2001). Figure copyright T. M. Achenbach and L. A. Rescorla. Reprinted by permission.

ples for CBCL Internalizing and Externalizing scores and for TRF and YSR Total Problems, Internalizing, and Externalizing scores. Most problem items also discriminated well between referred and general population samples, with 19 CBCL items having ORs ranging from 10.2 to 21.6. Sensitivity was 90% for identifying referred children based on a score > 95th percentile on any scale or syndrome of the CBCL, TRF, or YSR.

In Finland 598 adolescents who had participated in an epidemiological study 8 years earlier were assessed with the CBCL and the YSR (Helstelä, Sourander, & Bergroth, 2001). Adolescents were considered to be maladjusted if they had been referred for mental health services (N = 40) or if their parents reported, on a separate questionnaire, that they had "behavioral/emotional problems worse than those of other adolescents" (N = 31); the time frame for these judgments was not stated. Based on either referral for mental health services or parents' reports of "worse" problems, 55 adolescents were rated as maladjusted and 543 were considered adjusted. These two groups differed significantly on all CBCL problem scales. For example, mean Total Problems scores were 14.7 and 15.5 for nonmaladjusted boys and girls and 44.8 and 43.1 for maladjusted boys and girls, respectively. The OR for being in the maladjusted group, given a Total Problems score > 82nd percentile, was 14.4. Large ORs were also obtained for Internalizing (10.6) and Externalizing (10.2). In a related study by Helstelä and Sourander (2001), the maladjusted group included adolescents who reported, on a separate questionnaire, having more severe problems than their peers. The OR for YSR Total Problems score was 6.0, indicating that adolescents were six times more likely to fall in the maladjusted group if their YSR score was > 82nd percentile than if it was lower.

Another Finnish study assessed 2,316 18-year-olds entering military service (Sourander et al., 2004). The participants completed the YASR and reported on their use of mental health services in the past 12 months. ORs for use of mental health services in the past year if YASR scores were above versus below the 90th percentile were 9.0 for Total Problems, 5.1 for Externalizing, 8.1 for Internalizing, and from 2.2 (Intrusive) to 7.4 (Anxious/Depressed) on YASR syndromes. YASR Adaptive Functioning scale scores and YASR scores for drug and alcohol use were also significantly associated with use of mental health services (ORs of 2.8–4.0 for Adaptive Functioning, 6.3 for drug use, and 4.6 for alcohol use).

Sourander et al. (2005) reported additional findings for this cohort of Finnish military recruits. In a sample of 2,347 18-year-olds, 22.4% reported mild problems in response to the question "Do you have emotional, behavioral, or relational problems?" An additional 4%

reported moderate to severe problems, for a total of 26.4% reporting problems. The OR was 7.9 for having self-reported problems, given a YASR Total Problems score ≥ 90th percentile versus a score < 90th percentile. For Internalizing and Externalizing scores, ORs were 8.3 and 4.1, respectively. Seven YASR syndromes had significant ORs with self-reported problems (not Intrusive), with a range from 2.2 for Attention Problems to 8.7 for Anxious/Depressed.

As reported earlier, 4.7% of the 2,347 recruits obtained an ICD-10 diagnosis based on medical examinations. Of the diagnosed recruits, 63.7% had reported problems. On the other hand, most recruits with self-reported problems did not receive a diagnosis. This is evident from Sourander et al.'s report that 23.1% of the total sample of 2,347 met the cutpoint for self-reported problems but did not receive a diagnosis. Given the large difference in base rates for receiving a diagnosis versus having self-reported problems (4.7% vs. 26.4%), it is not surprising that most recruits with self-reported difficulties did not receive a diagnosis. It is noteworthy that ORs of YASR scores with self-reported problems, although substantial, were lower in every case than ORs of YASR scores with psychiatric diagnoses (e.g., 7.9 vs. 22.8 for YASR Total Problems score). This finding seems due to the fact that the self-reported problems group consisted largely of recruits with mild problems (22.4% of the total sample). In contrast, recruits with diagnoses (4.7% of the total sample) were probably more severely affected.

Schmeck et al. (2001) reported CBCL scores for 2,058 German 4- to 18-year-olds drawn from a national general population sample and for 2,058 clinically referred children matched on age, gender, and SES. Using a Total Problems score > 84th percentile as the cutpoint ($T > 60$), sensitivity and specificity were both 84%; accordingly, 84% of the sample were correctly identified as being in the nonreferred or referred group. Adding information from the individual syndrome scores did not improve prediction above using Total Problems scores alone. Schmeck et al. (2001) also reported an AUC of 92%, indicating that CBCL Total Problems score was an excellent predictor of referral status.

Fombonne (1992) compared CBCL scores for 437 French children attending mental health clinics with scores for 1,653 children from a general population sample, none of whom had been referred for mental health services. The two groups differed significantly on Total Problems, Total Competence, Internalizing, Externalizing, and 88 out of 118 problem items. The group difference on Total Problems was about 20 points, which corresponds to a d of 1.0, a large effect, according to J. Cohen (1988).

The association of referral status with TRF scores was tested in a sample of 396 nonreferred children and 408 children attending mental health clinics in Hawaii (Loo & Rapport, 1998). The mean Total Problems score for the nonreferred group was 15.1 versus 54.8 for the referred group (ES = 25%). Referred children had significantly higher TRF scores than nonreferred children on all syndromes except Aggressive Behavior, with the largest ESs on Anxious/Depressed (14%) and Attention Problems (18%).

Associations of SDQ Scores with Referral Status in Four Cultures

In an early SDQ study Goodman (1997) performed ROC analyses on SDQs completed by parents for 188 British children attending psychiatric clinics (63% male) and 158 British children attending dental clinics (53% male). The AUC for the SDQ Total Difficulties scores was 87%, indicating excellent discrimination between the two samples. For Total Difficulties scores on SDQs completed by teachers, the AUC = 85% for 146 psychiatric clinic attendees versus 39 dental clinic attendees.

Goodman (1999) compared SDQ scores for 467 British children in a community sample (52% male) versus 232 children attending one of three psychiatric clinics (68% male), using kappa as a measure of association. Kappas measure the percentage of agreement between two sets of yes/no classifications, corrected for chance agreement. They can range from –1.00 to +1.00. Between deviant versus nondeviant SDQ Total Difficulties scores and clinic versus community status, the kappas were .68 for parent reports (using a deviance cutpoint of 13), .56 for teacher reports (using a deviance cutpoint of 12), and .40 for self-reports (using a deviance cutpoint of 13). Using a cutpoint of ≥ 2 (definite) on a supplemental *overall difficulties* question (ranging from 0 for *none* to 3 for *severe*), kappas for referral status were .72 for parent reports, .63 for teacher reports, and .45 for self-reports. Averaged across all three kinds of raters, the highest mean kappa (.64) was obtained with the *impact score,* which is the sum of a rating of distress about "difficulties" and ratings of interference with life domains due to the "difficulties" (with ratings of *none* or *only a little* scored 0). For all three types of informant, this impact score differentiated clinic versus community children better than the SDQ Total Difficulties score, but discrimination was best when both the impact score and the Total Difficulties score were used.

Goodman, Meltzer, and Bailey (2003) compared self-report SDQ scores for 83 11- to 16-year-olds in a community sample and 116 age-matched children referred to a London mental health clinic. The mean Total Difficulties score was 1.4 standard deviations higher in the clinic sample than in the community sample (18.6 vs. 11.4). Based on a cutpoint at the 90th percentile (Total Difficulties score = 20), 31% of the clinic sample and 5% of the community sample scored in the deviant range. The AUC for differentiating between clinic and community samples based on Total Difficulties scores in an ROC analysis was 82%.

Koskelainen et al. (2000) tested the association between parent, teacher, and self-reports on the SDQ and parent-reported difficulties in 735 Finnish 7- to 15-year-olds. A child was considered to have difficulties if the parent gave a rating of 1 (*minor*), 2 (*definite*), or 3 (*severe*) on an item asking if the child had difficulties in emotion, concentration, behavior, or getting along with others. Using SDQ scores > 90th percentile as deviant, the ORs between SDQ deviance and having difficulties were 10.0 for parent reports, 3.2 for teacher reports, and 4.4 for self-reports. Koskelainen et al. (2000) also obtained parents' 0–2 ratings of whether they had sought child mental health services. For the 60% of children whose parents completed this item, the OR between parent-reported help seeking and parent-reported deviance on the SDQ was 8.7. Had the other 40% of parents completed the item, the results might have been different.

The association between SDQ scores obtained from parents and referral status was also tested in Germany, although the N was below our criterion of 300 (Klasen et al., 2000). Findings were reported for 163 German children attending psychiatric clinics (76% boys) and 110 German children in the community (52% boys). The AUC for SDQ parent-reported Total Difficulties was 91% and ranged from 78% (Peer Problems) to 97% (Conduct Problems) for the four SDQ subscales. AUC values were also reported for the CBCL for the same sample: 87% for CBCL Total Problems, ranging from 81% (Social Problems) to 96% (Externalizing). Additional analyses compared associations between SDQ and CBCL subscales and three global diagnostic categories (emotional disorders, conduct disorders, and hyperactivity/attention deficit disorders). Comorbidity was common, with 24% of the clinic sample having more than one of the diagnoses; 32% of the sample were excluded from these additional analyses because they did not receive any of the diagnoses. As would be expected, the AUCs were lower when predictions were measured for the three diagnostic categories than for referral status. For predicting the diagnostic categories, two comparisons yielded nonsignificantly higher AUCs for the CBCL (emotional disorder: 75 vs. 72%, and conduct disorder: 83 vs. 81%), whereas one comparison yielded a significantly higher AUC for the SDQ (hyperactivity/attention deficit disorder: 77 vs. 65%).

Bourdon et al. (2005) reported associations between SDQ scores and referral status for a sample of 9,878 4- to 17-year-olds in the United

States. Children with SDQ Total Difficulties raw scores ≥ 16 (90th percentile; N = 938, 9% of the sample) were significantly more likely to have received mental health services (OR = 12.2) or special education services (20.9) in the past year than children with scores < 90th percentile.

Use of Mental Health Services

Several studies have demonstrated that only a small fraction of children with high problem scores are actually referred for help. For example, Verhulst and van der Ende (1997) determined that only 3.5% of their general population sample of 2,227 Dutch 4- to 18-year-olds had been referred for help. This referred group constituted only 13% of the 428 children who scored in the deviant range on the CBCL Total Problems score. On the other hand, 71% of referred children scored in the deviant range on the CBCL. Factors significantly predicting referral included CBCL Total Problems score (OR = 8.2), parent-reported academic problems (OR = 3.0), change in family composition (OR = 4.1), one-parent family (OR = 2.6), and poor family functioning (OR = 2.0).

In another Dutch study 2,496 Rotterdam school children were assessed with the CBCL during routine medical examinations in 1989–1990. Their use of mental health services for the next 5 years was tracked using psychiatric case register records (Laitinen-Krispijn, van der Ende, Wierdsma, & Verhulst, 1999). Between 1 and 2% of the cohort received mental health services each year. By the end of 5 years, about 15% of those who had scored > 82nd percentile on Internalizing or Externalizing had received services. ORs for use of mental health services as a function of CBCL scores were highest for Attention Problems (7.1), Delinquent Behavior (5.9), Withdrawn (6.3), and Total Problems (4.6). These ORs decreased sharply over the 5-year period, indicating that parents either sought mental health services right away for these problems or never did within the 5-year period.

In Finland Sourander et al. (2004) reported that only 10% of 18-year-olds entering military service who had scored > 90th percentile on YASR Total Problems had used mental health services in the past year, whereas 48% of those who had used mental health services scored above this cutpoint. Overall, only 2.1% of the sample had sought mental health services in the past year.

Bourdon et al. (2005) reported that 32% of the 938 children in their U.S. study who scored > 90th percentile on SDQ Total Difficulties had used mental health services in the past 12 months. For the full sample with complete data (N = 9,878), 6.8% had used mental health services. When deviance on the SDQ was defined as parental response of "yes, definite" or "yes, severe" to the question of whether the child had experienced "overall difficulties" in the past year, 5% of the sample was identified (N = 518); 44% of this group had received mental health or special education services in the past year.

Summary of Associations between Referral Status and Scores on Empirically Based Scales

We found studies in six cultures that reported associations between scores on ASEBA scales and referral status. Although measures have varied across cultures, results indicated that ASEBA scores strongly discriminated between referred and nonreferred children. For example, referred groups obtained mean problem scores that were two to three times larger than scores obtained by nonreferred groups in Denmark, Finland, and the United States. Several studies reported ORs, with a range from 5 (YSR in the United States) to 14 (CBCL in the United States, YASR in Finland) for Total Problems scores. ESs on Total Problems scores for referral status were 15% (YSR), 36% (CBCL) in a U.S. national sample, and 25% for the TRF in a Hawaiian sample. Sensitivity with respect to referral status was 84% in Germany for deviance on the CBCL (AUC = 92%) and 90% in Denmark for deviance on the CBCL, YSR, or TRF. In Finland ASEBA scores also discriminated military recruits with self-reported or parent-reported problems from recruits without such problems.

Comparable associations have been reported for the SDQ in four cultures. For Total Difficulties scores, AUC values with respect to referral status ranged from 85% (teacher SDQ in the United Kingdom) to 91% (parent SDQ in Germany). In the United States, ORs for SDQ parent-reported Total Difficulties were 12 for mental health referral and 21 for special education services.

Studies conducted in both the Netherlands and Finland demonstrated that only 10–15% of individuals who obtained deviant scores on behavior checklists actually received mental health services, even when referral information over a period of several years was included. However, in the Bourdon et al. (2005) study conducted in the United States, 32% of children with SDQ scores > 90th percentile had received mental health services. Additionally, Verhulst and van der Ende (1997) reported that 3.5% of their Dutch general population sample assessed in 1993 had been referred for mental health services, whereas Bourdon et al. (2005) reported that 6.8% of their U.S. general population sample assessed in 2001 had received mental health services. These findings suggest that proportionately more children received mental health services in the U.S. in 2001 than in the Netherlands in 1993.

ASSOCIATIONS BETWEEN SCORES
ON EMPIRICALLY BASED SCALES AND LATER OUTCOMES

The most extensive longitudinal studies of associations between scores on the CBCL, TRF, and YSR and later outcomes have been conducted in the Netherlands and the United States. Highlights of these two major longitudinal studies are summarized in the following sections and in Table 5.3 and Figures 5.2 and 5.3.

South Holland Longitudinal Study

The South Holland sample consisted of 2,076 4- to 16-year-olds first assessed in 1983 (Time 1; Verhulst, Akkerhuis, & Althaus, 1985). Outcomes for this cohort have been reported for many different time intervals. We focus here on findings from the 6-year and 14-year outcome assessments.

Predictions from CBCL Scores

Verhulst and van der Ende (1992a) reported 6-year outcome data on 936 participants who were 4–11 years old at Time 1. Predictive rs across 6 years were .56 for Total Problems, .48 for Internalizing, .55 for Externalizing, and between .17 (Thought Problems) and .55 (Aggressive Behavior) for the eight CBCL syndromes (mean of .42 over the 11 scales). When Verhulst and van der Ende (1992a) used the 90th percentile as a cutpoint for deviance, ORs indicating continuity from Time 1 to the 6-year assessment were 9.0 for Total Problems, 10.1 for Internalizing, and 9.5 for Externalizing. Verhulst and van der Ende (1992b) reported that 33% of the children scoring > 90th percentile on CBCL Total Problems at Time 1 continued to score in this range at the 6-year assessment.

Hofstra et al. (2000) obtained parents' ratings on the Young Adult Behavior Checklist (YABCL; Achenbach, 1997) for 1,424 young adults in a 14-year outcome assessment of the South Holland sample. Findings were reported separately by gender for two age groups (ages 4–11 and ages 12–16 at Time 1). The 14-year predictive rs for Total Problems on the CBCL/YABCL averaged .43 across the four age and gender groups. As shown in Figure 5.2, the largest r was .54, for females who were 12–16 years old at Time 1. The 14-year rs ranged from .32 to .50 for Internalizing and from .34 to .56 for Externalizing across the four age and gender groups, with older girls again having the highest rs. When Hofstra et al. (2000) used the 82nd percentile cutpoint for deviance, 38–50% of those deviant at Time 1 on CBCL Total Problems

TABLE 5.3. Longitudinal Findings for Empirically Based Scales

Culture	Reference	N	Follow-up design	Longitudinal findings
Australia	Sawyer et al. (1996)	341	5-year: from age 5 to ages 10–11	rs (CBCL) = .54 (TP), .46 (I), .51 (E); 34% (TP), 42% (I), and 49% (E) remained deviant
Netherlands	Verhulst & van der Ende (1992a, 1992b)	936	6-year: from ages 4–11 to ages 10–17	rs (CBCL) = .56 (TP), .48 (I), .55 (E), .17–.55 syndromes; OR for deviance = 9.0 (TP), 10.1 (I), 9.5 (E); 33% deviant at Time 1 still deviant 6 years later
	Hofstra et al. (2000)	1,615	14-year: from ages 4–16 to ages 18–30	rs (CBCL/YABCL) = .43 (T), .32–.50 (I), .34–.56 (E); 41% deviant at Time 1 still deviant 14 years later
	Hofstra et al. (2002)	1,578	14-year: from ages 4–16 to ages 18–30	ORs = 1.9–6.1 for DSM diagnoses 14 years later (males) ORs = 1.8–10.5 for DSM diagnoses 14 years later (females)
	Hofstra et al. (2001)	802	10-year: from ages 11–19 to ages 21–29	rs (YSY/YASR) = .42 (T), .40 (I & E), .20–.39 syndromes If deviant in 1987: 22% (M), 23% (F) still deviant 10 years later and 30% (M), 43% (F) had ≥ 1 DSM diagnosis
	Bongers et al. (2003)	2,076	8-year: estimated growth curves from ages 4–18	Analyzed gender differences in intercept and slope of normative trajectories for boys and girls for CBCL TP, I, E, and eight syndromes
	Bongers et al. (2004)	2,076	8-year: growth curves from ages 4–18 for four types of externalizing behavior	Identified gender differences in trajectory groups (increasing, decreasing, consistently low, etc.) for aggression, status violations, property violations, and opposition subscales of externalizing behavior

		N	Follow-up	Findings
	Heijmans Visser et al. (2003)	1,286	6-year follow-up of clinic sample	ORs (CBCL > 82nd percentile) = 5.8 (TP), 2.8 (I), 8.1 (E) ORs (YSR > 82nd percentile) = 4.1 (TP), 4.2 (I), 7.0 (E) ORs (TRF > 82nd percentile) = 2.9 (TP), 2.8 (I), 5.7 (E)
	Heijmans Visser et al. (1999)	1,652	6-year follow-up of clinic sample	rs (CBCL: T1 to 6 years later) .51 (TP), .39 (I), .62 (E) rs (YSR: T1 to 6 years later) .47 (TP), .42 (I), .47 (E) rs (TRF: T1 to 6 years later) .45 (TP), .31 (I), .53 (E)
	Heijmans Visser et al. (2000)	544	10-year follow-up of clinic sample	rs (CBCL/YABCL) = .45 (TP), .33 (I), .51 (E), .26–.45 for eight syndromes rs (YSR/YASR) = .52 (TP), .48 (I), .53 (E), .25–.51 for eight syndromes
United States	Achenbach et al. (1995a, 1995b)	1,621	6-year: from ages 4–12 (ACQ) to ages 9–18 (CBCL, TRF, YSR)	rs (6 years, ACQ/CBCL) = .22–.53, mean .42; mean rs (3 years) = .57 (CBCL), .36 (TRF), and .44 (YSR) ESs (3 years) = 11–21% for predicting syndromes
	Achenbach et al. (1995c, 1995d)	767	6-year: from ages 11–16 to ages 19–22	rs (6 years, ACQ/YABCL) = .28–.53, mean .45 mean rs (3 years) = .59 (CBCL/YABCL), .48(YSR/YASR) ESs (3 years) = 13–29% for predicting syndromes
	Stanger et al. (1996)	1,103	6-year follow-up of clinic sample	rs (CBCL to CBCL) = .50 (TP), .43 (I), .58 (E) rs (CBCL to YABCL) = .51 (TP), .44 (I), .53 (E) ORs (CBCL to CBCL) = 5.2 (TP), 4.2 (I), 8.5 (E) ORs (CBCL to YABCL) = 4.2 (TP), 4.2 (I), 4.8 (E)
	Wadsworth and Achenbach (2005)	1,267	9-year: from ages 8–16 (ACQ) to ages 17–25	ORs (CBCL to YABCL) = 4.2 (TP), 4.2 (I), 4.8 (E) Increase in syndrome scores and cumulative prevalence of high scores over time for low SES

Note. TP, Total Problems; I, Internalizing; E, Externalizing; OR, odds ratio.

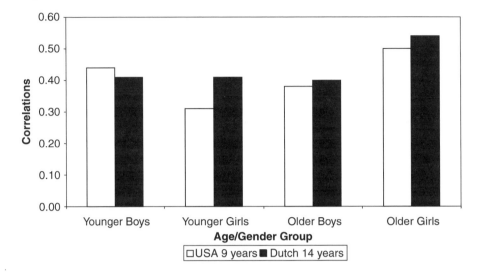

FIGURE 5.2. Predictive correlations for Total Problems in the United States and Dutch longitudinal studies. Data from Hofstra et al. (2000). Figure copyright T. M. Achenbach and L. A. Rescorla. Reprinted by permission.

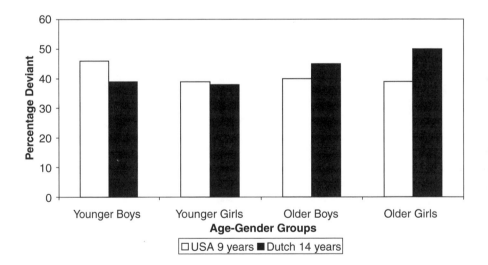

FIGURE 5.3. Percentage deviant at Time 1 still deviant at outcome on Total Problems in the United States and Dutch longitudinal studies. Data from Hofstra et al. (2000) and Rescorla et al. (2006). Figure copyright T. M. Achenbach & L. A. Rescorla. Reprinted by permission.

were deviant on YABCL Total Problems scores at the 14-year assessment (mean = 41%), as shown in Figure 5.3.

For 1,578 participants in the same longitudinal study, Hofstra et al. (2002) reported predictive associations from CBCL scores at Time 1 (ages 4–16) to DSM diagnoses made from the Composite International Diagnostic Interview (CIDI; World Health Organization, 1992) and portions of the Diagnostic Interview Schedule (DIS; Robins, Cottler, Bucholtz, & Compton, 1997) 14 years later (ages 18–30). Hofstra et al. (2002) defined deviance on Total Problems, Internalizing, and Externalizing as a score > 82nd percentile and deviance on syndromes as a score > 95th percentile. Based on deviance at Time 1 on Total Problems, ORs for any DSM diagnosis were 1.5 for males and 1.8 for females. When adjusted for associations with age at Time 1 and family SES, deviant Time 1 Delinquent Behavior scores for males predicted both mood disorders (OR = 6.1) and disruptive disorders (OR = 3.2) 14 years later. For females, deviant Time 1 Externalizing scores predicted both anxiety disorders (OR = 2.4) and disruptive disorders (OR = 10.4) 14 years later.

Predictions from YSR Scores

Predictive associations have also been reported for self-reports in Dutch follow-up studies (Hofstra, van der Ende, & Verhulst, 2001). Participants were 802 youths who completed the YSR in 1987 (at Time 3, when they were 11–19 years old), and who then completed the YASR in 1997 (Time 6) and were interviewed using the CIDI and portions of the DIS. Predictive rs over this 10-year period were .42 for Total Problems, .40 for Internalizing and Externalizing, and from .20 to .39 for the YSR/YASR syndromes. For predictions of YASR Total Problems, Internalizing, and Externalizing scores at Time 6 from their corresponding YSR scores 10 years earlier, ESs ranged from 13 to 19%. YASR syndromes were generally predicted best by their corresponding YSR syndrome. Using a YSR/YASR Total Problems score > 90th percentile as a cutpoint for deviance, 23% of males and 22% of females deviant at Time 3 were still deviant 10 years later. Participants who had YSR Total Problems scores > 90th percentile at Time 3 were almost twice as likely to have at least one DSM diagnosis 10 years later as those who were not deviant on the YSR at Time 3. Although many predictive relations were similar for females and males, there were some important gender differences. For example, high Total Problems scores in adolescence predicted a wider variety of psychiatric disorders in adulthood for females than for males.

Growth Curve Modeling

Using growth curve modeling, Bongers, Koot, van der Ende, and Verhulst (2003) compared 10-year developmental trajectories for CBCL scores in the South Holland longitudinal study. Internalizing, Anxious/Depressed, and Somatic Complaints scores were similar for boys and girls in childhood, but girls had higher scores in adolescence. On the Withdrawn syndrome, boys and girls initially obtained similar scores, and their scores increased at similar rates with age. For Externalizing and Aggressive Behavior, boys had higher initial scores than girls; scores decreased with age for both genders, but boys' scores declined more sharply. Boys had consistently higher scores than girls on Attention Problems across the 10-year period, but both genders showed increasing Attention Problems scores to age 11 and decreasing scores thereafter.

In the same sample, Bongers, Koot, van der Ende, and Verhulst (2004) examined individual differences in developmental trajectories for four types of externalizing behavior (aggression, oppositional behavior, property violations, and status violations). Bongers et al. (2004) constructed scales for these four types of behavior from CBCL items and identified trajectory subgroups for each scale. Aggression, for example, manifested three distinct trajectories: 81% of females and 60% of males were consistently low scorers, 15% of females and 29% of males were "low decreasers" (moderately high scores in childhood and low scores in adolescence), and 4% of females and 11% of males were "high decreasers" (high scores throughout the time period but some decrease from childhood to adolescence). A consistently low-scoring trajectory was also found for the other three scales (oppositional behavior, property violations, and status violations). For status violations, three trajectory groups of "increasers" were identified, varying in the magnitude of increase in adolescence. The most diverse trajectories were found for oppositional behavior.

Longitudinal Findings for Children Receiving Mental Health Services in the Netherlands

Ferdinand et al. (2003) reported 3-year outcomes for a referred sample of 6- to 12-year-olds ($N = 96$); at initial intake (Time 1), scores were obtained on the CBCL, the TRF, and the Semistructured Clinical Interview for Children and Adolescents (SCICA; McConaughy & Achenbach, 1994, 2000). The SCICA is administered by clinical interviewers who rate items similar to those of the CBCL and TRF. It yields scores on eight syndrome scales, many of which parallel those scored from the CBCL and TRF. At the 3-year follow-up (Time 2), Ferdinand et al. (2003) assessed four signs of disturbance: receipt of mental health services; parent report of wish for professional help for the child; judicial/police contacts; and school behavior problems, such as suspension, expulsion, truancy, misbehavior, and social problems.

Ferdinand et al. (2003) identified the best predictors of each sign of disturbance, after contributions of other significant predictors were taken into account. Time 1 scores on the SCICA Attention Problems syndrome, the CBCL Social Problems syndrome, and the TRF Aggressive Behavior syndrome best predicted receipt of mental health services between Time 1 and Time 2. The SCICA Aggressive Behavior syndrome was the best predictor of parent's wish for help. The TRF Social Problems syndrome was the best predictor of police/judicial contact. Lastly, the TRF Aggressive Behavior syndrome best predicted school problems. All ORs were relatively small (ORs 1.5).

Outcomes after 6 years for Dutch children receiving mental health services were reported by Heijmens Visser, van der Ende, Koot, and Verhulst (2003). They studied 1,286 children ages 4–18 who were initially assessed with the CBCL when they were seen for mental health services (Time 1) and were reassessed with the CBCL 6 years later (Time 2). Mean scores for all CBCL scales except Delinquent Behavior were much lower at Time 2 than at Time 1. Heijmans Visser et al. (2003) did not compare this decline in scores to what has been found over the same age periods in a Dutch general population sample. However, they stated that the decline of scores over 6 years in the clinic sample indicated some improvement in adjustment. Nevertheless, Time 2 scores for this clinic sample were still much higher than scores in the general population for their age and gender. For parent reports, ORs for persistence of deviance (> 82nd percentile) from Time 1 to Time 2 were 5.8 for Total Problems, 2.8 for Internalizing, and 8.1 for Externalizing. Corresponding ORs for persistence of deviance from Time 1 YSR to Time 2 YSR were 4.1 (Total Problems), 4.2 (Internalizing), and 7.0 (Externalizing). For the TRF, corresponding ORs were 2.9, 2.8, and 5.7.

For this same clinical sample of 1,286 children, Heijmens Visser, van der Ende, Koot, and Verhulst (1999) reported that 6-year predictive rs for Total Problems were .51 for the CBCL, .47 for the YSR, and .45 for the TRF. Heijmans Visser et al. (1999) also reported that predictive rs were significantly lower for Internalizing than for Externalizing scores on the CBCL ($r = .39$ vs. .62) and the TRF ($r = .31$ vs. .53), but not on the YSR ($r = .42$ vs. .47). Time 2 scores were significantly predicted by their Time 1 counterpart scores, but some Time 1 syndromes predicted multiple Time 2 scores. For example, Time 1 CBCL Anxious/Depressed scores positively predicted Time 2 CBCL Anxious/Depressed, Somatic Complaints, and Internalizing scores, but negatively predicted all other syndromes and Externalizing scores.

In addition, Heijmens Visser, van der Ende, Koot, and Verhulst (2000) reported young adult 10-year outcomes (Time 2) on the YASR and YABCL for 544 children and adolescents seen for mental health treatment at Time 1. Predictive rs from Time 1 CBCL to Time 2 YABCL scores were .45 for Total Problems, .33 for Internalizing, and .51 for Externalizing. Predictive rs from Time 1 YSR to Time 2 YASR scores were .52 (Total Problems), .48 (Internalizing), and .53 (Externalizing). Cross-informant predictive rs from the CBCL in childhood to the YASR in adulthood ranged from $r = .13$ for Thought Problems to $r = .34$ for Externalizing. Most Time 1 scores significantly predicted their counterpart scores 10 years later. In addition, some Time 1 scores predicted other problems at follow-up. For example, CBCL Social Problems scores at Time 1 predicted YABCL Internalizing, Externalizing, and Total Problems scores 10 years later. Similarly, Time 1 YSR Anxious/Depressed scores predicted Time 2 YASR Anxious/Depressed, Somatic Complaints, Aggressive Behavior, Internalizing, and Total Problems scores.

U.S. Longitudinal Findings

Several reports have presented longitudinal findings for a U.S. general population sample first assessed in 1986 at ages 4–16 (Time 1). For example, Achenbach et al. (1995a) reported 1992 (Time 3) 6-year outcomes at ages 9–18 for 1,621 participants. Time 1 scores were obtained on the ACQ (Achenbach et al., 1991). Across the 11 scales that were similar on the ACQ and the CBCL, the mean 6-year predictive r was .42, whereas the mean 3-year predictive r for the CBCL from 1989 to 1992 was .57 (Achenbach et al., 1995a). Three-year predictive rs were significant but slightly lower for the TRF (.36) and YSR (.44).

As in the Dutch longitudinal study, the strongest predictors in the U.S. longitudinal study of outcome syndrome scores tended to be earlier scores on the same syndromes, even after controlling for all other predictors (Achenbach et al., 1995a). Path analyses utilized syndrome scores that were averaged across informants (parent, teacher, and self) as both predictors and outcomes. When all other significant predictors were partialed out, Time 2 (1989) scores on many syndromes accounted for the largest percent of variance in Time 3 (1992) scores on the same syndromes: Withdrawn (ES = 18% for girls), Anxious/Depressed (ES = 18% for boys, 14% for girls), Social Problems (ES = 12% for boys), Attention Problems (ES = 10% for boys, 21% for girls), and Aggressive Behavior (ES = 17% for boys, 11% for girls).

From the same sample, Achenbach et al. (1995b) reported Time 1 and Time 2 predictors of six Time 3 signs of disturbance (receipt of mental health services, police contacts, suicidal behavior, academic problems, school behavior problems, and substance abuse). After other predictors were partialed out, Delinquent Behavior predicted more signs of disturbance than any other syndrome, including the following: school behavior problems and police contacts for both genders; mental health services and substance abuse for boys; and academic problems and suicidal behavior for girls. The Attention Problems syndrome predicted the second largest number of signs of disturbance. Stressful life experiences also significantly predicted most 1992 signs of disturbance, as did the presence of the same sign of disturbance in 1989, after partialing out other significant predictors.

Achenbach et al. (1995c) reported 1992 (Time 3) 6-year outcomes for 767 of their participants who were ages 19–22 at follow-up. Over the 6 years from Time 1 to Time 3, the mean r from CBCL to YABCL scores was .45. Over the 3 years from Time 2 to Time 3, the mean r from CBCL to YABCL scores was .59, whereas the mean r from YSR to YASR scores was .48. Path analyses indicated that the strongest predictors of adult syndromes for both genders were their earlier counterpart syndrome; for example, Withdrawn (ESs = 29% for males and 28% for females) and Somatic Complaints (ES = 13% for both genders). Adult Delinquent Behavior and Aggressive Behavior scores were predicted only by their counterpart syndromes for males (ESs = 25% and 27%, respectively). However, for females Attention Problems and Somatic Problems also predicted Delinquent Behavior, and Anxious/Depressed and Delinquent Behavior also predicted Aggressive Behavior.

Achenbach, Howell, McConaughy, and Stanger (1998) reported on Time 3 signs of disturbance in the same young adult sample. Low scores on the 1986 (Time 1) School scale significantly predicted dropping out of school (ESs = 14% for males, 28% for females). Unwed pregnancy was predicted by high 1986 Delinquent Behavior scores, low 1986 competence scores, ethnicity, and marital status of the subjects' parents. High Delinquent Behavior scores significantly predicted higher levels of substance use for both genders. Low School scores predicted later mental health services and police contacts for males and high levels of alcohol use and suicidal behavior for females.

Wadsworth and Achenbach (2005) tested the effects of parental SES on 9-year (Time 4) parent-reported outcomes for the 1,267 participants in the 1986 epidemiological sample who were 8–17 years old at Time 1. Syndrome scores for participants from middle- and upper-SES families tended to be consistent over the 9 years, whereas scores for participants from lower-SES families tended to increase over time. Additionally, individuals from lower SES families who were referred for mental health services had higher problem scores than referred individuals from middle- and high-SES families. The cumulative prevalence of high problem scores increased over time for individuals from low-SES families for Withdrawn, Thought Problems, Attention Problems, Delinquent Behavior, and Aggressive Behavior. For the Withdrawn syndrome, the increase in cumulative prevalence over time appeared to result partly from a lack of effective treatment, whereas for the other syndromes it appeared to reflect a pileup of new cases. For Anxious/Depressed, scores were significantly higher for low-SES individuals only at ages 18–27 (Time 4).

Figure 5.2 displays predictive rs for Total Problems scores over 9 years for the U.S. longitudinal sample and over 14 years for the Dutch longitudinal sample (Hofstra et al., 2000). Predictive rs were very similar in the two cultures (United States: .35–.50, the Netherlands: .34–.56). In both the United States and the Netherlands, the largest predictive rs were obtained for girls who were ages 12–16 at Time 1. Figure 5.3 displays the percentage of American young adults who had been deviant on the ACQ at Time 1 (> 82nd percentile on Total Problems) and were still deviant on the YABCL (> 82nd percentile) at the 9-year outcome assessment. Figure 5.3 also shows that the U.S. 9-year outcomes were very similar to the Dutch 14-year outcomes (Hofstra et al., 2000), with about 38–50% of the sample remaining deviant across age/gender groups in the two cultures.

Longitudinal Findings for Children
Receiving Mental Health Services in the United States

Stanger, MacDonald, McConaughy, and Achenbach (1996) reported 6-year outcome data for a sample of 1,103 children who had been referred for mental health services at two clinics in Vermont. At Time 1 intake, parents completed the CBCL. At follow-up, parents completed the CBCL for children ages 4–18 and the YABCL for young adults ages 19–27. Predictive rs from the CBCL at Time 1 to the CBCL or the YABCL at Time 2 ranged from .37 (Somatic Complaints) to .58 (Aggressive Behavior). When scores ≥ 90th percentile were used as the cutpoint for deviance on Internalizing, Externalizing, and Total Problems, ORs for persistence of deviance at Time 2 were highest for Externalizing (8.5 for the CBCL, 4.8 for the YABCL).

Australian Longitudinal Findings

Sawyer, Mudge, Carty, Baghurst, and McMichael (1996) reported 5-year follow-up data for 341 children in South Australia assessed at age 5 (Time 1) with the CBCL and at ages 10–11 (Time 2) with the CBCL, TRF, and YSR. Predictive rs were .54, .46, and .51 for Total Problems, Internalizing, and Externalizing on the CBCL. From the CBCL at Time 1 to the YSR and the TRF at Time 2, the highest predictive rs were for

Externalizing (.22 for YSR and .14 for TRF). With the 80th percentile as a cutpoint for deviance, 34%, 42%, and 49% of those deviant on CBCL Total Problems, Internalizing, and Externalizing at Time 1 were still deviant on these scales at Time 2.

Summary of Associations between Scores on Empirically Based Scales and Later Outcomes

Longitudinal studies using ASEBA scales have been a particularly rich area of research, especially in the Netherlands. Long-term longitudinal studies of large general population samples are very difficult to mount and sustain, but they are essential for answering fundamental questions about the development of psychopathology. It is especially valuable to have comparable longitudinal studies using the same instruments in multiple cultures, such as the Dutch and U.S. longitudinal studies. Results from these studies have been very similar. For example, in both cultures, the mean *r* for 6-year correlations of all CBCL scales was .42, and the strongest predictors of later syndrome scores were earlier scores on the same syndromes. The Dutch study revealed that 41% of individuals deviant on CBCL Total Problems at Time 1 were deviant on YABCL Total Problems 14 years later. For self-reports, 22% of males and 23% of females deviant on the YSR were deviant on the YASR 10 years later. Growth curve modeling of the Dutch data over a 10-year period has revealed a variety of different trajectory patterns for CBCL syndromes, with some striking differences by gender. In the U.S. longitudinal study, scores on Delinquent Behavior and Attention Problems as well as Time 1 School scale scores were the best predictors of various signs of disturbance 6 years later. Longitudinal stability has also been strong in Dutch and American follow-up studies of clinical samples, as measured by correlations and ORs.

GENETIC CORRELATES OF EMPIRICALLY BASED SCALE SCORES

Many studies have tested genetic and environmental correlates of empirically based scale scores. Some studies have compared scores for monozygotic (MZ) versus dizygotic (DZ) twins based on ratings by a single informant on a single scale at one time point. However, other studies have tested genetic models for multiple scale scores, multiple informants, or multiple time points. Still other studies have combined these approaches, such as by analyzing data from multiple informants at multiple time points. Our review summarizes findings from a sampling of these different kinds of studies. Table 5.4 presents findings from the genetic studies reviewed.

TABLE 5.4. Genetic Correlates of Empirically Based Scores

Culture	Reference	Sample	Measure analyzed	Genetic findings
Netherlands	Van der Valk et al. (2003)	Longitudinal sample of 1,575 twin pairs at ages 3 and 7	CBCL Internalizing CBCL Externalizing	For stability over time: A = 66%, C = 23%, E = 11%; C (boys/girls) = 13/8% at age 3, 26/35% at age 7 For stability over time: A = 55%, C = 37%, E = 8%; C (boys/girls) = 37/23% at age 3, 30/34% at age 7
	Bartels et al. (2004)	Longitudinal sample of 1,481 twin pairs at ages 3, 7, 10, and 12	CBCL Internalizing CBCL Externalizing	A = 59% at age 3 vs. 37% at age 12 C = 13% at age 3 vs. 37% at age 12 A (boys ages 3, 7, 10, 12) = 57%, 59%, 65%, 64% A (girls ages 3, 7, 10, 12) = 50%, 59%, 45%, 51%
	Rietveld et al., 2004	Longitudinal sample of 2,192 twins at ages 3, 7, 10, and 12	CBCL/2–3 Overactive at age 3 and CBCL/4-18 Attention Problems at ages 7, 10, and 12	A (boys ages 3, 7, 10, 12) = 50%, 33%, 41%, 40% D (boys ages 3, 7, 10, 12) = 22%, 39%, 31%, 30% E (boys ages 3, 7, 10, 12) = 28%, 28%, 28%, 30% A (girls ages 3, 7, 10, 12) = 41%, 57%, 48%, 54% D (girls ages 3, 7, 10, 12) = 33%, 16%, 25%, 18% E (girls ages 3, 7, 10, 12) = 26%, 27%, 27%, 28%
	Hudziak et al. (2005)	1,595 Dutch twin pairs at age 7	CPRS ADHD Index	A = 30%, D = 48%, E = 22%
	Boomsma et al. (2005)	Longitudinal sample of Dutch twin pairs at ages 3, 5, 7, 10, and 12; 9,025 pairs at age 3 and 2,363 pairs at age 12	CBCL/2–3 and CBCL/ 4–18 Anxious/ Depressed	For common variance between parents: A (3, 5, 7, 10, 12) = 76%, 60%, 67%, 60/53%, 48% Maternal unique variance: A (3, 5, 7, 10, 12) = 59%, 38/47%, 39%, 36%, 27% Paternal unique variance: A (3, 5, 7, 10, 12) = 19%, 27/22%, 14%, 19%, 29% Total variance for mothers: A (3–12) = 69–37% Total variance for fathers: A (3–12) = 59%–42%
Norway	Gjone, Stevenson, and Sundet (1996)	526 MZ, 389 DZ; ages 5–9, 12–15	CBCL Internalizing CBCL Externalizing	A = 43%, C = 31% A = 83%, C = 7%

136

Location	Study	Sample	Measure	Results
	Gjone and Stevenson (1996); Gjone, Stevenson, Sundet, and Eilertsen (1996)			For common variance between Internalizing and Externalizing: C = 23–53% for age/gender groups A= 73%, 76%, 79%, 75% for age/gender groups E = 27%, 24%, 21%, 25% for age/gender groups
Taiwan	Kuo et al. (2004)	279 twin and sibling pairs ages 12–16	CBCL Attention Problems CBCL Competence and Problem scales	Girls' Total Competence: A = 64%, C = 13%, E = 23% Boys' Total Competence: A = 17%, C = 64%, E = 19% Girls' Total Problems: A = 71%, C = 5%, E = 24% Boys' Total Problems: A = 41%, C = 43%, E = 16% Girl' Internalizing: A = 44%, C = 29%, E = 27% Boys' Internalizing: A = 8%, C = 68%, E = 23% Girls' Externalizing: A = 71%, C = 0%, E = 29% Boys' Externalizing: A = 0%, C = 64%, E = 36% Girls' Attention Problems: A = 70%, D = 0%, E = 30% Boys' Attention Problems: A = 70%, D = 12%, E = 16%
United Kingdom and Sweden	Eley et al. (1999)	1,022 Swedish twin pairs ages 7–9 and 529 British twin pairs ages 8–16	CBCL Aggressive CBCL Delinquent Correlation between Aggressive and Delinquent	Ranges for boys and girls in Sweden and United Kingdom: A = 53–75%, C = 7–16%, E = 18–31% Ranges for boys and girls in Sweden and United Kingdom: A = 14–41%, C = 37–54%, E = 22–32% Swedish/British boys: A = 38/25%, C = 53/56%, E = 9/19% Swedish/British girls: A = 72/88%, C = 18/6%, E = 10/6%
United Kingdom	Arsenault et al. (2003)	1,116 British twin pairs at age 5	CBCL Aggressive and Delinquent Behavior TRF Aggressive and Delinquent Behavior Latent factor	A = 69%, E = 31% A = 76%, E = 24% Common antisocial variance: A = 82%, E = 18%

Note. TP, Total Problems; I, Internalizing; E, Externalizing; A, additive genetic influences; C, shared, common environmental influences; D, dominance genetic influences; E, unshared environmental influences.

137

In behavior genetic modeling, statistical procedures are used to estimate the effects genetic factors (i.e., the *genotype*) and environmental factors on the manifestation of a trait (i.e., the *phenotype*). Most of the genetic studies we review employed the *ACE* model. In the ACE model, scores for MZ and DZ twins are analyzed to yield estimates of three kinds of effects. We refer to one kind of effect as *heritability*, which is the percentage of total variance in a trait that is attributable to genetic factors. The letter *A* is used to refer to heritability because ACE models test genetic effects that are *additive* in nature, as explained below. The letter C in the ACE model refers to a second kind of effect, which is the variance attributable to shared or common environmental factors. These are factors that influence all the children in a family more or less equally. Finally, the letter *E* in the ACE model refers to the third kind of effect, which is the variance attributable to nonshared environmental factors. These nonshared environmental factors are specific to each child in a family rather than being common to all the children.

To understand additive genetic effects, it is necessary to have a basic understanding of genes. Organisms typically have two *alleles* for most of their genes. Alleles are alternate forms at the same gene location. For each gene, an organism normally inherits one allele from the mother and another allele from the father. Alleles for any given gene typically take one of two forms, which geneticists label with upper case and lower case letters. For example, the two alleles comprising the gene for flower color might be labeled X = red and x = white. For any given gene, an organism can be *homozygous* (i.e., both alleles are the same, such as XX or xx), or *heterozygous* (i.e., the two alleles are different, such as Xx). When a genetic effect is additive, the phenotype of a trait is determined by adding the effects of each allele of the gene. For example, plants that are XX will have red flowers, plants that are Xx will have pink flowers, and plants that are xx will have white flowers.

Although many behavior genetic studies equate heritability with additive genetic effects, some studies also include *dominance* genetic effects in their statistical models. Dominance genetic effects (represented in genetic models by the letter *D*) occur when the homozygous dominant allele (XX) and the heterozygous pair (Xx) have the same phenotype and only the homozygous recessive pair has a different phenotype. Genetic dominance is often illustrated using eye color, because the allele for brown eyes is dominant and the allele for blue eyes is recessive. So, people who are homozygous dominant (XX, i.e., two brown alleles) or heterozygous (Xx, i.e., one brown and one blue allele) have brown eyes, whereas only people who are homozygous recessive (xx, i.e., two blue alleles) have blue eyes.

For statistical reasons beyond the scope of this chapter, analyses using MZ and DZ twins to estimate genetic and environmental effects cannot currently test for both dominance and shared environment in the same model. Therefore, when researchers choose to estimate both additive (A) and dominance (D) genetic effects, they omit C (shared environment), and the resulting model is not ACE but ADE, where D stands for dominance genetic effects. Researchers typically opt for an ADE rather than an ACE model when shared environmental effects appear to be negligible. They test shared environmental effects by comparing the correlations between scores for MZ twins with the correlations between scores for DZ twins. If the MZ correlations are more than twice as large as the DZ correlations, researchers may conclude that shared environmental effects are negligible and that dominance genetic effects should be tested. If they draw these conclusions, they may choose to replace C with D.

Genetic Correlates of the Internalizing and Externalizing Scales

Gjone, Stevenson, Sundet, and Eilertsen (1996) analyzed genetic and environmental influences on CBCL Internalizing and Externalizing scores in 526 MZ and 389 DZ younger (ages 5–9) and older (ages 12–15) Norwegian twin pairs. Across both ages and genders, heritability (A) was larger for Externalizing (83%) than for Internalizing (43%). Shared environmental variance (C) was correspondingly smaller (7 vs. 31%). For reasons they did not explain, Gjone et al. did not appear to include nonshared environmental variance (E) in their model.

Further analyses of this Norwegian twin sample (Gjone & Stevenson, 1997) applied the ACE model to the common (i.e., shared) variance between Internalizing and Externalizing. For the common variance between Internalizing and Externalizing, shared environmental variance was the largest component in the model (C = 23–53% across age/gender groups).

In behavior genetics research, a twin who manifests the condition of interest in that research is often referred to as an *index* twin. When an index twin's co-twin also manifests the condition of interest, the twins are referred to as *concordant* for the condition. A central element of behavior genetics research is to compare *concordance rates* for MZ and DZ twins. The concordance rate is generally higher for MZ than for DZ twins when heritability is high for a condition. However, the concordance rate is similar for MZ and DZ twins when heritability is low.

In the Gjone and Stevenson (1997) study, the conditions of interest were deviance on the CBCL Internalizing and Externalizing scales. Therefore, Gjone and Stevenson classified each twin as deviant (score ≥ 1 *SD* above the sample mean) or nondeviant (score < 1 *SD* above sample mean) on Internalizing and Externalizing. Twins could be "pure" Internalizers (i.e., they had deviant scores only for Internalizing), "pure" Externalizers (i.e., they had deviant scores only for Externalizing), *comorbid* (i.e., they were deviant on both Internalizing and Externalizing), or nondeviant (deviant on neither scale). The concordance rate in this study was thus the percentage of twins who were deviant when their index co-twin was deviant.

Gjone and Stevenson (1997) found that MZ twins had a much higher concordance rate than DZ twins when the index twin was a pure Internalizer or a pure Externalizer. However, when the index twin was comorbid (i.e., was deviant on both Internalizing and Externalizing), MZ and DZ concordance rates were more similar. Thus, both the ACE findings and the MZ–DZ concordance rates indicated that genetic influences were stronger among individuals who were deviant on only the Internalizing or Externalizing scale than among individuals who were deviant on both scales. In contrast, shared environmental influences were stronger among individuals who were deviant on both the Internalizing and Externalizing scales.

Van der Valk, van den Oord, Verhulst, and Boomsma (2003) tested genetic and environmental correlates of CBCL Internalizing and Externalizing scores for 1,575 Dutch twin pairs rated by mothers at age 3 and again at age 7. For Internalizing scores, the effect of shared environment (C) was smaller at age 3 than at age 7 (boys: 13 vs. 26%; girls: 8 vs. 35%). For Externalizing scores, the effect of shared environment was more similar at the two ages (boys: 37 vs. 30%; girls: 23 vs. 34%). For Internalizing, predictive *r*s between ages 3 and 7 were .35 for boys and .41 for girls; 66% of this stability was attributable to heritability, 23% to shared environmental factors, and 11% to nonshared environmental factors. For Externalizing, predictive *r*s were .55 for boys and .53 for girls, with 55% of this stability attributable to heritability, 37% to shared environmental factors, and 8% to nonshared environmental factors.

Genetic and environmental mechanisms associated with Internalizing and Externalizing scores were examined longitudinally at ages 3, 7, 10, and 12 in 1,481 Dutch twin pairs (Bartels et al., 2004). As shown in Figure 5.4a, heritability for Internalizing scores decreased with age (A = 59% at age 3, 37% at age 12), whereas shared environmental effects increased with age (C = 13% at age 3, 37% at age 12). For Externalizing (Figure 5.4b), heritability changed less with age and was some-

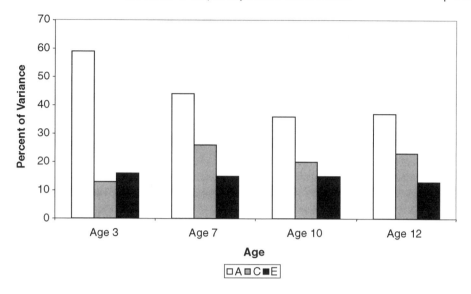

FIGURE 5.4a. ACE results for Internalizing scores of Dutch twins at ages 3, 7, 10, and 12. Data from Bartels et al. (2004). Figure copyright T. M. Achenbach and L. A. Rescorla. Reprinted by permission.

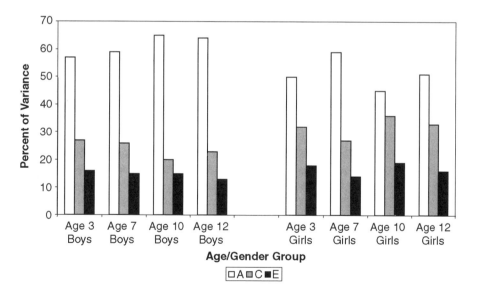

FIGURE 5.4b. ACE results for Externalizing scores of Dutch twins at ages 3, 7, 10, and 12. Data from Bartels et al. (2004). Figure copyright T. M. Achenbach and L. A. Rescorla. Reprinted by permission.

what greater for boys than girls at most ages. For both Internalizing and Externalizing, stability across age was explained largely by effects of heritability and shared environment, whereas change across age was largely explained by effects of nonshared environment.

Genetic Correlates of the Attention Problems Syndrome

In the same Norwegian sample described previously for Internalizing and Externalizing, Gjone, Stevenson, and Sundet (1996) assessed genetic and environmental influences on the CBCL Attention Problems syndrome in 526 MZ and 389 DZ younger (ages 5–9) and older (ages 12–15) twin pairs. The AE model provided the best fit for both genders in both age groups. Heritability estimates (A) were 73–79% across the four age/gender groups.

Rietveld, Hudziak, Bartels, Beijsterveldt, and Boomsma (2004) examined genetic and environmental influences on problems of overactivity and attention in a longitudinal sample of 2,192 Dutch MZ and DZ twins at ages 3, 7, 10, and 12. They analyzed CBCL/2–3 Overactive Behavior scores at age 3 and CBCL/4–18 Attention Problems scores at ages 7, 10, and 12. As would be expected, boys had higher scores than girls at all four ages. In these Dutch twin pairs, the *r*s between Attention Problems scores for MZ twins were more than twice as large as the *r*s between Attention Problems scores for DZ twins (e.g., MZ r = .66 vs. DZ r = .13 at age 3). Rietveld et al. (2004) therefore decided that shared environmental effects were negligible and that dominance as well as additive genetic effects should be estimated. Thus, they used an ADE model, which included both A (the additive genetic parameter) and D (the dominance parameter) as heritability parameters. As shown in Figure 5.5, heritability (A + D) ranged from 70–74% for all age/gender groups. Nonshared environmental influences (E) accounted for the rest of the variance. Longitudinal associations (i.e., stability across time) were also largely accounted for by genetic factors (A + D), with nonshared environmental influences ranging from only 8–24%.

Genetic Correlates of ADHD Measured by the CPRS

Hudziak et al. (2005) examined genetic correlates of mothers' ratings on the CPRS ADHD Index in a sample of 1,595 Dutch twin pairs at age 7. The ADHD Index is a 12-item scale that Conners (2001) found to be the best CPRS measure of DSM-IV ADHD. Hudziak et al. (2005) reported heritability of 78%, comprised of 30% additive genetic factors (A) and 48% dominance genetic factors (D). Nonshared environmental

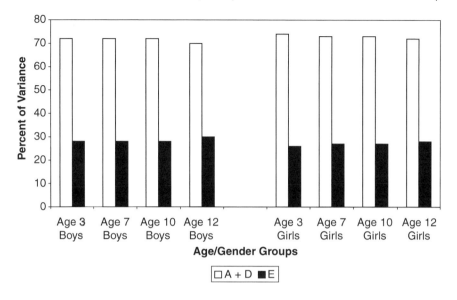

FIGURE 5.5. ADE results for Attention Problems in Dutch twins at ages 3, 7, 10, and 12. Data from Rietveld et al. (2004). Figure copyright T. M. Achenbach and L. A. Rescorla. Reprinted by permission.

variance (E) was 22%. Genetic and environmental influences were similar for boys and girls.

Genetic Correlates of Aggressive Behavior and Delinquent Behavior Syndromes

Several studies have examined genetic and environmental correlates of CBCL Aggressive and Delinquent Behavior scores. For example, Eley, Lichtenstein, and Stevenson (1999) compared genetic models for 1,022 Swedish twin pairs (ages 7–9) and 529 British twin pairs (ages 8–16). As shown in Figure 5.6, genetic influences (A) were larger and shared environmental (C) influences were smaller for Aggressive Behavior than for Delinquent Behavior in both Sweden and Britain. Genetic influences (A) were zero for Delinquent Behavior for boys in Britain.

The r between Aggressive Behavior and Delinquent Behavior was .56 for boys and .61 for girls in Sweden and .56 and .55 for boys and girls, respectively, in Britain. These bivariate rs measure the common (i.e., shared) variance between Aggressive and Delinquent Behavior. Eley et al. (1999) applied the ACE model to these bivariate rs. For boys, shared environment (C) had the largest influence on the common vari-

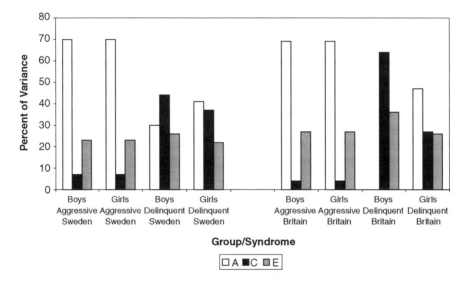

FIGURE 5.6. ACE results for Aggressive Behavior and Delinquent Behavior syndromes in Swedish and British twins. Note that there is no bar for A for boys Delinquent Britain because such influences were zero. Data from Eley et al. (1999). Figure copyright T. M. Achenbach & L. A. Rescorla. Reprinted by permission.

ance between Aggressive Behavior and Delinquent Behavior in both cultures (Sweden: C = 53%; Britain: C = 56%). For girls, however, genetic factors (A) had the largest influence on the common variance between Aggressive Behavior and Delinquent Behavior in both cultures (Sweden: A = 72%; Britain: A = 88%). Thus, the common variance between Aggressive Behavior and Delinquent Behavior was much more heritable in girls than in boys. Eley et al. (1999) noted that shared environment had a much greater influence for boys than for girls on the common variance between aggressive and unaggressive antisocial behavior, despite the fact that shared environmental influences were modest for both genders for Aggressive Behavior. In discussing their findings, Eley et al. (1999) suggested that girls have "higher resistance" than boys to antisocial behavior. This means that girls tend to be less likely to exhibit antisocial behavior than boys, so that when they do so it is probably because attributes "internal" to the individual (i.e., genetic factors) drive the behavior. As evidence for this hypothesis, Eley et al. (1999) noted that concordance for criminality is higher in female co-twins than in male co-twins.

Arsenault et al. (2003) examined genetic and environmental effects on measures of antisocial behavior at age 5 obtained from four sources totaling 1,116 British twin pairs. A composite measure of antisocial behavior was derived from mothers' ratings on the CBCL Aggressive Behavior and Delinquent Behavior syndromes (plus some additional antisocial items). A similar composite was derived from teachers' ratings on the TRF. Examiners' ratings and children's self-reports elicited in a puppet interview comprised the two additional measures of antisocial behavior. Heritability (A) was 69% for the CBCL composite score and 76% for the TRF composite score. Arsenault et al. also found that genetic factors accounted for most of the common variance among the four measures of antisocial behavior (A = 82%). Thus, 82% of the variance in pervasive, cross-situational antisocial behavior was heritable. Arsenault et al. concluded that the unique variance (i.e., the variance left in each measure after the common variance between the four measures was removed) was not measurement error but reflected genuine genetic and nonshared environmental effects specific to each measure.

Genetic Correlates
of the Anxious/Depressed Syndrome

A longitudinal study examined mothers' and fathers' ratings of Dutch twins on the CBCL Anxious/Depressed syndrome at ages 3, 5, 7, 10, and 12, with Ns ranging from 9,222 pairs at age 5 to 2,363 pairs at age 12 (Boomsma, van Beijsterveldt, & Hudziak, 2005). For ratings by both mothers and fathers, heritability of Anxious/Depressed scores declined with age. When the variance common to mothers' and fathers' ratings was analyzed, heritability (A) declined with age (from 76 to 48%). When unique, rater-specific variance was analyzed, heritability (A) was higher in mothers' ratings than in fathers' ratings at most ages. The authors concluded that heritability for Anxious/Depressed declines with age, and that differences between parents reflect each parent's unique perspectives on his or her children's functioning, rather than unreliability or biases.

Genetic Correlates of CBCL Competence
and Problem Scores among Taiwanese Youths

Kuo, Lin, Yang, Soong, and Chen (2004) tested genetic effects on all CBCL scales separately by gender for Taiwanese 12- to 16-year-olds. Samples were much smaller than in other genetic studies reviewed here: 194 MZ twin pairs (108 female, 86 male) and 85 DZ twin and sibling pairs (27 female, 35 male). Kuo et al. (2004) reported that heritability was much higher for girls than for boys for Total Competence, Total Problems, Externalizing, and Internalizing. Heritability for Attention Problems was identical for girls and boys. Although the gender differences in this Taiwanese study are intriguing, they must be viewed as very tentative because of the small samples. Replication with larger samples is clearly needed.

Summary of Genetic Studies
Using Empirically Based Scales

Many genetic studies of empirically based scale scores have been published, resulting in an exponentially expanding international database in which to examine genetic and environmental correlates of problems reported for children. The comparability of ASEBA syndromes across informants and age periods makes these syndromes particularly useful for genetic studies. The studies varied widely in terms of the scales analyzed and the complexity of their designs (e.g., multiple time points, multiple raters, multiple scales). Nonetheless, some major conclusions can be drawn from this rapidly growing body of research. Findings indicated large influences of heritability on the Attention Problems, Anxious/Depressed, and Aggressive Behavior syndromes (i.e., in most studies, A > 70%). Similarly high heritability was found for the CPRS ADHD Index. It is noteworthy that heritability was lower for Delinquent Behavior than for Aggressive Behavior (e.g., Eley et al., 1999). Heritability parameters often varied by gender. For example, the common variance between Aggressive Behavior and Delinquent Behavior was much more heritable for girls than for boys in both Sweden and the United Kingdom (Eley et al., 1999). Heritability also varied by age. For example, heritability declined with age for CBCL Anxious/Depressed scores based on ratings of Dutch twins by their mothers and fathers. Furthermore, the variance unique to different informants was not due to measurement error or rater bias but validly captured different genetic and environmental variances (Arsenault et al., 2003; Boomsma et al., 2005).

SCORES OBTAINED BY IMMIGRANT CHILDREN
ON EMPIRICALLY BASED INSTRUMENTS

Children of immigrants constitute an increasingly large percentage of the population in many countries. An important aspect of globalization is the increase in migration, both legal and illegal, from countries with widespread poverty to countries that offer more economic opportunities. Political, ethnic, and religious persecution as well as wars and famine are also driving millions from their home cultures to seek opportunities in new cultures. Immigrant families tend to have higher birthrates than indigenous families in host cultures, further accelerating population shifts. For all these reasons, the number of immigrant children being served by educational, legal, medical, mental health, and social welfare systems is increasing rapidly in many cultures. Consequently, a growing research area is assessment of the mental health needs of children of immigrants. Numerous studies using empirically based assessment instruments have been done in the Netherlands, but studies have also been done in other countries, including Israel, Australia, the United States, and Norway.

CBCL, TRF, and YSR Studies of Turkish Immigrants in the Netherlands

Several studies have assessed children of Turkish immigrants in the Netherlands. An initial study compared CBCL scores for 833 Turkish children living in the Netherlands with those of 2,081 Dutch children from a general population sample and 3,127 Turkish children from a general population sample in Ankara, Turkey (Bengi-Arslan, Verhulst, van der Ende, & Erol, 1997). Turkish immigrant children had higher scores than Dutch children on 6 of the 11 CBCL problem scales, with the largest ESs on Anxious/Depressed (16%) and Internalizing (10%). Turkish immigrant children also had slightly higher scores than Turkish children in Ankara, but all ESs were < 1%. Thus, parents of Turkish children in the Netherlands reported many more problems than parents of Dutch children, but only slightly more than parents of Turkish children in Ankara. Markedly higher scores were obtained on the Anxious/Depressed syndrome by both groups of Turkish children than by Dutch children. Bengi-Arslan et al. (1997) speculated that the high Anxious/Depressed scores may reflect children's reactions to child-rearing practices in Turkish families, which are characterized by strict demands for obedience, harsh verbal criticism, physical punishment, and threats, including threats of punishment by God.

Bengi-Arslan et al. (1997) also reported that Turkish immigrant children scored lower than Dutch children (ES = 2%) and Ankara children (ES = 3%) on the School scale of the CBCL. Some Turkish immigrant children do not learn to speak Dutch until they enter school, and their parents tend to have lower educational attainment than Dutch parents, both of which might contribute to lower school performance.

On the other hand, Turkish immigrant children obtained higher scores than Dutch (ES = 7%) and Ankara (ES = 1%) children on the Social scale.

A comparison of TRF scores for 524 Turkish immigrant students versus 1,625 Dutch students was reported by Crijnen, Bengi-Arslan, and Verhulst (2000). No significant differences were found between Turkish students and Dutch students on any of the 11 TRF problem scales. Higher problem scores were reported for students from lower-SES families than from higher-SES families in both cultural groups. Because proportionately more Turkish families were lower SES, Turkish students' TRF problem scores might have been slightly lower than Dutch students' scores if SES differences were partialed out.

An especially interesting aspect of the Crijnen et al. (2000) study was that 221 of the Turkish immigrant students were also rated on the TRF by teachers of Turkish background, who instructed them during part of the school day. Ratings by these Turkish teachers yielded scores on Anxious/Depressed that were significantly higher than scores obtained by Dutch students rated by Dutch teachers (ES = 20%). As a consequence of these higher Anxious/Depressed scores, Turkish students rated by their Turkish teachers also scored higher than Dutch students on Internalizing (ES = 11%) and Total Problems (ES = 5%). Crijnen et al. (2000) argued that the high scores for Turkish teachers' ratings of immigrant students on Anxious/Depressed reflect several factors. First, when they enter school, Turkish immigrant students quickly master conversational Dutch, but their language proficiency for academic work is limited. On the other hand, their parents expect them to conform to school demands and to excel academically, resulting in pressure for academic success that they struggle to meet. Dutch teachers do not appear to be aware that this gap between expectation and performance creates anxiety about failure in the students. However, because Turkish teachers share the students' cultural heritage and converse with them in their own language, they are better able to detect these worries and anxieties.

YSR scores obtained by 363 Turkish immigrant youths and 1,098 Dutch youths were compared by Murad, Joung, van Lenthe, Bengi-Arslan, and Crijnen (2003). Turkish girls obtained higher YSR problem scores than Dutch girls on Withdrawn, Anxious/Depressed, Social Problems, Internalizing, and Total Problems, even after accounting for other significant predictors, such as school attainment, parent education, family factors, and life stress factors. The largest difference between Dutch and Turkish YSR scores was for Withdrawn (OR = 2.8). Turkish boys scored higher than Dutch boys on Withdrawn and Anxious/Depressed and lower than Dutch boys on Delinquent Behavior, after controlling for other significant predictors, with the largest OR being for Withdrawn (2.0). Murad et al. (2003) suggested that lower YSR Delinquent Behavior scores for Turkish boys than Dutch boys may reflect lower actual levels of antisocial behavior. However, these lower scores may also reflect underreporting of antisocial behavior by Turkish boys out of fear of reprisal by the authorities.

Factors associated with individual differences in CBCL scores among 833 Turkish immigrants were examined by Sowa, Crijnen, Bengi-Arslan, and Verhulst (2000). Parents completed the CBCL in Turkish and also completed a 55-item questionnaire administered by a Turkish-speaking interviewer. Being a second-generation rather than a first-generation immigrant and participating in a Koran course were associated with lower scores on Delinquent Behavior. By contrast, problems in school, parental divorce, incarceration of a family member, family mental health problems, and parental arguments were associated with higher Delinquent Behavior scores. Higher Attention Problems scores were associated with repeating a grade, problems at school, parental divorce and arguments, traffic accidents, and/or incarceration of family members. Higher Anxious/Depressed scores were associated with gender (higher for girls), problems at school, parental arguments, incarceration of a family member, theft/fire in the home, and family financial or employment problems.

CBCL, TRF, and YSR Studies of Moroccan Immigrants in the Netherlands

Several studies of Moroccan immigrants in the Netherlands have been reported by Stevens and her colleagues. For example, Stevens et al. (2003) compared CBCL, TRF, and YSR scores for 819 Moroccan immigrants, 833 Turkish immigrants, and 2,227 Dutch children. On the CBCL, Moroccan immigrant parents reported significantly fewer problems than Turkish immigrant parents on six of the eight syndrome scales (largest ES = 20% on Anxious/Depressed) and significantly fewer problems than Dutch parents on Attention Problems (ES = 1%). On the YSR, Moroccan youths reported fewer problems than Turkish youths on all syndromes except Delinquent Behavior (largest ES = 9% on Anxious/Depressed) and fewer problems than Dutch youths on five syndromes (largest ES = 6% on Attention Problems).

TRF scores presented a different picture. Teachers rated Moroccan students higher than Turkish students on Attention Problems (ES = 2%), Delinquent Behavior (ES = 4%), and Aggressive Behavior (ES = 5%). Teachers also rated Moroccan students higher than Dutch students on these same syndromes: Attention Problems (ES = 2%), Delinquent Behavior (ES = 8%), and Aggressive Behavior (ES = 5%). Thus, Moroccan parents and youths reported fewer problems than were reported for Turkish and Dutch youths, whereas teachers reported more problems for Moroccan students than for either Turkish or Dutch students. This pattern of discrepancies in how Moroccan youths are viewed by different informants might contribute to a feeling of alienation on the part of Moroccan parents and youths with respect to Dutch society.

Striking gender differences in associations between acculturation status and scores on the CBCL and YSR for 387 Moroccan immigrants were reported by Stevens, Vollebergh, Pels, and Crijnen (2006). Based on an acculturation status interview, the youths were classified as integrated (i.e., highly attached to both Moroccan and Dutch cultures), ambivalent (i.e., moderate attachment to both Moroccan and Dutch cultures), or separated (i.e., highly attached to Moroccan culture but not to Dutch culture). Within the sample, 47% were integrated (48% of whom were girls), 13% were ambivalent (74% of whom were girls), and 40% were separated (49% of whom were girls). Problem scores for boys did not differ significantly across the acculturation status groups. For girls, however, both the CBCL and YSR yielded higher problem scores for the ambivalent acculturation group than for the integrated or separated groups. Furthermore, the association between ambivalent acculturation and problem scores was significantly mediated by level of parent–child conflict. Specifically, Moroccan immigrant adolescent girls who were torn between identifying with Moroccan culture and with Dutch culture had high levels of parent–child conflict, which then led to increased problems of both an internalizing and an externalizing nature.

Stevens, Vollebergh, Pels, and Crijnen (in press) tested associations between CBCL and YSR problem scores and parent-reported parenting practices for 727 Moroccan immigrant youths. For both boys and girls, parents of youths were more likely than parents of younger children to report being low in affection, responsiveness, monitoring, and use of explanations during discipline. Furthermore, parents reported this style of parenting more often for boys than for girls. For children, CBCL Total Problems, Internalizing, and Externalizing scores were higher in families using high levels of punishment and discipline than in families using low or medium levels. There were few other significant associations between parenting style and CBCL problems for children. However, for youths, low parental affection was associated with higher CBCL and YSR scores on virtually all problem scales. In addition, low parental responsiveness was associated with higher CBCL Total Problems and Internalizing scores. Furthermore, parents who reported low monitoring and high discipline had youths with higher CBCL Total Problems and higher YSR Internalizing and Externalizing scores. Lastly, youths whose parents granted more autonomy had higher CBCL Internalizing scores.

YSR Findings for Russian Immigrants in Israel

Ponizovsky, Ritsner, and Modai (1999) used the YSR to assess suicidal ideation and suicide attempts as well as other problems in 406 Russian Jewish immigrants to Israel, 203 Jewish youths in Russia, and 104 Israeli adolescents. Significantly more immigrant youths endorsed YSR item *91. I think about killing myself* than their Russian counterparts (11 vs. 4% respectively), but the 11% prevalence for immigrant youths did not differ significantly from the 9% prevalence for their Israeli peers. Similar results were reported for YSR item *18. I deliberately try to hurt or kill myself* (10% by immigrants, 4% by Jewish youths in Russia, 9% by Israelis). Ninety-five percent of the immigrants with suicidal ideation had made a suicide attempt. Immigrants reporting suicidal ideation obtained higher scores on all YSR syndromes than immigrants not reporting suicidal ideation.

The immigrant group as a whole obtained significantly higher YSR scores than their Israeli peers only on Social Problems and Attention Problems, whereas they obtained significantly higher scores than their Russian peers on all syndromes except Social Problems and Attention Problems. For both immigrants and Israelis, but not for Russians, those with suicidal ideation had higher scores for obsessiveness, hostility, sensitivity, depression, anxiety, and paranoid ideation on a distress inventory. Immigrants with suicidal ideation did not differ from immigrants without suicidal ideation on length of time in Israel, but they reported significantly more problems with the Hebrew language, their health, the Israeli climate, Israeli peers, their own families, and their own personality traits. Ponizovsky et al. (1999) interpreted their findings as consistent with the migration-convergence hypothesis; that is, the immigrants appeared to be more similar to their Israeli peers than to their Russian peers in suicidal symptoms and in general behavioral and emotional adjustment.

SDQ Scores for Diverse Immigrants in Norway

Oppedal, Røysamb, and Heyerdahl (2005) collected self-report SDQ data from 1,295 10th-grade youths in Oslo from immigrant families; 52% of the youths were first-generation and 48% were second-generation immigrants. The immigrant youths came from 11 different cultures of origin, with samples ranging from $N = 45$ (Iraq) to $N = 541$ (Pakistan). No comparisons between the ethnic groups and Norwegian youths were reported, nor were SDQ scores interpreted in relation to any normative benchmarks.

First-generation immigrant girls reported significantly more difficulties than second-generation girls on the SDQ Total, Emotional, Peer, and Hyperactivity scales. In contrast, second-generation immigrant boys reported more difficulties than first-generation boys on SDQ Total, Conduct, and Hyperactivity scales. Although no ESs were provided for these comparisons, the published data enabled us to calculate Cohen's d for the first- versus second-generation differences; ds for SDQ Total Difficulties score were .35 (girls) and .19 (boys). The data also indicated that second-generation girls had higher host culture competence and lower perceived discrimination than first-generation girls, but no difference was found for first- versus second-generation boys on host culture competence or perceived discrimination. When these two acculturation factors were accounted for, the gender × generation interaction was no longer significant.

Significant ethnic group differences were reported for all SDQ problem scales, but no ESs were reported. Adolescents from Morocco, India, and Somalia obtained the lowest SDQ Total Difficulties scores. Significantly higher scores were obtained by adolescents from Turkey, Pakistan, Latin America, Iraq, Iran, and Vietnam. Adolescents from groups seeking work opportunities (e.g., Pakistanis) did not appear to have lower SDQ scores than refugees from wars (e.g., Iraqis). Significant differences among ethnic groups were reported for a variety of acculturation factors, but no clear pattern was evident for acculturation across the 11 different ethnic groups. Total SDQ scores had rs of .23 with reported ethnic identity crises and of .32 with reported experiences of racism. High levels of host culture competence and family values had very small but significant negative rs with SDQ Total Difficulties scores (both −.10).

Summary of Findings for Immigrant Children on Empirically Based Scales

Several studies of immigrant children's adjustment, assessed with empirically based scales, have been conducted with Turkish samples in the Netherlands. These studies found that Turkish immigrant children had higher problem scores than Dutch children on the CBCL, particularly on Internalizing problems, but that their scores were only slightly higher than those reported for Turkish children living in Turkey

(Bengi-Arslan et al., 1997). When rated by their *Dutch* teachers, Turkish immigrant students' scores did not differ significantly from Dutch students' scores. However, when rated by their *Turkish* teachers, Turkish immigrant students had much higher Anxious/Depressed scores than Dutch students rated by Dutch teachers. Crijnen et al. (2000) attributed these patterns to Turkish students' anxiety about meeting parental expectations for school achievement. On the YSR, Turkish youths had significantly higher problem scores than Dutch youths on several scales.

For Moroccan immigrants in the Netherlands, CBCL and YSR problem scores were lower than those for Turkish and Dutch youth, whereas TRF problem scores were higher than those for Turkish and Dutch youth (Stevens et al., 2003). This discrepancy between informants in how Moroccan youths are perceived might contribute to Moroccan parents' and youths' feeling of alienation from Dutch mainstream culture, as represented by the school. Stevens et al. (in review) also reported important gender differences, notably that Moroccan girls with ambivalent acculturation had higher CBCL problem scores than girls with integrated or separated acculturation, whereas Moroccan boys' CBCL problem scores did not differ across acculturation types.

For a different immigrant group, Ponizosky et al. (1999) reported that Russian immigrants in Israel had much higher YSR problem scores than Russian Jewish youths who had not emigrated, but that they were comparable to Israeli youths except for higher scores on Social Problems and Attention Problems. Oppedal et al. (2005) reported that youths from different immigrant groups in Norway varied in SDQ scores, but no ESs for these differences were reported. Whether the immigrant families were seeking work opportunities or were refugees did not appear to affect SDQ scores.

SUMMARY

We summarized studies of seven kinds of correlates of children's scores on ASEBA scales: SES, marital status of parents, diagnoses, referral status, longitudinal outcomes, genetic factors, and immigration. Less research on these topics has been conducted using the Conners' scales and the SDQ, but these studies were summarized where relevant.

Across 15 cultures, low SES was reported to be associated with higher problem scores, with ESs of 1–5%. Low SES was also consistently associated with lower competence scores, but fewer studies analyzed competence scores.

The effect of parental marital status on children's problem scores has been examined in surprisingly few studies meeting our criteria, despite the fact that marital status is easy to assess. Findings indicate that children in divorced and single-parent families tend to obtain higher problem scores than children in intact families.

Studies testing associations of ASEBA scales, the CPRS and CTRS, and the SDQ with DSM or ICD diagnoses in several cultures have typically indicated high sensitivities and large ORs. Predictions tended to be more accurate when more stringent criteria for psychiatric caseness were employed, most likely because these criteria reduced the disparity in base rates between diagnoses and deviance using the rating forms. Discriminative validity was evident in these associations (i.e., syndromes predicted best in relation to diagnoses involving similar kinds of problems), but significant associations were often found between multiple syndromes and diagnoses, probably owing to comorbidity.

Studies in six cultures indicated that ASEBA scores strongly discriminated between referred and nonreferred children: Mean scores were much higher in referred than nonreferred groups. Similarly strong associations were reported for the SDQ in four cultures.

Longitudinal studies using empirically based scales over a 14-year period in the Netherlands and over a 9-year period in the United States have yielded very similar results. In both cultures, the mean predictive r for 6-year correlations of all CBCL scales was .42, and the strongest predictors of later syndrome scores were earlier scores on the same syndrome. In the U.S. longitudinal study, scores on Delinquent Behavior and Attention Problems as well as Time 1 School scale scores were the best predictors of various signs of disturbance six years later.

Numerous genetic studies have demonstrated high heritability for several ASEBA syndromes. Notably, heritability appears to be much higher for Aggressive Behavior than for Delinquent Behavior. Heritability patterns vary by gender and age as well as by type of problem. Several studies have demonstrated that variance unique to different informants is not due to measurement error or rater bias but validly reflects different genetic factors.

Turkish immigrant children in the Netherlands had significantly higher CBCL problem scores than Dutch children, particularly on Internalizing problems, but only slightly higher CBCL scores than Turkish children living in Turkey. When rated by their Turkish but not their Dutch teachers, Turkish immigrant students had much higher Anxious/Depressed scores than Dutch students. For Moroccan immigrants to the Netherlands, scores on the CBCL and YSR were lower than those for Turkish and Dutch youth, whereas scores on the TRF were higher than those for Turkish and Dutch youth. Ambivalence about acculturation appears to increase problem scores for Moroccan girls but not for Moroccan boys. Russian Jewish immigrants in Israel obtained significantly higher YSR scores on all syndromes except Social Problems and Attention Problems than Russian Jewish youths who had not emigrated. Russian Jewish immigrant youths obtained higher scores than their Israeli peers only on these same syndromes. Russian Jewish immigrants endorsed suicidal items on the YSR at comparable rates to Israeli peers but at higher rates than Jewish youths in Russia. A study using the SDQ with 11 immigrant groups in Norway indicated significant differences across groups, but comparisons with Norwegian youths and ESs were lacking. Reasons for emigrating (e.g., looking for work vs. fleeing war) did not appear to affect SDQ scores.

CHAPTER 6

Multicultural Findings on Patterns of Problems in Empirically Based Assessment Instruments

In this chapter we review multicultural research on patterns of problems identified via empirically based assessment instruments. The research includes multiple factor analyses of ASEBA instruments, the CTRS (Conners, 1969; Goyette et al, 1978), and the SDQ (Goodman, 2001). For our literature review, we gave priority to studies that met the criteria listed in Chapter 4, p. 69.

METHODOLOGICAL CONSIDERATIONS

Research on patterns of problems typically employs factor-analytic methods. In recent decades, factor-analytic methodology has changed dramatically, as seen most notably in the widespread use of confirmatory factor-analytic (CFA) procedures to test factor models. Prior to the development of CFA, factor analysis was primarily used to derive factor structures from bivariate associations among variables. As previously noted, this type of factor analysis is called exploratory factor analysis (EFA). In EFA a matrix of correlations among the items of an instrument is computed. A particular factor-analytic algorithm is then used to derive a limited number of *factors* from this matrix of correlations. Factors are sets of items that tend to co-occur (i.e., to be mutually associated with each other). The output of a factor analysis consists of a listing of coefficients of association between every item and each of the factors. These coefficients, called *factor loadings*, can range from −1.00 to +1.00 and are analogous to correlation coefficients. Researchers typically choose a minimal factor loading, such as .30, as a cutpoint for retaining items on factors. They then give each factor a name to summarize the items that have loadings above the designated cutpoint on that factor. For example, factor analysis of ASEBA forms usually generates a factor containing a set of co-occurring somatic problems, such as vomiting, headaches, nausea, and stomachaches without known medical cause. This factor is descriptively designated as Somatic Complaints.

Another step in EFA is *rotation* of the retained factors. Rotation involves transforming the factor loadings in order to simplify the factor-analytic results. Different factor rotation methods employ different transformations to accomplish this simplification.

In an EFA researchers typically inspect all the factors and their item loadings in order to choose how many factors to retain. Factors that account for a very small amount of total variance or that have very few items that load above the cutpoint are usually not retained.

EFA is often used to identify sets of co-occurring items in an instrument that is being developed. EFA is also sometimes used to determine whether the factors identified in one sample are found in a new sample. The new sample may be drawn from the same culture or from a different culture. Researchers using EFA to test the replicability of factors in the new sample typically compare the new EFA results with the original EFA results in terms of the number of factors obtained and the loadings of items on those factors.

CFA has become increasingly popular as a method for testing factor models. CFA is used to test the degree to which a data set fits a particular model. The model can be derived by EFA or by other means, such as from theoretical assumptions. CFA can test the same model in many data sets, such as testing a syndrome model in data from multiple cultures. The model to be tested typically specifies which items load on which factors. Researchers can choose from a variety of CFA procedures in testing a factor model. They also have many choices of *fit indices*—statistics that indicate how well a model fits the data. For some fit indices, such as the comparative fit index (CFI; Bentler, 1990), good fit is indicated by a result above a critical value. For other fit indices, such as the root mean square error of approximation (RMSEA; Browne & Cudeck, 1993), good fit is indicated by a result below a critical value. Because different fit indices test different aspects of a CFA's results, they may not always agree. The best evidence that a specific model fits the data is that multiple fit indices indicate good fit.

Factor-analytic techniques have many permutations. Each choice among these permutations can influence the analytic results. When researchers conduct EFA or CFA in one culture to test factor structures derived in other cultures, their results may differ from the original results if they choose options that differ from the original options. Methodological differences are therefore important to consider when reviewing factor-analytic findings from different cultures for the same instruments. In the following section we summarize some of the important choices researchers make in factor analysis.

Methodological Choices in Factor Analysis

For both EFA and CFA, one of the first choices is the sample to be analyzed. Samples from general populations may contain many individuals who have few problems (e.g., they have many items rated 0). If a sample includes many people with ratings of 0 on most of the problem items, then associations among those problem items may be hard to find. Similarly, some items on an instrument may be rarely endorsed (e.g., most people receive ratings of 0 on those particular items). Including items on which most people are rated 0 is apt to reduce associations among items. In general population samples, problem items often have a *positive skew*, which reflects the fact that most individuals obtain low ratings (e.g., ratings of 0) and only a small percentage of individuals obtain higher ratings (e.g., ratings of 1 or 2). To reduce the skew, item ratings can be dichotomized (e.g., scored as 0 vs. 1 and 2) before correlations among the items are computed.

Many statistical choices can influence the results of factor analyses. Although the technical details of these choices are beyond the scope of this book, some of the choices should be noted. One choice is the type of correlation to use. Pearson r indicates the degree of association between two continuous variables. In contrast, a tetrachoric correlation is calculated for two dichotomous variables but estimates what r would be if the underlying variables were continuous. A polychoric correlation is similar to a tetrachoric correlation, but it is computed from > 2 rating categories (such as a 0, 1, 2 scale). Another choice is the type of factor rotation to use: Varimax rotations produce factors that are "orthogonal" (i.e., uncorrelated with each other), whereas oblimin and promax rotations produce factors that are "oblique" (i.e., correlated with each other). Yet another choice is the mathematical estimation procedure used: Maximum likelihood (ML), unweighted least squares (ULS), and weighted least squares (WLS) methods are the main methods used in the studies we review.

In EFA, choices must also be made about how to assign items to factors, because some items may load above the selected cutpoint (e.g., > .30) on more than one factor. These items are said to be *cross-loading*. Researchers can allow cross-loading items or can assign every item to only one factor. They often do this by inspecting each cross-loading item's loadings on the different factors and then assigning the item to the factor on which it has its highest loading.

THE 1983, 1991, AND 2001 ASEBA SYNDROME MODELS

Many factor-analytic studies of the CBCL, TRF, and YSR have compared the 1991 eight-syndrome model (Achenbach, 1991a) with factors obtained using translations of ASEBA instruments. However, other studies have tested the syndrome model reported by Achenbach and Edelbrock (1983). Still others have tested the 2001 eight-syndrome model (Achenbach & Rescorla, 2001). We therefore summarize the important similarities and differences between the 1983, 1991, and 2001 versions of the syndrome model.

Achenbach and Edelbrock (1983) derived separate factors from CBCL data for ages 4–5, 6–11, and 12–16. Data were obtained for children attending 42 mental health clinics, mostly in the eastern United States (N = 2,300). Items with endorsement rates < 5% were excluded separately for each age/gender group. EFA was applied to Pearson correlations, and two kinds of rotation were used. Data for each age/gender group were analyzed separately. Analogous procedures were used to derive syndromes for the TRF (Achenbach & Edelbrock, 1986) and the YSR (Achenbach & Edelbrock, 1987). The effect of these analytic choices was that some syndromes were common across forms and age/gender groups, whereas other syndromes were not. For example, an Aggressive syndrome was found for every age/gender group on all three instruments, whereas a Sex Problems syndrome was found only on the CBCL for girls ages 4–5 and ages 6–11.

The 1991 cross-informant syndromes (Achenbach, 1991a) were derived for ages 4–5, 6–11, and 12–18 (11–18 for the YSR). Data were ratings of children attending 52 clinics in the eastern, southern, and midwestern United States (N = 4,455), including children whose data contributed to the 1983 syndromes. Items were excluded for a particular age/gender group if they were endorsed for < 5% of children in that group. EFAs were applied to Pearson correlations and varimax rotations were performed for each age/gender group, first for all items on each instrument that were reported for ≥ 5% of children on that instrument and then for the 89 items common to the CBCL, TRF, and YSR. Items were retained on a factor if they loaded $\geq .30$, except for Aggressive Behavior, where a cutpoint of $\geq .40$ was used because of the large number of items loading $\geq .30$. Items were allowed to load on more than one factor.

This factor-analytic process yielded eight syndromes that were consistent across the CBCL, TRF, and YSR; hence Achenbach (1991a) called them *cross-informant* syndromes. These eight cross-informant syndromes were then factor analyzed in what is termed a *second-order factor analysis*. Based on this second-order factor analysis, three syndromes loaded on the second-order Internalizing grouping (Withdrawn, Somatic Complaints, Anxious/Depressed), two syndromes loaded on the second-order Externalizing grouping (Delinquent Behavior and Aggressive Behavior), and three syndromes did not load differentially on either Internalizing or Externalizing (Social Problems, Thought Problems, and Attention Problems).

As described in Chapter 2, the 2001 versions of the ASEBA syndromes resulted from analytic procedures that differed from those used to derive the 1983 and 1991 versions of the syndromes. The forms analyzed contained a few new items (six on the CBCL and YSR, three on the TRF). Items with endorsement rates $< 5\%$ in most age/gender groups were excluded from the factor analyses. The sample included children from a U.S. national general population sample and from U.S., English, and Australian clinics. To be included in the factor-analytic sample, forms had to have Total Problems scores above the median for the U.S. general population sample ($N = 4,994$ for the CBCL, 4,437 for the TRF, and 2,551 for the YSR). Four age/gender groups were analyzed for the CBCL and TRF (ages 6–11 and 12–18 for each gender) and two were used for the YSR (ages 11–18 for each gender), for a total of 10 age/gender groups across the three instruments.

As described by Achenbach and Rescorla (2001), two factor extraction methods were applied to Pearson correlations, and two rotation methods (varimax and oblimin) were used. Factors found in most analyses were further analyzed by applying single-factor WLS procedures to tetrachoric correlations of 0 versus 1 and 2 ratings. For example, an Aggressive Behavior factor was found in virtually all analyses. All items loading on this factor in any analysis were included in the single-factor WLS analysis for Aggressive Behavior of data for each of the 10 age/ gender samples. Finally, the factors were tested in a single CFA for each form, with the age/gender groups combined. For example, the CFA for the CBCL tested the fit of an eight-syndrome model to the 96 items that loaded on any of the eight syndromes found in the EFA phase. The RMSEAs were .06 for the CBCL, .05 for the YSR, and .07 for the

TRF (using a seven-syndrome model for the TRF, with a separate CFA for the Attention Problems syndrome and its two subscales). Although different studies specify different RMSEA critical values for "good fit," most specify critical values ≤ .08. Thus, the RMSEAs obtained for the 2001 CFAs were considered to indicate good fit.

Achenbach and Rescorla (2001) assigned each cross-loading item to only one syndrome. Each item that had a significant and positive loading ≥ .20 on more than one factor in ≥ 5 analyses was identified. The item was then assigned to the factor on which the item had the highest mean loading across all the analyses.

Despite many differences in samples, items, and factor-analytic procedures, the 2001 syndromes were very similar to the 1991 syndromes and were given similar names: Anxious/Depressed, Withdrawn/Depressed (formerly Withdrawn), Somatic Complaints, Social Problems, Thought Problems, Attention Problems, Rule-Breaking Behavior (formerly Delinquent Behavior), and Aggressive Behavior. The changes in names for two of the syndromes were based primarily on loadings of some of the new items on those factors (e.g., *5. There is very little he/she enjoys* on the former Withdrawn syndrome, and *28. Breaks rules at home, school, or elsewhere* on the former Delinquent Behavior syndrome).

Most items were assigned to the same factor in 2001 as in 1991. Correlations between scores on the 1991 syndromes and the 2001 syndromes ranged from .87 to 1.00. Furthermore, second-order factor analysis of the 2001 syndromes resulted in the same syndromes being assigned to the Internalizing and Externalizing groupings as in 1991.

TESTING THE ASEBA EIGHT-SYNDROME MODEL IN THE UNITED STATES

In an early CFA study of the 1991 eight-syndrome model, Dedrick, Greenbaum, Friedman, Wetherington, and Knoff (1997) analyzed CBCL data for 631 American children ages 8–18. The children, participants in the National Adolescent and Child Treatment Study, were classified as having "serious emotional disturbance." Dedrick et al. (1997) applied ULS to polychoric correlations among the CBCL items that comprised the 1991 eight-syndrome model. The CFI (Bentler, 1990), the Tucker–Lewis nonnormed index (TLI; Tucker & Lewis, 1973), and the Bentler-Bonett normed fit index (BBI; Bentler & Bonnett, 1980) all exceeded the critical value of .90. The RMSEA of .079 was below the critical value of .08, also indicating acceptable fit. The mean factor loading across all items and factors was .57. Noting that several of the items with low loadings were those loading on more than one factor in the 1991 Achenbach model, Dedrick et al. suggested that allowing cross-loading items may be unwise. Overall, Dedrick et al. concluded that the CFA results supported the 1991 eight-syndrome model and yielded findings similar in most respects to those reported by Achenbach (1991a).

TESTS OF THE 1983 OR 1991 SYNDROME MODELS IN OTHER CULTURES

Tests of the 1983 or 1991 CBCL syndrome models have been reported in data from five cultures (the Netherlands, Korea, Thailand, France, and Australia). The studies varied with respect to the CBCL factor model tested (1983 or 1991) as well as the statistical procedures used. We review these studies in the following section.

Factor Analyses of Dutch CBCL, TRF, and YSR Data

A test of the 1991 CBCL cross-informant syndrome model was conducted on a Dutch sample (De Groot, Koot, & Verhulst, 1994). The sample included 4,674 children referred to 25 mental health centers in the province of South Holland from 1982 to 1991. In half the sample, EFA was used to derive factors from Dutch scores on the items comprising the U.S. 1991 cross-informant syndrome model. In the other half of the sample, CFA was used to test both the factor model derived from the first half of the Dutch sample and the U.S. factor model.

The EFA procedures differed from those used by Achenbach (1991a) in several ways, including the type of correlation and the method of rotation used, as well as the treatment of cross-loading items. Despite these procedural differences, the EFA yielded essentially the same eight syndromes. Pearson correlations between scores obtained on the Dutch and U.S. versions of the syndromes ranged from .82 for Social Problems to .99 for Somatic Complaints and Anxious/ Depressed. The items were almost identical on the Dutch and U.S. Somatic Complaints and Anxious/Depressed syndromes, whereas only four items were the same on the Social Problems syndrome.

For the CFA, both the Dutch and U.S. factor models were tested in the second half of the Dutch sample using ULS on polychoric correlations. Three fit indices were used: GFI (goodness of fit index), AGFI (adjusted goodness of fit index), and RMR (root mean square of the residual). For both the Dutch and U.S. models, GFI = .885, AGFI = .878, and RMR = .096. Further results indicated that 87 of the 94 factor loadings for the Dutch factor solution and 81 of the 91 loadings for the U.S. factor solution were replicated in this Dutch validation sample. Based on these results, De Groot et al. (1994) concluded that the cross-informant syndrome model derived in the United States was strongly supported by the Dutch data.

DeGroot, Koot, and Verhulst (1996) conducted CFAs on TRF and YSR ratings of children assessed in six mental health clinics in South Holland. TRFs were obtained for 2,442 5- to 18-year-olds, and YSRs were obtained for 1,139 11- to 18-year-olds. The same statistical procedures were used as by De Groot et al. (1994), namely, EFA with half of the sample and CFA with the other half. For both the TRF and the YSR, polychoric correlations and promax rotation were used. ULS was then used to test both the Dutch and the U.S. factor models, using GFI, AGFI, and RMR as fit indices.

For the TRF, all eight U.S. syndromes were replicated in the Dutch EFA. Correlations between the U.S. and Dutch versions of the syndromes ranged from .91 for Delinquent Behavior to 1.00 for Somatic Complaints. CFAs for the TRF indicated very similar levels of fit for the U.S. versus Dutch syndrome models (U.S./Dutch: GFI = .85/.86, AGFI = .84/.86, RMR = .128/.120). Five TRF items failed to load ≥ .30 on the Dutch factors, whereas 13 items failed to load ≥ .30 on the U.S. factors.

For the YSR, De Groot et al.'s (1996) EFA yielded only six factors. One difference from the U.S. eight-syndrome model was that Anxious/Depressed and Withdrawn were combined into a single factor in the Dutch results. A second difference was that Delinquent Behavior and Aggressive Behavior comprised one factor in the Dutch EFA. Correlations between the four factors that were similar in the Dutch and the U.S. solutions ranged from .86 for Attention Problems to 1.00 for Somatic Complaints. CFAs of the Dutch and U.S. YSR syndrome models indicated very similar levels of fit (U.S./Dutch: GFI = .87/.88, AGFI = .86/.87, RMR = .098/.092). Four items failed to load ≥ .30 on their assigned syndrome for the U.S. model, whereas 10 items failed to load on their assigned syndrome for the Dutch model.

Albrecht, Veerman, Damen, and Kroes (2001) also tested the 1991 U.S. eight-syndrome model in the Netherlands. Albrecht et al. (2001) used CFA on CBCL data for 846 children and adolescents rated by group care workers in residential psychiatric and child welfare institutions. They applied ULS to polychoric correlations. All three fit indices indicated acceptable fit to the U.S. model (GFI = .86, AGFI = .85, RMR = .081). Alternative models, such as a one-factor model and an uncorrelated eight-factor model, yielded unsatisfactory fit to the data. Albrecht et al. (2001) also found good fit for the Internalizing and Externalizing factors (GFI = .989, AGFI = .976, RMR = .053).

Factor Analysis of Korean CBCL Data

Oh and Ha (1999) performed EFA with varimax rotation on CBCLs obtained for 834 children ages 6–11 attending psychiatric clinics in Korea. Items were excluded if reported for < 5% of the sample. A factor loading cutpoint of ≥ .30 was used for all factors except Aggressive Behavior, for which ≥ .40 was used. Oh and Ha replicated five of the 1983 CBCL syndromes: Aggressive Behavior, Delinquent Behavior, Somatic Complaints, Attention Problems, and Social Withdrawal. The items comprising the Korean and U.S. versions of these syndromes were similar, and correlations between the two versions of the syndromes were reported to be high. The Korean EFA also yielded an Emotional Lability factor. This factor included a mixture of Internalizing and Externalizing problem items (e.g., *45. Nervous*; *75. Shy*; *86. Stubborn*; *87. Moody*; *88. Sulks a lot*; *9. Hot temper*). Oh and Ha suggested that this factor may reflect the fact that Korean children are expected to suppress negative emotions and that they may engage in passive–aggressive behaviors when such suppression is unsuccessful.

Factor Analysis of Thai CBCL Data

Weisz, Weiss, Suwanlert, and Chaiyasit (2003) performed EFA on CBCLs obtained for 924 children ages 6–11 attending mental health clinics in Thailand. They compared both the 1983 and 1991 U.S. syndrome models with Thai results. Their EFA, which excluded problem items reported for < 5% of the sample, applied ML and a promax factor rotation, which differed from the methods used to derive the 1983 and 1991 syndromes. Weisz et al. (2003) also performed second-order factor analysis using the syndromes as inputs. Similarity between the Thai and U.S. versions of syndromes was measured using *concordance kappa*, a measure of agreement corrected for chance that can range from –1.00 to +1.00. A concordance kappa for each item was computed from a 2 × 2 matrix indicating whether the item loaded or did not load on the Thai versus the U.S. version of the same syndrome.

The EFA of the Thai data yielded syndromes that were somewhat similar to the U.S. syndromes of Aggressive Behavior, Anxious/Depressed, Withdrawn, Somatic Complaints, Delinquent Behavior, and Attention Problems. However, only 17% of the concordance kappas met Landis and Koch's (1977) threshold for "substantial or almost perfect agreement" (> .61), whereas 17% showed "moderate agreement" (.41–.60) and 56% showed "slight to fair" agreement (.00–.40). Mean concordance kappa for Externalizing items was "fair" (.31), whereas mean concordance kappa for Internalizing items was "moderate" (.55).

Weisz et al. (2003) concluded that the CBCL syndromes did not fit the Thai data very well, which they attributed to cultural differences between the United States and Thailand. However, major differences between the Thai factor-analytic procedures and those used to derive the 1983 and 1991 syndromes may have contributed to the differences in the results.

Factor Analysis of French CBCL Data

Berg, Fombonne, McGuire, and Verhulst (1997) performed EFA on CBCL ratings of the items comprising the 1991 eight-syndrome model for 776 4- to 16-year-old children from a French clinical sample as well as 2,215 4- to 16-year-olds from De Groot et al.'s (1994) Dutch clinical sample. Berg et al. (1997) applied EFA to Pearson rs, used a promax rotation, set .30 as the minimum factor loading, and prohibited cross-loading items. The French and Dutch data were analyzed separately. The EFA yielded seven factors that corresponded well to seven of the syndromes in the 1991 U.S. eight-syndrome model. A factor corresponding to Thought Problems was not obtained. Only 43 of the items had loadings of $\geq$ .30 on these seven factors. After the 43-item, seven-factor model was rotated, CFA was used to measure the fit of the model to the data from which it was derived. All fit indices, which included GFI, AGFI, and CFI, exceeded .90, indicating good fit. Correlations between factor scores based on the 43-item, seven-factor model and those derived from the 1991 eight-syndrome model were large for both the French and the Dutch data (range from .75 for Social Problems in the French data to .97 for Aggressive Behavior in both samples). Berg et al. (1997) concluded that the homogeneity of their samples appeared to have led to low intercorrelations between items, which in turn led to fewer items loading on most factors than had been found in the 1991 U.S. data.

Factor Analysis of Australian CBCL Data

Heubeck (2000) tested the 1991 eight-syndrome model as well as several other models using CBCL data for 2,237 children ages 4–17 assessed in mental health clinics in Sydney, Australia. Heubeck also conducted analyses using Achenbach's (1991a) U.S. clinical sample. All analyses applied ULS factor estimation to polychoric correlations. Heubeck concluded that the eight-syndrome model provided a better fit to the Australian and U.S. data than a one-factor model. The RMSEA was slightly worse for the Australian sample (.092) than for the U.S. sample (.085). Between 89 and 93% of the items loaded > .30 on their assigned factor. Six of the eight syndromes replicated quite well in the Australian sample, with the best replication for Somatic Complaints, Anxious/Depressed, and Aggressive Behavior. The syndromes that replicated least well in Australia were Social Problems and Attention Problems. Five of the most problematic items were those that cross-loaded on more than one syndrome in the Achenbach (1991a) model.

MULTICULTURAL TESTS
OF THE 1991 EIGHT-SYNDROME MODEL

The most comprehensive test of the 1991 eight-syndrome model was conducted by Hartman et al. (1999). CBCL and TRF data from general population and/or clinical samples in Greece, the Netherlands, Israel, Norway, Portugal, and Turkey were subjected to ML analysis of Pearson rs and ULS analysis of polychoric correlations. Two versions of each model were tested, one using only the items common to syndromes on both the CBCL and the TRF (the "common item" version) and the other using all items loading on each syndrome on either the CBCL or the TRF (the "full cross-informant" version). The CFA allowed for correlations between syndromes.

ML results for 14 samples (eight for the CBCL and six for the TRF) for the common-item and full cross-informant versions indicated that the 28 RMSEAs ranged from .042 to .067 (mean of .054), all within the range of .03–.07 that Hartman et al. specified for good fit. Most other indices also indicated good fit in these 28 analyses. Nonetheless, Hartman et al. concluded that the eight-syndrome model was not confirmed in these ML analyses.

Hartman et al. also analyzed their samples using ULS estimation with polychoric correlations. As the authors noted, polychoric correlations may be distorted when cell frequencies are low. Although cell frequencies were not reported, subsequent analyses of most of these data sets by Achenbach, Dumenci, Erol, and Roussos (2000) revealed many empty cells and cells with very low frequencies. This resulted from Hartman et al.'s failure to exclude items reported for < 5% of the sample, contrary to the procedure used by Achenbach (1991a, 1991b). Had Hartman et al. used this 5% exclusion rule, between 1 item and 28 items would have been excluded from the various samples (mean of 11 items for the common-item version and mean of 14 items for the full cross-informant version).

Hartman et al. (1999) noted that the item scores were skewed and that the use of polychoric correlations might be problematic because "the assumption of underlying bivariate normality of the variables may be unrealistic." Subsequent analysis of most of the data sets analyzed by Hartman et al. confirmed that every item was significantly skewed (Achenbach et al., 2000). Hartman et al. also cautioned that inadequate fit based on the indices they used might "result from violation of the factor analytic requirement of multivariate normality of the variables." Despite these cautions, Hartman et al. chose to evaluate their fit indices using stricter criteria (i.e., 99% null hypothesis intervals) than they cited earlier in their paper as indicating good fit or than recommended by Browne and Cudeck (1993) for RMSEA. It is not surprising, therefore, that the RMSEAs for their ULS analyses failed to meet this extremely stringent criterion of .010–.035. Based on these findings, Hartman et al. concluded that the eight-syndrome model was not confirmed.

TESTS OF THE 2001 EIGHT-SYNDROME MODEL IN TURKISH SAMPLES

Dumenci, Erol, Achenbach, and Simsek (2004) used CFA to test the 2001 eight-syndrome model in three Turkish samples: (1) a general population sample of 5,195 children ages 6–18; (2) a clinical sample of 963 children ages 6–18; (3) and a sample of 3,498 children ages 6–18 that included children from the general population and clinically referred children who had Total Problems scores above the general population median, comparable to the U.S. sample used by Achenbach and Rescorla (2001). In explaining their methodology, Dumenci, Erol, et al. (2004) ruled out using ULS, because it is not the most efficient estimator of model parameters, although it has the advantage of not requiring normally distributed items. They also ruled out ML, because it assumes normally distributed item scores, which are seldom found for problem items. Instead, Dumenci et al. chose to use *weighted least squares with the mean- and variance-adjusted fit statistic* (WLSMV), which they explained is the most appropriate method for use with ordinal data that are not normally distributed. Based on Yu and Muthén's (2002) recommended options, they used RMSEA with a cutpoint of .06 as their primary test of model fit. All analyses used tetrachoric correlations between scores of 0 versus 1 and 2 for the 96 items on the Turkish translation of the 1991 CBCL that loaded on the 2001 factors in the U.S. syndrome model. Each item was assigned to the syndrome that it measured in the eight-syndrome model, and no cross-loading items were allowed.

RMSEAs for all three Turkish samples met the criterion for good fit (general population sample RMSEA = .041; clinical sample RMSEA =

.057; combined general population and clinical samples RMSEA = .054). In contrast, when a one-factor model was tested against the same items, the RMSEA exceeded .06 for the clinical and the combined samples. The RMSEA for the one-factor model in the general population sample was below .06 (RMSEA = .051), but it was larger than the RMSEA of .041 for the eight-syndrome model. It is notable that the best model fit was obtained in the general population sample. Dumenci et al. also found that 99% of the items had significant (p < .01) and substantial positive factor loadings on the syndromes to which they were assigned. The median factor loading of .60 was comparable to the median loading of .62 reported by Achenbach and Rescorla (2001) for the U.S. sample on which the eight-syndrome model was derived.

Dumenci, Erol, et al. (2004) noted that the eight syndromes were intercorrelated (median r = .66, range .13–.92), as was found in the U.S. data (Achenbach & Rescorla, 2001). The intercorrelations indicate that a general psychopathology factor is tapped by all the syndromes, analogous to the CBCL Total Problems score. Dumenci et al. stressed that, although many of the rs between syndromes were substantial, all were at least six standard errors below 1.00, indicating discrimination among the eight syndromes. Dumenci et al. further noted that correlations between the two Externalizing syndromes (.92) and among the three Internalizing syndromes (median = .59, range .31–.85) indicated replication of these second-order factors in the Turkish data.

MULTICULTURAL TESTS
OF THE 2001 EIGHT-SYNDROME MODEL

The most comprehensive tests of the ASEBA eight-syndrome model have been done by Ivanova and colleagues, who conducted CFAs for the CBCL (Ivanova et al., 2006a), the TRF (Ivanova et al., 2006b), and the YSR (Ivanova et al., 2006c).

Testing the 2001 Eight-Syndrome Model on CBCL Data from 30 Cultures

Ivanova et al. (2006a) tested the correlated eight-syndrome U.S. model using CFA for CBCL data from general population samples of 6- to 18-year-olds from 30 cultures (N = 58,030). Cultures represented Asia, Africa, Australia, the Caribbean, Europe, the Mediterranean, the Middle East, and North America. Rescorla et al. (2006a) reported distributions of CBCL problem scale scores for children ages 6–16 from these same samples, as summarized in Chapter 4.

Ivanova et al. (2006a) conducted CFA using WLSMV on tetra-choric correlations (ratings of 0 vs. 1 and 2), the same procedure used by Dumenci, Erol, et al. (2004) to test Turkish data against the 2001 eight-syndrome model. Because most of Ivanova's samples were assessed with the 1991 CBCL, the CFA was applied to the 96 items from the 1991 CBCL that loaded on the 2001 eight-syndrome model. RMSEA was used as the primary index of model fit, with values ≤ .06 taken to indicate good fit, based on recommendations by Yu and Muthén (2002). The TLI and the CFI were used to provide additional fit information. As recommended by Browne and Cudeck (1993), TLI and CFI values ≥ .90 were taken to indicate good fit, whereas values of .80–.89 were taken to indicate acceptable fit.

Ivanova et al. (2006a) obtained RMSEAs ranging from .026 for China to .055 for Ethiopia. The eight-syndrome model thus fit well for all 30 cultures. For 21 of the 30 cultures, the RMSEA was ≤ .040, indicating particularly good model fit. The TLI indicated acceptable-to-good model fit for all cultures except Ethiopia, whereas the CFI indicated acceptable-to-good model fit for all cultures except Ethiopia, Germany, Hong Kong, and Lithuania.

Ivanova et al. (2006a) reported that all 96 items loaded significantly on their predicted factors for 27 of the 30 cultures. For two cultures, one item failed to load significantly on its predicted factor. For Ethiopia, six items failed to load significantly on their predicted factors. Median factor loadings across the eight syndromes ranged from .51 in Ethiopia to .71 in Australia. Median item loadings averaged across all 30 cultures were lowest for Thought Problems (.57) and highest for Aggressive Behavior (.69).

Testing the 2001 Eight-Syndrome Model on TRF Data from 20 Cultures

In deriving the 2001 syndromes for the TRF, Achenbach and Rescorla (2001) found that the Attention Problems syndrome could be hierachically modeled as subsuming correlated Inattention and Hyperactivity–Impulsivity subfactors. Because it embodies the variance shared by the two subfactors, the Attention Problems factor can be viewed as operationalizing a construct that involves problems of both inattention and hyperactivity–impulsivity. Each of the two subfactors reflects somewhat different manifestations of the underlying liabilities represented by the superordinate Attention Problems factor. Individuals may obtain deviant problem scores on either or both of the subfactors. The greater differentiation of the Attention Problems syndrome scored from the TRF than from the CBCL and YSR may reflect the greater

number of TRF items that tap attention problems and a greater aware-
ness of distinctions between different kinds of attention problems on
the part of teachers than parents and youths.

To test the 2001 TRF model, Ivanova et al. (2006b) performed CFAs
on TRFs completed for the 30,030 6- to 15-year-olds from the 20 cultures
other than the United States whose scale scores were summarized in
Chapter 4 and have been detailed by Rescorla et al. (in press). Because
most of the samples were assessed with the 1991 TRF, the CFAs were
applied to the 109 problem items that are on both the 1991 and 2001 TRF
and that loaded on the 2001 syndrome model. For the test of the seven
syndromes other than Attention Problems, RMSEAs ranged from .034
for Japan to .076 for Poland. For the test of the Attention Problems syndrome and its two subsyndromes, the RMSEAs ranged from .037 for
China to .069 for Poland. All the RMSEAs were in the range considered
to represent good to acceptable fit. Median factor loadings for the problem items ranged from .65 in the Lithuanian sample to .75 in the Japa-
nese sample. Averaged across all the samples, the median factor loadings
for items comprising each syndrome ranged from .64 for Social Problems to .77 for Withdrawn/Depressed and Somatic Complaints.

Testing the 2001 Eight-Syndrome Model on YSR Data from 23 Cultures

Ivanova et al. (2006c) applied CFAs to YSRs completed by 30,243 11- to
18-year-olds from 23 cultures. The YSR scale score distributions for 11-
to 16-year-olds from these same samples were summarized in Chapter 4
and have been reported in detail by Rescorla et al. (2006c). CFA was
applied to the 89 problem items that the 1991 and 2001 YSR have in
common and that loaded on the 2001 eight-syndrome model. Ivanova
et al. found that the RMSEAs ranged from .035 for Ethiopian youths to
.050 for Jamaican youths, indicating good fit for all 23 cultures. Median
factor loadings for the problem items ranged from .53 in the Greek
sample to .67 in the Finnish sample. Averaged across all the samples,
the median factor loadings for items comprising each syndrome
ranged from .55 for Attention Problems to .63 for Anxious/Depressed
and Somatic Complaints. The results thus strongly supported the eight-
syndrome model in self-ratings by youths from 23 very diverse cultures.

SUMMARY OF TESTS OF ASEBA SYNDROME MODELS

Bicultural tests of the 1983 and 1991 ASEBA syndrome models have
been conducted using data from the Netherlands, Korea, Thailand,
France, and Australia. Although the factor-analytic procedures differed

from those used to derive the models in the United States, results of these studies generally supported the basic models. EFA and CFA studies conducted in the United States (Dedrick et al., 1997), the Netherlands (De Groot et al., 1994), Korea (Oh & Ha, 1999), and Australia (Heubeck, 2000) provided substantial support for the 1991 eight-syndrome model, despite some anomalous results in each study. Hartman et al. (1999) used two different kinds of CFA to test the 1991 eight-syndrome model in multiple cultures. Although their RMSEAs were all in the range specified for good fit, Hartman et al. (1999) interpreted their findings as failing to support the 1991 syndromes.

In testing the 2001 eight-syndrome model, Dumenci, Erol, et al. (2004) obtained good fit in all three of their Turkish samples. The most comprehensive tests of the 2001 eight-syndrome model have been reported by Ivanova et al. (2006a, 2006b, 2006c). The results for the CBCL in 30 cultures, the TRF in 20 cultures, and the YSR in 23 cultures indicated good fit for the model across very diverse cultures. Most items in most cultures loaded significantly on their predicted syndromes, and median item loadings across cultures were substantial for all syndromes.

FACTOR-ANALYTIC STUDIES OF THE CTRS

Several bicultural studies have tested the factor structure of the CTRS in cultures other than the United States. Some studies tested the 5-factor model derived from the 39-item CTRS (Conners, 1969), which included Hyperactivity, Inattentive–Passive, Conduct Problems, Tension–Anxiety, and Sociability. Other studies tested the 28-item model (Goyette et al., 1978), which included Hyperactivity, Conduct Problems, and Inattentive–Passive. We review these studies in the following sections.

Factor Analysis of Italian CTRS Data

In an early study O'Leary et al. (1985) applied EFA and varimax rotation to ratings on the 39-item CTRS (Conners, 1969) for 344 second- to fourth-graders in 14 schools of Northern Italy. In one set of analyses, the authors imposed a maximum of six factors. In the other set of analyses, they did not impose a maximum number of factors but required every retained factor to have at least three items with loadings > .40. This latter set of analyses also yielded six factors. Three of these six factors were similar for boys and girls (Inattention, Interpersonal Problems, and Anxiety/Passivity). However, the items on these factors differed somewhat by gender. With respect to the other three factors, Hyperactivity and Conduct Problems formed a single factor for boys, whereas they comprised two separate factors for girls. A Delinquency factor was obtained for boys but not for girls. Factors designated as Depression were obtained for both genders, but the items loading on these factors were quite different.

Factor Analysis of Hong Kong CTRS Data

Luk et al. (1988) reported results from an EFA with varimax rotation of CTRS ratings of 914 6- to 12-year-olds attending public schools in Hong Kong. Four factors were obtained that differed from those reported by Conners (1969) in two major ways. First, items from the U.S. Conduct Problems and Hyperactivity factors loaded on a single factor in the Hong Kong data. Second, the Hong Kong data yielded a factor tapping problems in social relations, such as being isolated and unpopular.

Leung, Luk, and Lee (1989) performed EFA with varimax rotation of ratings on the 39-item CTRS for 1,746 6- to 12-year-olds attending special schools in Hong Kong. These schools served children with disabilities, such as blindness, deafness, other physical handicaps, mental retardation, and emotional maladjustment. Eight factors emerged, which the authors considered to demonstrate a "broad similarity" with the five factors Conners reported for the United States. The Hong Kong Hyperactivity–Inattention factor combined the Hyperactivity and Inattentive–Passive factors found by Conners. Two different Conduct Problems factors emerged, each sharing some items with the Conners Conduct Problems factor. Only 1 factor (Sociability) was identical to the original American factor. A Passivity factor contained some items that had loaded on the Inattentive–Passive factor in the United States.

Factor Analysis of Greek CTRS Data

Roussos et al. (1999) conducted EFA with varimax rotation and CFA on ratings from the 28-item CTRS to test Goyette et al.'s (1978) four-factor model for 852 6- to 12-year-old Greek students. The Greek data yielded four factors, three of which corresponded closely to their U.S. counterparts (Hyperactivity, Conduct Problems, and Inattentive–Passive). Overall, 24 out of 28 items loaded highest on the factor to which they were assigned in Goyette et al.'s analyses. In the CFA for both models, the RMR of .05 indicated good fit. However, the GFI and AGFI indicated relatively weak fit for both the Goyette et al. model and the Greek model (Goyette/Greek: GFI = .73/.79, AGFI = .69/.75). Therefore, Roussos et al. concluded that the fit of both models to the Greek data was less good than is desirable. They also reported similar results from comparable analyses for 209 children attending psychiatric clinics.

Summary of Tests of CTRS Factor Models

Bicultural studies of both the CTRS 1969 five-factor model and the 1978 four-factor model have been reported. These studies provided mixed support for the factor structures identified in the United States. O'Leary et al. (1985) reported six rather than five factors for an Italian translation of the 39-item CTRS, but only three factors were similar for boys and girls. Luk et al. (1988) reported replication of two U.S. factors for the CTRS in a Hong Kong sample. Conduct Problems and Hyperactivity items loaded on a single factor, and a fourth factor tapping social problems was found. Leung et al. (1989) reported eight factors for children attending special schools in Hong Kong, with only one U.S. factor (Sociability) replicating perfectly. Roussos et al. (1999) reported that 24 out of 28 items loaded highest on their assigned factor in EFA of Greek data from a school-based sample. CFAs testing both the U.S. model and the Greek model against the Greek data yielded GFI and AGFI values indicating poor fit, but the RMR indicated good fit for both models.

FACTOR-ANALYTIC STUDIES OF THE SDQ

As described in Chapter 2, Goodman (2001) factor analyzed ratings on the 25-item SDQ for British children obtained from parents ($N = 9,998$) and teachers ($N = 7,313$). Self-ratings were also analyzed for 3,983 11- to 15-year-olds. In the analysis of parent ratings, all SDQ items had their highest loadings on scales to which Goodman (1997) had previously assigned them, which he designated as Emotional Symptoms, Conduct Problems, Hyperactivity, Peer Problems, and Prosocial Behavior. In the analyses for teacher and self-ratings, two items had loadings on other scales that exceeded or approximated their loadings on their assigned scale.

Factor Analysis of Finnish SDQ Data

Koskelainen et al. (2001) factor analyzed SDQ self-ratings for 1,458 Finnish 13- to 17-year-olds. For each gender, two different EFAs with varimax rotation were conducted. The authors imposed a five-factor solution for the first EFA, whereas they imposed no limit on the number of factors for the second EFA. For girls, the five-factor solution yielded factors that corresponded to Goodman's (1997) five scales, although two Hyperactivity items and one Peer Problems item loaded highest on other factors. For boys, four factors were similar to Goodman's scales, except that one Peer Problems item loaded highest on another factor. Four of the five Conduct Problems items loaded higher on other factors. The EFA without constraint on the number of factors yielded three factors that appeared to measure externalizing behavior (Conduct Problems and Hyperactivity items), internalizing behavior (Emotional Symptoms and Peer Problems items), and prosocial behavior.

Factor Analysis of Congolese SDQ Data

Kashala, Elgen, Sommerfelt, and Tylleskar (2005) conducted EFA with varimax rotation on teachers' ratings of a French translation of the SDQ obtained for 1,187 children ages 7–9 attending schools in Kinshasa, capital of the Democratic Republic of Congo. The EFA yielded five factors, with 16 out of 25 items having their highest loadings on their assigned factor. For Emotional Symptoms and Prosocial Behavior, all five items loaded highest on their assigned factor. For Hyperactivity and Conduct Problems, three of five assigned items loaded highest on their respective factors, but the other two items on each scale had their highest loadings on other factors. The five Peer Problems items all loaded on other factors.

Factor Analysis of German SDQ Data

Woerner et al. (2004) conducted EFA with varimax rotation on parent SDQs obtained for the 930 6- to 16-year-old children comprising the German normative sample. The sample was recruited as part of a nationwide survey on weight and eating habits. The EFA yielded five factors, with all 25 items having their highest loadings (all > .40) on their designated scale.

Becker, Woerner, et al. (2004) conducted EFA with varimax rotation on teachers' SDQ ratings of 543 5- to 17-year-olds attending a mental health clinic in Göttingen, Germany. The EFA yielded five factors. No details were provided about item loadings, but Becker et al. reported a "high degree of concordance" with the original SDQ scales. For this same clinical sample, Becker et al. also conducted CFA for parent SDQs. They reported good fit for the five-factor model (AGFI = .85, RMR = .07). Finally, Becker et al. conducted EFA with varimax rotation on parent SDQs for their clinical sample plus the German standardization sample (total N = 1,686). This EFA yielded five factors, with all 25 items reportedly loading on their assigned scale. Becker, Hagenberg, et al.

(2004) reported an EFA with varimax rotation for 214 self-report SDQs obtained from the same Göttingen clinical sample. Five factors were extracted, with the factor loadings reportedly showing "a high conformance with the original SDQ scales."

Factor Analysis of Norwegian SDQ Data

Rønning et al. (2004) applied CFA to self-report SDQs obtained from 4,167 11- to 16-year-olds in 66 schools in Norway. No significant gender differences were found. Only one of the four fit indices used clearly indicated good fit (GFI = .98). The RMSEA was reported to be .47, but it was described later in the paper as indicating good fit, suggesting that RMSEA might actually have been .047. The other two indices were not within the bounds of good fit. The CFI of .82 was below the critical value of .90, whereas the standardized root mean square residual (SRMR) of .11 exceeded the critical value for good fit. Overall, Rønning et al. described the fit as "questionable," noting that many items had high correlations not only with items on their assigned factor but also with items from other factors.

Factor Analysis of Dutch SDQ Data

Muris, Meesters, Eijkelenboom, and Vincken (2004) applied EFAs to self-report SDQs obtained from 1,111 children in the Netherlands, with the sample divided into two age cohorts (8- to 10-year-olds and 11- to 13-year-olds). Results were similar for the two age cohorts. Using principal components analysis and oblimin rotation, the best solution contained four factors: Emotional Symptoms, Hyperactivity–Inattention, mixed Peer and Conduct Problems, and Prosocial (containing the Prosocial scale items plus several reverse scored items from other scales). Results using varimax rotation were similar. A two-factor solution was also considered satisfactory, with all problem items loading on one factor and all prosocial and positively worded items loading on a second factor. Muris et al. (2004) concluded that a four-factor structure fit the data better than Goodman's (2001) five-factor solution.

Factor Analysis of U.S. SDQ Data

The 5-factor SDQ model derived in the United Kingdom was tested on a U.S. national probability sample of 9,574 4- to 17-year-olds (Dickey & Blumberg, 2004). Two different EFA procedures were applied to half the sample. The results of one procedure indicated good replication for three factors. For the Conduct Problems and Peer Problems factors, respectively, two and three of the five assigned items had higher loadings on other factors. The second EFA procedure yielded three correlated factors, which Dickey and Blumberg termed "externalization problems," "internalization problems," and "prosocial problems." They tested this three-factor model on the second half of the U.S. sample using two different CFA methods. Both methods yielded good fit for the three-factor model (GFIs of .97 and .94; RMRs of .06 and .04).

Dickey and Blumberg suggested that one reason their PCA results differed somewhat from those of Goodman (2001) may have been rewordings of some items to reflect American rather than British usage. They also noted that all eight items on the Prosocial Problems factor found in their three-factor solution had positive wording (i.e., "generally obedient"), unlike most other SDQ items. They therefore suggested that these eight items may reflect a "positive construal" factor that reflects parents' willingness to attribute positive qualities to their children. They also noted that their three-factor solution was very similar to the solution reported by Koskelainen et al. (2001) for Finnish SDQ ratings.

Summary of Tests of the SDQ Factor Model

Factor-analytic studies of the SDQ have been conducted in Finland, Norway, Germany, the Congo, the Netherlands, and the United States, as well as the United Kingdom. Results in some cultures have provided substantial support for the SDQ five-factor model, whereas results in other cultures have failed to support the model. Studies conducted in Germany using both a general population and a clinical sample replicated the SDQ five-factor model (Becker, Hagenberg, et al., 2004; Becker, Woerner, et al., 2004; Woerner et al., 2004). Using EFA with teacher SDQs from the Congo, Kashala et al. (2005) obtained five factors, but only 16 out of 25 items had their highest loadings on their assigned factor. Rønning et al. (2004) reported inconsistent support for the SDQ five-factor model in their CFA of self-report data obtained from Norwegian adolescents, leading them to describe the fit as "questionable." Muris et al. (2004) obtained a four-factor solution for Dutch self-report SDQ data. In Finland, when Koskelainen et al. (2001) did not prescribe the number of factors, EFA of the parent SDQ yielded externalizing, internalizing, and prosocial factors. Very similar EFA results were obtained by Dickey and Blumberg (2004) in a U.S. sample. When they tested this three-factor internalizing–externalizing–prosocial model using CFA on the second half of their sample, they found that all indices indicated good fit.

SUMMARY

Bicultural tests of the 1983 and 1991 ASEBA syndrome models in five cultures generally supported the basic model, despite the use of different factor-analytic procedures in many studies. Hartman et al. (1999) tested the 1991 eight-syndrome model in multiple cultures. Although their RMSEAs were all in the range specified for good fit, Hartman et al. interpreted their findings as failing to replicate the 1991 syndromes. Dumenci, Erol, et al. (2004) used CFA to test the 2001 eight-syndrome model in three Turkish samples. RMSEAs indicated good fit in all three samples. The most comprehensive tests of the 2001 ASEBA eight-syndrome model have been reported by Ivanova et al. (2006a, 2006b, 2006c). Results for the CBCL in 30 cultures, the TRF in 20 cultures, and the YSR in 23 cultures indicated good fit for the model across very diverse cultures. Most items in most cultures loaded significantly on their assigned syndrome, and median item loadings across cultures were substantial for all syndromes.

Factor-analytic studies of the CTRS in Italy, Hong Kong, and Greece have generally supported the factor structure obtained in the United States, but some differences in the number and/or the composition of the factors were also reported. EFA and/or CFA results for the SDQ in Finland, the Congo, Germany, Norway, the Netherlands, and the United States have been mixed. Whereas results in Germany and the Congo generally supported the SDQ five-factor model, results in Norway provided inconsistent support for the five-factor model, results in the Netherlands supported a four-factor model, and results in the United States and Finland indicated that a three-factor internalizing–externalizing–prosocial model provided a closer fit to the data than the five-factor U.K. model.

CHAPTER 7

Multicultural Findings on the Prevalence of Diagnostically Based Disorders

In Chapter 3 we presented ways in which the diagnostically based approach has been used to develop assessment procedures for making diagnoses. In this chapter we present findings on the prevalence of diagnostically defined disorders in different cultures.

THE NATURE OF DIAGNOSTICALLY BASED PREVALENCE STUDIES

Diagnostically based prevalence studies have assessed disorders mainly with diagnostic interviews comprised of questions designed to obtain yes/no answers as to whether a child meets criteria for particular diagnoses. In studies that are designed to estimate the prevalence rates of disorders within a particular culture, diagnostic interviews are administered to samples of children and/or parents chosen to be representative of that culture.

One-Stage versus Two-Stage Epidemiological Designs

Studies of the prevalence rates of disorders assessed with diagnostic interviews have differed with respect to whether they used "one-stage" or "two-stage" designs (also called "one-phase" and "two-phase" designs). In *one-stage* designs, diagnostic interviews are used to assess all individuals in a sample. In *two-stage* designs, by contrast, low-cost assessment procedures are used in Stage 1 to screen all individuals in a sample. The low-cost assessment procedures are intended to distinguish between individuals who are most likely to be "cases" (i.e., to meet criteria for diagnoses) because they have high problem scores versus individuals who are likely to be noncases (i.e., they do not meet criteria for diagnoses). In Stage 2 of two-stage designs, most individuals who were identified as potential cases in Stage 1, plus a small proportion of individuals who were identified as potential noncases, are assessed with diagnostic interviews.

The purpose of two-stage designs is to avoid the cost of administering expensive diagnostic interviews to the entire sample while still obtaining good estimates of prevalence rates by interviewing the most likely cases, plus some ostensible noncases in order to determine what proportion of ostensible noncases are really cases. Most two-stage studies find that some individuals identified as potential cases by screening procedures fail to meet diagnostic criteria when interviewed. Conversely, some individuals identified as potential noncases by screening procedures do meet diagnostic criteria when interviewed. Because only those who are chosen for the Stage 2 subsamples can ultimately receive diagnoses, complex statistical formulas must be applied to the findings from the different subsamples to estimate the prevalence of disorders in the population as a whole.

The possible cost-saving advantage of interviewing only subsamples in two-stage studies may be offset by the greater complexity and reduced accuracy of estimating population prevalence rates, as compared to one-stage studies. Furthermore, the savings achieved by using fewer diagnostic interviews in two-stage studies may also be offset by the costs of finding, contacting, and visiting the members of the subsamples a second time in order to administer the diagnostic interviews. Another important consideration is that the ultimate completion rate for Stage 2 diagnostic interviews is usually reduced by refusals and by the unavailability of some selected individuals who had participated in the Stage 1 screening.

Diagnostic Interviews

The interview used most widely in epidemiological studies of children's disorders has been the Diagnostic Interview Schedule for Children (DISC; Costello et al., 1982; Shaffer et al., 2000), which we described in Chapter 3. Since the DISC was initially developed in the early 1980s, different versions have been developed for making diagnoses according to DSM-III, DSM-III-R, and DSM-IV criteria. In addition to the differences necessitated by changes in diagnostic criteria from one edition of the DSM to another, there have been numerous variations in the interview algorithms, wording of questions, and methods for determining whether diagnostic criteria are met.

Because so many diagnoses have been included in the DSM-III, DSM-III-R, and DSM-IV, time constraints and other logistic considerations have limited most epidemiological studies to subsets of DSM diagnoses. Different subsets of diagnoses have been reported in different studies, and the methods for making the diagnoses have also differed. For example, some studies have used data from only a single informant, whereas other studies have used data from children and their parents. A few studies have used data from teachers as well.

We have not found any published statistical comparisons between prevalence rates for diverse diagnoses of children from multiple cultures who were similarly assessed with the same version of the DISC. In lieu of direct multicultural comparisons, we consider DISC studies that have potential implications for multicultural assessment of psychopathology from the diagnostically based perspective. However, we found one report of statistical comparisons between prevalence rates for two DSM diagnoses made in two cultures with the DISC (Bird et al., 2001). We also found statistical comparisons between prevalence rates for more diverse diagnoses made in two cultures with the Development and Well-Being Assessment (DAWBA; Fleitlich-Bilyk & Goodman, 2004), a diagnostic interview that we described in Chapter 3.

CRITERIA FOR STUDIES OF PREVALENCE

The paucity of published studies that used the same instrument to make the same diagnoses in the same way for representative samples from multiple cultures limits possibilities for rigorous multicultural comparisons of prevalence rates for diagnostically defined disorders. However, to shed as much light as possible on multicultural aspects of psychopathology from the diagnostic perspective, we give priority to findings from studies that met the criteria specified in Chapter 4, including peer-reviewed publications, representative samples with $N \geq$ 300, and appropriate statistical analyses. In addition, prevalence findings had to be based on DSM or ICD diagnostic criteria that were operationalized in terms of the standardized interviews that we reviewed in Chapter 3.

PREVALENCE RATES OBTAINED IN DIAGNOSTICALLY BASED STUDIES

At this writing, the DISC and the DAWBA are the only instruments for which we have found published studies of prevalence rates for diagnoses of children's disorders in more than one culture. We first describe the DISC prevalence studies and then summarize findings across studies. We then present DISC findings from the Dunedin Longitudinal Study that are relevant to ascertaining prevalence rates for diagnostically defined disorders in different cultures (McGee, Feehan, Williams, & Anderson, 1992). Thereafter, we present DAWBA findings and other findings related to multicultural comparisons of diagnoses.

One-Stage Epidemiological Studies Using the DISC

We begin with one-stage studies, which have been designed to use the DISC with all eligible participants who were selected for epidemiological samples. We then present two-stage studies, which differ from one-stage studies in that they used low-cost screening procedures at Stage 1 to identify potential cases and noncases to be assessed with the DISC at Stage 2.

Methods for Epidemiology of Child and Adolescent Disorders Study

The Methods for Epidemiology of Child and Adolescent Disorders Study (MECA) was intended to improve methods for determining the prevalence of disorders among 9- to 17-year-olds (Lahey et al., 1996). In 1991 and 1992, 1,523 eligible caretaker–youth pairs were identified in general population samples from Atlanta, Georgia; New Haven, Connecticut; San Juan, Puerto Rico; and Westchester County, New York. Parent and youth versions of the DISC-2.3 for DSM-III-R were administered to 1,285 (84.4%) of the caretaker–youth pairs.

Shaffer et al. (1996) reported prevalence rates "for the 10 most prevalent disorders that were not eliminated in DSM-IV and for 'Any Substance Use' disorder" (p. 870). According to the DISC-P (P = parent) alone, 30.3% of the youths met DSM-III-R criteria for at least one disorder. According to the DISC-Y (Y = youth, but the DISC-Y is also known as the DISC-C, where C = child), 32.2% of the youths met DSM-III-R criteria for at least one disorder. When disorders were counted as present if criteria were met according to either the DISC-P or DISC-Y, the prevalence rate was 50.6%, indicating minimal overlap between diagnoses based on parent interviews and those based on youth interviews. (Unless otherwise noted, the prevalence rates that we cite in the following sections include diagnoses based on reports by parents, plus diagnoses based on reports by their children. In other words, a diagnosis was counted as present if all the diagnostic criteria were met according to the parent's report, or according to the child's report, or according to reports by both the parent and child.)

In addition to MECA, other studies have also found very high prevalence rates of diagnoses for general population samples assessed with the DISC. Consequently, measures of impairment are often added to the diagnostic criteria in order to distinguish between children who qualify for DSM diagnoses but do not appear impaired versus children who qualify for diagnoses and have varying degrees of impairment (e.g., Bird et al., 1988). When Shaffer et al. added impairment criteria by requiring a Children's Global Assessment Scale (CGAS; Shaffer et al., 1983) score < 71 (designated by Shaffer et al. as "mild impairment"), the prevalence rate based on the DISC-P and DISC-Y diagnoses fell from 50.6 to 24.7%. Applying a more stringent CGAS cutpoint of < 61 (designated as "moderate impairment") reduced the prevalence rate to 12.8%. Shaffer et al. then added various criteria for "diagnosis specific impairment"—that is, endorsement of impairment items related to a diagnosis for which DSM criteria were met. When criteria were added for diagnosis-specific impairment, the prevalence rates dropped to 20.9% for a CGAS cutpoint < 71 and 11.5% for a CGAS cutpoint < 61. However, as Shaffer et al. pointed out, these prevalence data do not indicate the likely prevalence of disorders in the United States, because they were based on samples in four localities that were "not generally representative of the United States" (pp. 869–870).

Comparison of MECA Diagnoses
for Puerto Rican versus Mainland Children

Bird et al. (2001) compared prevalence rates for MECA diagnoses of CD and ODD obtained for children in the San Juan, Puerto Rico, sample with those obtained in the U.S. mainland sample. To make their comparisons, Bird et al. divided the mainland sample into the following three ethnic groups: Hispanics, African Americans, and children who were neither Hispanic nor African American. Because the mainland samples for Hispanic (N = 52) and African American (N = 189) children fell below our criterion of N = 300, we report only the comparisons between the San Juan sample (N = 301) and the mainland sample (N = 668) that excluded Hispanic and African American children. The prevalence rates for CD did not differ significantly (San Juan = 4.1%, mainland = 5.4%), but ODD was significantly ($p < .01$) less prevalent in the San Juan sample (3.0%) than in the mainland (8.0%) sample. When antisocial behaviors were grouped into levels of severity, San Juan children also obtained significantly lower scores than mainland children.

Quebec Child Mental Health Survey

Using the DISC-2.25, which was an earlier version of the DISC-2.3 than was used in MECA, the Quebec Child Mental Health Survey (QCMHS) assessed nine DSM-III-R diagnostic categories in a probability sample of 2,400 6- to 14-year-olds living in the province of Quebec, Canada, during 1992 (Breton et al., 1999). The DISC was administered to parents and 12- to 14-year-olds by lay interviewers. Because children younger than 12 failed to understand many DISC questions (Breton et al., 1995), 6- to 11-year-olds were assessed with the "Dominic," a cartoon-based interview designed to obtain data for seven diagnostic categories. With parents' consent, phone interviews were conducted with the teachers of 6- to 11-year-olds to assess disruptive behavior disorders. The overall response rate for families was 83.5%.

Based on parent and child reports of symptoms, plus reports of impairment by parents and 12- to 14-year-olds in response to DISC questions, the overall prevalence rate for any of the nine categories of DSM disorders was 32.4%. The rate was 19.9% according to parents' reports alone and 15.8% according to child reports alone. Because the teachers' telephone interviews identified considerably more cases of ADHD than did the parent or child interviews, the overall prevalence rate would have been higher if these teacher-identified cases were included. Although 87% of the assessments were done in French and 13% in English, prevalence rates were not reported separately for Francophones versus Anglophones.

Australian National Survey of Mental Health and Well-Being

In the Australian National Survey of Mental Health and Well-Being (ANSMHWB), parents in a national probability sample of 3,597 6- to 17-year-olds were administered the ADHD, CD, and Depressive Disorder modules of a DSM-IV version of the DISC, called the DISC-IV (Sawyer et al., 2001). The completion rate was 86% for households that were contacted, that were identified as containing an eligible child, and that agreed to participate.

It was found that 15% of the Australian 6- to 17-year-olds met criteria for at least one of the three DSM-IV diagnostic categories that were assessed. The 15% prevalence rate would have been lower if the DSM-

IV impairment criteria had been applied. On the other hand, the authors pointed out that "if a wider range of disorders had been investigated, a higher prevalence of mental disorders would have been identified" (Sawyer et al., 2001, p. 807). The prevalence rate would also have been higher if diagnoses from child interviews had been available to add to the diagnoses made from parent interviews.

Puerto Rican DSM-IV Study

In the Puerto Rican DSM-IV Study (PRDSM-IVS), Canino et al. (2004) used a DSM-IV version of the DISC to assess an islandwide probability sample of 1,886 4- to 17-year-olds. Lay interviewers administered a Spanish translation of the DISC-P to one parent of each child. A different lay interviewer administered a Spanish DISC-C to each 11- to 17-year-old. The completion rate was 90.1%. For the 14 diagnostic categories assessed, the prevalence rate was 19.8% for any diagnosis, based on the DISC-P for the 52% of children who were too young for the DISC-C and based on either the DISC-P or DISC-C for the 11- to 17-year-olds.

When Canino et al. applied the DSM-IV criteria for impairment specific to each diagnosis, the overall prevalence rate for any diagnosis fell to 16.4%. When a CGAS score < 69 was required instead of the DSM-IV criteria for impairment, the prevalence rate fell to 7.5%. And when both the DSM-IV impairment criteria and the CGAS score < 69 were required, the prevalence rate fell further, to 6.9%.

In summary, one-stage epidemiological studies using the DISC have included the MECA study of children in three U.S. east coast areas and San Juan, Puerto Rico; the QCMHS in Quebec, Canada; the ANSMHWB in Australia; and the PRDSM-IVS in Puerto Rico. All four studies used the DISC to make DSM diagnoses of children in their entire respective samples. However, major methodological differences probably contributed to differences in prevalence rates for diagnoses of ≥ 1 DSM disorder, which ranged from 15% in the Australian ANSMHWB to 50.6% in MECA. Table 7.1 summarizes findings for the prevalence of ≥ 1 DSM diagnosis from these studies as well as from the two-stage studies that are detailed in the following sections.

Table 7.2 summarizes findings for the prevalence of more specific groups of diagnoses from studies that provided sufficiently comparable data. Just as there is wide variation in the prevalence rates for any diagnosis, there is also wide variation in the rates for specific categories of diagnoses. For example, the rates for any anxiety disorder ranged from 3.7% in a British sample to 39.5% in MECA. As with the rates for any diagnosis, the many methodological differences between the studies may well have contributed to the differences in rates for specific diagnoses.

Two-Stage Epidemiological Studies Using the DISC

We found three two-stage studies from different cultures. All three used the CBCL and other ASEBA forms to identify potential cases and noncases in Stage 1, followed by administration of the DISC to make DSM diagnoses in Stage 2.

Dutch National Study

In what appears to be the only published two-stage study of DISC-based diagnoses in a national sample, Stage 1 screening of Dutch 4- to 18-year-olds was performed in 1993 by home interviewers who asked parents to complete the CBCL and 11- to 18-year-olds to complete the YSR (Verhulst et al., 1997). With parental permission, TRFs were mailed to teachers for completion. The CBCL was completed for 2,227 (82.2%) of the 2,709 eligible children for whom parental informants were reached. Stage 2 was designed to estimate the prevalence of DSM-III-R diagnoses for 13- to 18-year-olds by administering Version 2.3 of the DISC-P to parents and the DISC-C to youths.

Of the 853 parents who completed the Stage 1 CBCL for 13- to 18-year-olds, 780 (91.4%) consented to be reapproached for Stage 2 interviews. Candidates for the Stage 2 DISC were selected by identifying 200 youths whose standardized Total Problems scores averaged across the Stage 1 CBCL, TRF, and YSR were > 75th percentile (potential cases) and 112 randomly selected youths whose standard scores averaged across the Stage 1 CBCL, TRF, and YSR were < 75th percentile (potential noncases). From the 312 youths thus selected for the Stage 2 assessment, the DISC-P was completed for 274 (87.8%) and the DISC-C was completed for 272 (87.2%). The net Stage 2 completion rate for parents was 66.0%, computed as follows: 82.2% (the percentage of the 2,709 eligible children whose parents completed the Stage 1 CBCL) × 91.4% (the percentage of the 853 13- to 18-year-olds with CBCLs whose parents consented to be reapproached for Stage 2) × 87.8% (the percentage of consenting parents who actually completed the DISC-P) = 66.0%.

The Stage 2 interviews yielded a 21.8% prevalence rate for any DSM-III-R disorder (from the 23 that were assessed) based on the DISC-P and 21.5% based on the DISC-C. Despite the similarity of these prevalence rates, the DISC-P and DISC-C agreed in assigning diagnoses to only 4% of the youths. When diagnoses were counted as present

TABLE 7.1. Prevalence of Any DSM Diagnosis Found in Different Cultures According to the DISC and DAWBA

Study	Location	Sample	Completion rate[a]	Ages	Diagnoses	Prevalence[c]
MECA						
Shaffer et al. (1996)	3 U.S. areas and San Juan, Puerto Rico	One-stage; general population; 1,269 parent and child interviews	84.4%	9–17	11 DSM-III-R DISC-2.3	Total = 50.6% CGAS < 71[d] = 24.7% CGAS < 61[d] = 12.8%
QCMHS						
Breton et al. (1999)	Quebec, Canada	One-stage; provincewide; 2,400 parent and child interviews	83.5%	6–14	9 DSM-III-R DISC-2.25 Dominic for children ages 6–11	Total = 32.4%
ANSMHWB						
Sawyer et al. (2001)	Australia	One-stage; nationwide; 3,597 parent interviews	86% of those contacted; 70% estimated for all eligibles	6–17	3 DSM-IV DISC-IV	Total = 15%
PRDSM-IVS						
Canino et al. (2004)	Puerto Rico	One-stage; islandwide; 1,886 parent interviews, 911 child interviews	90.1%	4–17	14 DSM-IV DISC-IV	Total = 19.8% DSM-IV impairment = 16.4% CGAS > 69 = 7.6% DSM-IV impairment and CGAS < 69 = 6.9%
DNS						
Verhulst et al. (1997)	Netherlands	Two-stage, nationwide; 853 Stage 1 274 parent interviews 272 child interviews	66.0%	13–18	23 DSM-III-R DISC-2.3	Total = 35.5% CGAS < 71 = 14.1% CGAS < 61 = 7.9%

PRCPES						
Bird et al. (1988)	Puerto Rico	Two-stage; islandwide; 777 Stage 1 386 parent and child interviews	80.9%	4–16	Every DSM-III[b] diagnosis 1985 DISC Psychiatrists' judgments	Total = 49.5% CGAS < 71 = 33.9% CGAS < 61 = 17.9%
ZESCAP						
Steinhausen et al. (1998)	Zurich, Switzerland	Two-stage; cantonwide; school-based; 2,043 Stage 1 399 parent interviews	41.8%	6–17	15 DSM-III-R DISC-2.3	Total = 22.5%
DLS						
McGee et al. (1992)	Dunedin, New Zealand	One-stage; longitudinal study of birth cohort; 750 child interviews	72.3%	11, 15	10 DSM-III 1982 DISC at age 11; shortened 1982 DISC at age 15	Total: Age 11 = 8.8% Age 15 = 19.6%
Taubaté–British						
Fleitlich-Bilyk and Goodman (2004)	Taubaté, Brazil; Britain	One-stage; Taubaté schools 1,251 parent interviews, plus teacher questionnaires and youth interviews; British national s7,611 parent interviews, plus teacher questionnaires and youth interviews	Taubaté 88.6% Britain 77.3%	7–14	14 DSM-IV DAWBA	Taubaté = 12.7% Britain = 9.7%

Note. Studies are listed in the order in which they were presented in the text of this chapter.

[a]For one-stage studies, the completion rate was the percent of identified eligible children for whom diagnostic interviews were completed (Shaffer, Breton, Sawyer, Canino, McGee, Fleitlich-Bilyk studies); for two-stage studies, the completion rate was the percent of identified eligible children for whom the Stage-1 screening questionnaires were completed multiplied by the percent of children selected for the Stage-2 diagnostic interviews, for whom the interviews were actually completed (Bird, Steinhausen, Verhulst studies).

[b]Bird et al. (1988) stated that psychiatrists assigned "every psychiatric disorder for which criteria were met" (p. 1122). Other than stating that mental retardation and specific developmental disorders could not be diagnosed with the data obtained, they did not specify the number of diagnostic categories that were used.

[c]Prevalence = the percent of children identified as having ≥ 1 DSM diagnosis. CGAS, Children's Global Assessment Scale; CGAS < 71 indicates the percent of children who had ≥ 1 DSM diagnosis plus CGAS scores < 71 ("probable" disorders); CGAS < 61 indicates the percent who had ≥ 1 DSM diagnosis plus CGAS scores < 61 ("definite" disorders).

[d]Tables 3 and 4 in Shaffer et al. (1996) indicate CGAS ≤ 70 and ≤ 60 (i.e., < 71 and < 61), but text alternates between "less than 70 or 60" and "70 or less" (pp. 870, 874).

TABLE 7.2. Prevalence of Specific Categories of DSM Diagnoses Found in Different Cultures According to the DISC and DAWBA

Study	Prevalence of diagnoses in %					
	ADHD	Any anxiety	Any mood[a]	Any disruptive[b]	Conduct disorder	Oppositional defiant disorder
MECA						
Shaffer et al. (1996)	6.5	39.5	8.8	14.3	5.8	7.1
QCMHS[c]						
Breton et al. (1999)	5.0	14.7	1.6	3.1	0.4	2.8
ANSMHWB						
Sawyer et al. (2001)	11.2	NR	3.0	NR	3.0	NR
PRDSM-IVS						
Canino et al. (2004)	8.9	9.5	4.1	12.6	2.6	6.0
DNS						
Verhulst et al. (1997)	2.6	23.5	7.2	7.9	6.0	1.3

PRCPES						
Bird et al. (1988)	16.1	NR	8.7	NR	NR	14.8
ZESCAP						
Steinhausen et al. (1998)	5.3	11.4	0.7	6.5	NA	2.1
DLS (ages 11, 15)						
McGee et al. (1992)	1.7, 1.2	NR	1.4, 4.0	NR	2.0, 5.7	1.3, 2.0
Taubaté, Brazil–British						
Fleitlich-Bilyk and Goodman (2004)	1.8	5.2	1.0	7.0	2.2[d]	3.2
Ford et al. (2003)	2.4	3.7	0.8	5.0	1.5[d]	2.3[d]

Note. Studies are those that are summarized in Table 7.1 plus Ford et al. (2003) data from 5- to 15-year-old British sample from which 7- to 14-year-olds were drawn for comparison with Taubaté sample. NR, data not reported.

[a]In some studies, mood disorders included only depressive disorders.

[b]Disruptive disorders included ADHD, CD, and ODD, except the QCMHs and Taubaté–British studies, which excluded ADHD.

[c]Rates for the QCMHS include parent reports only; rates for child and teacher reports were listed separately by Breton et al. (1999).

[d]Because the Fleitlich-Bilyk and Goodman (2004) comparison of Taubaté versus British prevalence rates did not report specific British rates for CD and ODD, the rates listed here are for 5- to 15-year-olds, from the same British national sample as the 7- to 14-year-olds whose rates for other diagnoses were compared with rates for Taubaté 7- to 14-year-olds.

if they were made from either the DISC-P or DISC-C, the prevalence rate of any DSM-III-R diagnosis projected to the population of Dutch 13- to 18-year-olds was 35.5%. To add impairment to DSM-III-R criteria for disorders, Verhulst et al. (1997) used the DISC interviewers' ratings on the CGAS (Shaffer et al., 1983). When a CGAS score < 71 (designated by Verhulst et al. as "probable" disorders) was required, the prevalence rate fell from 35.5 to 14.1% of Dutch 13- to 18-year-olds. When a more stringent CGAS score of < 61 (designated as "definite" disorders) was required, the prevalence rate fell to 7.9% of Dutch 13- to 18-year-olds.

Puerto Rican Child Psychiatry Epidemiological Study

The most direct cross-cultural comparison with the Dutch national study is afforded by a two-stage study done in Puerto Rico (Bird et al., 1988). Stage 1 began in 1985 when interviewers visited households that had previously been chosen for a study of adult psychopathology. Parents of randomly selected 4- to 16-year-olds completed the CBCL, and teachers completed the TRF.

In Stage 2, DSM-III versions of the DISC-P and DISC-C were used to assess children who had scored in the clinical range on either the CBCL or TRF (potential "cases"), plus a 20% random sample of children who had scored in the normal range on both the CBCL and TRF (potential "noncases"). Child psychiatrists administered the DISC-P and DISC-C. During the interviews, the psychiatrists were allowed to clarify ambiguous responses through additional questions and unstructured probes. If the structured DISC did not seem likely to provide accurate information, the psychiatrists could complete the interview without the structured format. Because computerized diagnostic algorithms were not yet available, the psychiatrists used their clinical judgment to weight the information from each parent and child to decide which DSM-III symptom criteria were met and to apply DSM-III rules for making diagnoses. If doubts arose about the appropriate diagnoses for a case, the case was discussed with other child psychiatrists until consensus was reached. Any DSM-III diagnosis could be applied, although Bird et al. pointed out that a lack of psychometric testing precluded accurate ascertainment of mental retardation and specific developmental disorders (p. 1122).

For the 843 children identified as eligible for the study, Stage 1 assessments were completed for 777 (92.2%). Among the children selected for Stage 2, 386 (87.7%) completed the Stage 2 assessment. The net completion rate was thus 92.2% × 87.7% = 80.9%. Among the children assessed at Stage 2, the prevalence rate for any DSM-III diagnosis was 49.5% according to data combined from parents and their children. When CGAS ratings of impairment were added to DSM-III diagnoses, the prevalence rate fell from 49.5 to 33.9% for "probable" disorders (CGAS < 71) and dropped to 17.9% for "definite" disorders (CGAS < 61). If we compare these Puerto Rican rates of 49.5%, 33.9%, and 17.9% with the Dutch rates of 35.5%, 14.1%, and 7.9%, respectively, we might be tempted to conclude that disorders defined by the DSM are substantially less common among Dutch than Puerto Rican children. However, before we can draw any conclusions about differences between the cultures, we need to consider the following methodological differences that could have affected the obtained prevalence rates:

1. The lower net completion rate of 66.0% in the Netherlands versus 80.9% in Puerto Rico could have resulted in a loss of more "cases" in the Netherlands, because parents whose children have the most problems may be the least likely to consent to surveys (e.g., Steinhausen, Winkler Metzke, Meier, & Kannenberg, 1998, p. 267).
2. In the Puerto Rican study, the psychiatrist interviewers were allowed to depart from the structured format of the DISC. In addition, they used their clinical judgment to decide whether the combination of parent and child reports met criteria for DSM diagnoses. By contrast, the Dutch study used computerized algorithms to generate diagnoses separately from DISC-P and DISC-C interviews administered by separate lay interviewers.
3. Although the CBCL and TRF were used in Stage 1 of both studies to identify potential cases and noncases, the studies used different cutpoints on the scores to select potential cases and noncases for the Stage 2 DISC interviews.
4. The Dutch study used 23 DSM-III-R diagnostic categories, whereas the Puerto Rican study permitted all DSM-III diagnostic categories, although it did not report the number of categories actually used.
5. The Stage 2 diagnoses in the Dutch study were made for 13- to 18-year-olds versus 4- to 16-year-olds in the Puerto Rican study.

There may really be differences between the rates of DSM-defined disorders in the Netherlands versus Puerto Rico. However, the many methodological differences between these careful studies of probability samples preclude firm conclusions about whether the rates of DSM-based disorders really differ significantly between the Netherlands and Puerto Rico.

Zurich Epidemiological Study

The Zurich Epidemiological Study of Child and Adolescent Psychopathology (ZESCAP) assessed 6- to 17-year-olds who were attending school in the Canton of Zurich, Switzerland during 1994 (Steinhausen et al., 1997, 1998). The ZESCAP was similar to the Dutch and Puerto Rican two-stage studies (Bird et al., 1988; Verhulst et al., 1997) in that it used the CBCL and YSR at Stage 1 to identify potential cases and noncases. It was also similar to the Dutch study in using the DISC-2.3 administered by lay interviewers to make DSM-III-R diagnoses of the Stage 2 sample. However, unlike the Dutch study, YSRs for the ZESCAP were administered to groups of students in schools and CBCLs were distributed by teachers in envelopes for students to take to their parents. After completing the CBCL, the parents were to mail it to the researchers. Also, only parents were interviewed in the ZESCAP, and they were queried regarding only 15 diagnostic categories, whereas the Dutch study interviewed parents and youths separately regarding 23 diagnostic categories.

CBCLs were obtained for 2,043 students, with a completion rate of 73.5% of the target sample. Based on DISC-P interviews with 399 parents, the ZESCAP yielded an estimated prevalence rate of 22.5% for DSM-III-R disorders in the population of 6- to 17-year-olds attending school in Zurich. This finding was similar to the 21.8% prevalence rate found in the Dutch study for 23 diagnostic categories assessed with the DISC-P. However, it was considerably less than the 35.5% prevalence rate found when DISC-C diagnoses were included in the Dutch prevalence rate. In addition to the lack of DISC-C interviews, the ZESCAP prevalence rate may have been reduced by the low net completion rate of 41.6% (73.5% at Stage 1 × 56.6% at Stage 2 = 41.6%), because, as Steinhausen et al. (1998, p. 267) reported, nonparticipants may have been at elevated risk for disorders because they obtained higher problem scores in teachers' ratings than participants did.

In summary, two-stage epidemiological studies using the DISC have included the Dutch National Study (DNS) in the Netherlands, the Puerto Rican Child Psychiatry Epidemiological Study (PRCPES) in Puerto Rico, and the ZESCAP in Zurich. As shown in Table 7.1, the prevalence rates for any DSM diagnosis ranged from 22.5% in the

ZESCAP to 49.5% in the PRCPES. Although the range of prevalence rates is not quite as broad as in the one-stage studies summarized in Table 7.1, major variations in net completion rates were introduced by differential attrition from the Stage 1 screening procedures to the Stage 2 DISC interviews.

Dunedin Longitudinal Study Using the DISC

A longitudinal study carried out in Dunedin, New Zealand, may have implications for multicultural studies of DSM diagnoses made from the DISC, even though it did not systematically select a sample to be representative of a larger population. The Dunedin Longitudinal Study (DLS) began with 1,037 children who were born in a single hospital in 1972 and 1973 (McGee et al., 1992). When the participants were 11 years old, they were interviewed by a single child psychiatrist using the 1982 version of the DISC-C (Costello et al., 1982).

At age 15, the participants were interviewed again, this time with a shortened version of the DISC-C. To equate the DISC data obtained at ages 11 and 15, the authors analyzed only the DISC items that were used at both ages. Rating forms completed by parents were used to confirm problems reported by their children, although differences between the items rated at ages 11 and 15 necessitated complex algorithms for linking the parents' ratings to their children's DISC responses. DISC data and parents' ratings were available at both ages for 750 (72.3%) of the original sample of 1,037 children.

For the 10 diagnostic categories that were analyzed, more than twice as many youths met criteria for DSM-III diagnoses at age 15 (19.6% of the sample) as at age 11 (8.8% of the sample). For diagnoses that were confirmed by parents' ratings, there was little change in the total prevalence rate from age 11–15 for boys, but a substantial increase in diagnoses for girls. For diagnoses based on self-reports that were not confirmed by parents, both genders showed fourfold increases from age 11–15, including statistically significant increases in diagnoses of nonaggressive conduct disorders and depressive disorders.

The lack of parent DISCs, plus methodological differences between age 11 and 15 assessments, limit the possibilities for explaining the sharp increase in the percentage of youths meeting criteria for DSM-III diagnoses. Nevertheless, the findings suggest that developmental changes in the base rates of problems on which DSM diagnoses are based, especially problems that may be unknown to parents, need to be considered in determining how to define disorders in each culture.

Findings with the DAWBA

As we reported in Chapter 3, the DAWBA is intended to make diagnoses by having clinicians judge responses obtained from structured interviews administered by nonclinicians (Goodman, Ford, Richards, et al., 2000). Other than the DISC, the DAWBA is the only structured diagnostic interview for which we have found published reports of prevalence rates of child diagnoses in at least two cultures. Furthermore, it is the only structured diagnostic interview for which we have found a direct statistical comparison between prevalence rates of diverse diagnoses in at least two cultures.

The statistical comparison was between DSM-IV diagnoses made in a probability sample of children living in England, Scotland, and Wales versus a sample of children attending schools in Taubaté, a municipality of about 220,000 residents in southeastern Brazil (Fleitlich-Bilyk & Goodman, 2004; Ford et al., 2003). The British children were selected from the approximately 90% of 5- to 15-year-olds for whom postal codes were listed in a British government register for child benefits. A probability sample of 14,250 children was drawn from 475 of the 9,000 British postal codes. From the sample of 14,250 children, 790 were ineligible because they could not be traced, were in foster care, had died, or were outside the target age range. For the remaining 13,460 children in the sample, DAWBA interviews were administered to parents of 10,405 (77.3%). Self-report interviews were also administered to 4,115 11- to 15-year-olds. Teachers completed questionnaires regarding ADHD and conduct–oppositional problems for 8,382 of the children who were attending school.

The Brazilian children were chosen from samples of Taubaté "mainstream" schools that agreed to participate. From the participating schools, 1,504 7- to 14-year-olds were selected by stratified random sampling. Of the 1,504 selected children, 92 were excluded because of errors or moves to other schools. Diagnostic data were ultimately obtained for 1,251 (88.6%) of the 1,412 eligible children, based on parent DAWBA interviews plus self-report interviews with the 11- to 14-year-olds and questionnaires completed by teachers. The DAWBA questions were described as being "closely related to DSM-IV and ICD-10 diagnostic criteria" and as focusing "on current rather than life-time problems" (Fleitlich-Bilyk & Goodman, 2004, p. 729). Because the Taubaté sample included only 7- to 14-year-olds, they were compared with British 7- to 14-year-olds from the Ford et al. (2003) sample.

After adjusting for oversampling of certain kinds of schools, the authors estimated a prevalence rate of 12.7% for any of 14 DSM-IV diagnoses among 7- to 14-year-olds attending schools in Taubaté. This finding compared with an estimated prevalence rate of 9.7% for British 7- to 14-year-olds. Although the difference between 9.7% and 12.7% may seem small, it did indicate that significantly more Taubaté than British 7- to 14-year-olds qualified for DAWBA diagnoses. The largest difference in prevalence rates was for the combination of oppositional and conduct disorders, for which the 7.0% rate found in Taubaté was significantly higher than the 5.0% found in Britain.

Implications of the British versus Taubaté Comparisons

Although there are far fewer published studies of the DAWBA than of the DISC, DICA, or K-SADS, the DAWBA findings are worth considering because they appear to provide the only statistical comparison of prevalence rates for diverse DSM diagnoses obtained by children living in different cultures. It is possible that the statistically significant difference between the 9.7% rate estimated for British children versus the 12.7% rate estimated for Taubaté children reflects a true difference between the percentages of children in the two cultures who have disorders, as defined by the DAWBA version of DSM-IV criteria. However, the following factors could have differentially affected the estimates of the prevalence rates:

1. The British estimate was based on a national population sample, whereas the school-based Taubaté sample omitted children who were not attending the mainstream schools that agreed to cooperate. These sampling differences could have had unknowable effects on the estimated prevalence rates.
2. The net completion rate of 88.6% for parental DAWBA interviews in Taubaté was substantially higher than the 77.3% completion rate in Britain. Children who are selected but are then not assessed in epidemiological surveys may tend to be at greater risk for disorders than most of the children who are actually assessed (e.g., Steinhausen et al., 1998).
3. SES, cultural, and language differences between Britain and Taubaté could have affected respondents' answers to the DAWBA questions.

Despite the factors that argue against accepting the difference between the British and Taubaté prevalence rates at face value, the relatively small size of the difference suggests that use of the same standardized diagnostic procedure may yield fairly similar prevalence rates in at least two cultures.

Comparisons with DISC Findings

As summarized in Table 7.1, our review of four DISC epidemiological studies that based diagnoses on multi-informant data yielded prevalence rates for DSM diagnoses that ranged from 32.4% in the QCMHS to 50.6% in MECA, with a mean of 42.0% (Bird et al., 1988; Breton et al., 1999; Shaffer et al., 1996; Verhulst et al., 1997). (Canino et al., 2004, reported a prevalence rate of 19.8% for a sample of 4- to 17-year-olds in which the parent DISC was used for all ages and the child DISC was also used for the 11- to 17-year-olds.) In the studies that augmented DISC criteria with impairment criteria based on CGAS scores, a CGAS cutpoint < 71 resulted in prevalence rates ranging from 14.1% in the DNS to 33.9% in the PRCPES, with a mean of 24.2% (Bird et al., 1988; Shaffer et al., 1996; Verhulst et al., 1997). With a CGAS cutpoint < 69, Canino et al. (2004) obtained a prevalence rate of 7.6%. When a CGAS cutpoint < 61 was imposed, the range was from 7.9% in the DNS to 17.9% in the PRCPES, with a mean of 12.9%. When taken at face value, the prevalence rates for DSM diagnoses based on the DISC were thus far higher (range = 19.8–50.6%, mean = 42.0%) than when based on the DAWBA (9.7 and 12.7%, mean = 11.2%). With a CGAS cutpoint < 71, the DISC prevalence rates remained substantially higher (range = 14.1–33.9%, mean = 24.2%) than the DAWBA rates. However, when more severe CGAS cutpoints of < 69 and < 61 were imposed, the DISC prevalence rates (range = 7.6–17.9%, mean = 12.9%) approximated the DAWBA rates.

Several factors could have contributed to the differences between the prevalence rates obtained with DSM-III, DSM-III-R, and DSM-IV versions of the DISC and the DAWBA. Some possible contributors to the differences in obtained prevalence are the following:

1. The DISC rates for DSM-III and DSM-III-R diagnoses may have been higher than the DISC and DAWBA rates for DSM-IV diagnoses because more explicit impairment criteria are included in the DSM-IV versions of some diagnostic categories than in the DSM-III and DSM-III-R versions.

2. DAWBA diagnoses were made by psychiatrists who considered current problems reported to nonclinicians by informants. Although the diagnoses in the PRCPES were also made by psychiatrists, they personally administered the DISC interviews and could depart from the DISC structure when they felt that it would improve the assessment. By contrast, the MECA, QCMHS, and DNS derived diagnoses from algorithms applied

separately to parent and child interviews administered by nonclinicians.

3. The DISC studies spanned different age ranges than the 7- to 14-year age range that was used for the Taubaté versus British comparison.

4. Sampling, cultural, language, and procedural differences, as well as differences in the numbers of diagnostic categories, the DSM criteria, and the completion rates, could have contributed to the differences between the DISC and DAWBA findings.

Prevalence findings for psychopathology inevitably depend on many methodological factors. Much remains to be done to develop and apply methodology for documenting multicultural similarities and differences in diagnostically based assessment of psychopathology. A particularly salient issue concerns the degree to which diagnoses of psychopathology should be determined by judgments of whether children's functioning is impaired by the particular behavioral and emotional problems that are specified by the DSM diagnostic criteria. It is usually quite difficult for interviewees to accurately report whether each of the DSM's criterial symptoms *causes* impairment. For example, a parent might affirm that a child "has been physically cruel to animals," which is a criterial symptom for CD. However, the parent may not be able to accurately report whether this "behavior causes clinically significant impairment in social, academic, or occupational functioning." This is typical of the judgments required by DSM-IV (American Psychiatric Association, 2000, p. 99). And if the interviewee reports cruelty to animals but cannot accurately state that the cruelty *causes* impairment, should the cruelty be discounted?

The DSM model for psychopathology requires that each criterial feature be judged as present versus absent and that disorders be judged as present versus absent according to whether the requisite diagnostic criteria are, or are not, met. This present-versus-absent model for diagnoses is based on physical diseases where particular tissue pathology, symptoms, signs, and/or physical pathogens define particular diseases. Although DSM-IV requires that each symptom cause impairment in order to be judged present, people who are diagnosed as having physical diseases may not necessarily be impaired by the disease at the time when they are diagnosed. Does this mean that lack of impairment should preclude a diagnosis? Both for purposes of helping individuals and for research on epidemiology, etiology, prevention, course, treatment, and outcome, judgments of physical pathology differ in crucial ways from judgments of impairment. For example, if HIV test results could only be considered positive after individuals are already impaired by each symptom of HIV, little could be done to prevent people with HIV from developing AIDS. Furthermore, little could be learned about the true prevalence of HIV, risk factors, or effective treatment.

As of this writing, no methods for detecting tissue pathology or physical pathogens are included in the DISC or DAWBA procedures for determining the presence of child psychopathology. Instead, the DISC and DAWBA diagnostic criteria must be judged on the basis of informants' reports of behavioral and emotional problems, including the intensity, frequency, duration, consequences, and age of onset of the problems. Many of the criterial problems are displayed to some degree by many children at some time in their lives. Furthermore, many of the problems are correlated with each other and may be difficult to separate decisively into different diagnoses that must each be judged as present versus absent. Because current diagnostic criteria must be assessed in terms of verbal reports of children's behaviors and emotions, efforts to operationalize diagnoses require assessment procedures that can translate what informants can remember and report into yes/no judgments of diagnostic criteria.

CROSS-CULTURAL DIFFERENCES IN DIAGNOSTIC DECISIONS

Until more studies apply the same standardized diagnostic procedures to representative samples of children from multiple cultures, estimates of multicultural differences in prevalence rates for diagnostically based disorders may need to depend on indigenous diagnostic practices. To shed light on possible cultural variations in diagnostic practices, Prendergast et al. (1988) compared diagnoses made by psychiatrists from the United Kingdom and the United States. The psychiatrists' diagnoses were based on case histories of 41 6- to 11-year-old boys who were referred to U.K. or U.S. mental health services mainly for problems of hyperactivity. Many of the U.K. boys had received ICD-9 diagnoses of hyperkinetic disorder, whereas many of the U.S. boys had received DSM-III diagnoses of attention deficit disorder (ADD). The psychiatrists read case histories for all 41 boys. They also viewed videotaped excerpts of interviews with eight boys from each country.

Research and clinical psychiatrists from both countries participated. They were first trained to use the ICD-9 and DSM-III. They then studied each case and used a standard list of symptoms to indicate the symptoms they judged to be present. Thereafter, they diagnosed each case according to the ICD-9 and DSM-III criteria.

The main findings follow:

1. The research psychiatrists achieved moderate agreement with each other on major diagnostic categories, with kappas of .60–.77 (mean = .66) for ICD-9 diagnoses and .40–.83 (mean = .69) for DSM-III diagnoses.
2. Among clinical psychiatrists, agreement on diagnoses was considerably lower, with kappas of .20–.39 (mean = .30) for ICD-9 diagnoses and .05–.33 (mean = .24) for DSM-III diagnoses.
3. Viewing videotapes did not improve diagnostic agreement.
4. For both the research and clinical psychiatrists, agreement on the presence of particular symptoms was generally low and was not related to whether the psychiatrists agreed on the diagnoses.
5. U.K. psychiatrists made proportionally fewer diagnoses of hyperkinetic disorder and ADD than U.S. psychiatrists, especially when using ICD-9.
6. There were fewer ICD-9 diagnoses of hyperkinetic disorder than DSM-III diagnoses of ADD, especially by U.K. psychiatrists.

The differences between the diagnoses made by U.S. and U.K. psychiatrists who were trained on the same diagnostic systems, who were given the same data, and who came from two similar cultures that share the English language suggest that indigenous diagnoses may not be a sufficient basis for comparing the rates of actual disorders in different cultures.

In addition to differences in diagnostic practices, there may also be cultural variations in mental health professionals' perceptions of children's problems. As an example, when viewing videos of four 8-year-old boys, mental health professionals from China and Indonesia rated the boys as being significantly more hyperactive and disruptive, according to DSM-III-R criteria, than did mental health professionals from Japan and the United States (Mann et al., 1992). This finding suggests that different thresholds for perceiving problem behaviors may contribute to cultural differences in diagnoses, even when trained mental health professionals use the same diagnostic rules.

CONCLUSIONS FROM DIAGNOSTICALLY BASED FINDINGS

As shown in Table 7.1, the prevalence rates for DSM diagnoses made from the DISC and DAWBA ranged from 8.8% for 11-year-olds in the DLS to 50.6% for 9- to 17-year-olds in the MECA samples drawn from Atlanta, New Haven, San Juan, and Westchester County. Should we conclude that there really are sixfold differences in the true prevalence of diagnostically defined disorders among the cultures studied? A six-fold difference has also been found in prevalence rates for DSM-IV diagnoses of adults interviewed in 14 countries, ranging from a 4.3% prevalence rate in Shanghai, China, to 26.4% in a U.S. national sample (WHO World Mental Health Survey Consortium, 2004). An important reason for doing multicultural studies is certainly to identify differences as well as similarities in the prevalence of psychopathology. Unfortunately, methodological differences among the studies listed in Table 7.1 limit the conclusions to be drawn about multicultural variations in diagnostically based childhood disorders, as outlined in the following section.

Methodological Differences

Because each study differed from most other studies in multiple ways, it is hard to precisely pinpoint specific methodological factors that might explain the large differences in findings among the studies reviewed. However, to advance multicultural studies of diagnostically based disorders, it would be helpful to standardize methodologies as much as possible when assessing children from different cultures. To highlight areas in which standardization might be improved, we now consider methodological differences in sampling procedures, the ages of the children, the use of multiple informants, the diagnostic criteria, and the analytic methods.

Sampling Procedures

A major difference among the sampling procedures was in whether they were one- or two-stage designs. Six of the studies summarized in Table 7.1 were one-stage, whereas three were two-stage. (The DLS is listed among the six one-stage studies because it did not diagnose a subsample from an initial screening sample. However, because it was a longitudinal study rather than a prevalence study, we do not consider it here.)

Advantages of one-stage designs are that (1) they avoid attrition from Stage 1 to Stage 2 and (2) they can base prevalence estimates on the entire sample of children who are initially assessed. Advantages of two-stage designs are that (1) they use costly diagnostic interviews only for the Stage 2 assessments and (2) they may be able to do more intensive assessments of their Stage 2 samples than would be practical in one-stage studies. Although use of a one-stage versus two-stage design was not the only factor affecting completion rates, Table 7.1 shows that completion rates for one-stage prevalence studies ranged from 77.3% for the British sample of the British–Taubaté comparison to 90.1% for the Puerto Rican PRDSM-IVS. The mean completion rate for the one-stage prevalence studies was 85.0%. (If the Australian ANSMHWB estimate of a 70% completion rate for all possible eligibles is used instead of the 86% rate for identified eligibles who agreed to participate, the mean would be 82.4%.) By comparison, the completion rates for the three two-stage studies ranged from 41.8% for the Zurich ZESCAP to 80.9% for the PRCPES, for a mean of 62.9%.

Important sampling differences also include (1) the sampling "frames," that is, the operational definitions of populations from which the samples were drawn, and (2) the methods for drawing the samples from the frames. To obtain a fully representative sample of children, the least biased strategy is typically to use probability sampling. Probability sampling applies random selection procedures to ensure that every individual in the sampling frame has about the same probability of being selected. In practice, probability sampling is often done in stages whereby particular localities are randomly selected, neighborhoods are then randomly selected within the selected localities, and individuals are selected by stratified random sampling within the selected neighborhoods.

If official records are available for all the children in a population, these records can serve as a sampling frame from which children are selected by stratified random sampling. Of the studies listed in Table 7.1, the Dutch DNS sample and the British sample of the British–Taubaté comparison were selected by multistage random sampling from official records for entire countries, although the British sample was drawn only from the 90% of children for whom postal codes were listed in a register of child benefits. The QCMHS used this type of sampling for the province of Quebec, Canada, whereas the PRCPES sample was drawn from an updated version of an islandwide probability sample previously used for a prevalence study of adult disorders. The ANSMHWB sampled clusters of households within census districts. The ZESCAP sample was drawn by stratified random sampling from all types of schools in the canton of Zurich, Switzerland, whereas the Taubaté portion of the British–Taubaté comparison was drawn from cooperating mainstream schools. The ZESCAP and Taubaté samples thus omitted children who were not attending the local schools that were sampled. Because the MECA sample was obtained by different methods in the four participating localities, its prevalence rates are not generalizable to a particular population.

Although probability sampling from entire populations is important for obtaining accurate prevalence estimates, high completion rates are also needed to warrant confidence in the results obtained from even well-designed probability samples. Multiple studies have reported that children with high levels of problems are more likely to be missed than children with lower problem levels (Cox, Rutter, Yule, & Quinton, 1977; Steinhausen et al., 1998; Verhulst, Koot, & Berden, 1990). Thus, the effects of sampling variations on the prevalence rates summarized in Table 7.1 may include differences in the sampling designs (e.g., particular permutations of probability vs. nonprobability sampling); the sampling frames (e.g., total populations vs. schools); completion rates (which ranged from 41.8 to 90.1% in the Table 7.1 studies); and the unknown proportions of children with relatively high versus low problem levels who may have been missed.

Ages of the Children

As shown in Table 7.1, the prevalence studies spanned different age ranges, with the broadest being 4–17 years in the PRDSM-IVS and the narrowest being 13–18 years in the DNS. Only the ANSMHWP and ZESCAP spanned the same ages. As indicated by the large increase in DISC-C prevalence rates found for the same DLS youths interviewed at ages 11 and 15, age differences could contribute to the differences in prevalence rates shown in Table 7.1. Not only the ages spanned but the proportion of children at each age, as well as age-related differences in assessment methods, may affect the obtained prevalence estimates. For example, for adolescents, self-reports of problems have been obtained via structured diagnostic interviews. For younger children, self-reports have either not been obtained or have been obtained by less direct methods, such as the Dominic cartoons used in the QCMHS and the less structured administration of the DISC in the PRCPES.

Multiple Informants

Low levels of agreement have been found between diagnoses derived separately from structured interviews with children and their parents (Breton et al., 1999; Jensen et al., 1999; Shaffer et al., 1996; Verhulst et al., 1997). Consequently, the total number of diagnoses based on parent plus child interviews has typically been almost twice as high as the number based only on parent interviews or only on child interviews. The addition of data from teachers may further affect estimated prevalence rates. However, teacher data have typically been obtained by questionnaires regarding only a few disruptive behaviors, rather than by interviews that include all criteria for diverse disorders. Among the prevalence studies listed in Table 7.1, only the ANSMHWP and the

ZESCAP based diagnoses solely on the DISC-P, although the ZESCAP's Stage 1 selection procedure included the YSR. The ANSMHWP's prevalence rate of 15% and the ZESCAP's prevalence rate of 22.5% were lower than the prevalence rates obtained when diagnoses were combined from multiple informants, except for the British–Taubaté comparison, in which psychiatrists mentally combined DAWBA multi-informant data to make diagnoses. Thus, not only the use of multi-informant data but the ways in which such data are used to make diagnoses may affect the estimated prevalence rates.

Diagnostic Criteria

Official nosologies have shaped diagnostically based assessment instruments, data collection procedures, and methods for translating data into diagnoses. Because the DSM and ICD have not specified assessment operations for determining the presence versus absence of disorders (other than IQ tests for mental retardation), diagnostic interviews such as the DISC and DAWBA are used to operationalize diagnostic criteria in terms of questions that are asked of parents and children. The changes in diagnostic criteria from DSM-III to DSM-III-R and DSM-IV have necessitated different versions of the interviews. Even for a particular edition of the DSM, there have been multiple versions of some interviews, such as the DISC, which have differed in the questions that were asked, the follow-up probes, and the algorithms for deciding whether criteria were met for each feature of each diagnosis and for each diagnosis as a whole.

The times spanned by diagnostic questions have also differed; for example, the DAWBA focuses on current diagnoses, whereas the DISC may include lifetime diagnoses, potentially yielding higher prevalence estimates than would be obtained only for current diagnoses. Moreover, the number of diagnoses assessed has varied widely from three in the ANSMHWB to 23 in the DNS and "every psychiatric disorder for which criteria were met" in the PRCPES (Bird et al., 1988; p. 1122).

In addition to differences in the assessment instruments and data collection procedures, prevalence studies have differed in how they translated their data into diagnoses. The most direct translations into diagnoses have been made by applying separate computerized algorithms to DISC responses obtained from each informant. This procedure was used to generate DSM diagnoses in the MECA, QCMHS, ANSMHWB, PRDSM-IVS, DNS, and ZESCAP studies.

Two studies based their prevalence estimates on psychiatrists' judgments of data obtained from interviews with parents and children. In Stage 2 of the PRCPES, child psychiatrists personally administered the DISC-C and DISC-P. Based on information from both interviews, the psychiatrists then used their clinical judgment to decide whether a child met DSM-III criteria for each feature and then for each diagnosis. When necessary, a child was discussed with other child psychiatrists until consensus was reached. It was found that 49.5% of the children met criteria for at least one DSM-III diagnosis. Subsequent application of CGAS cutpoints reduced this rate.

In the other study that used psychiatrists' judgments of multi-informant data, the data obtained from DAWBA interviews administered by nonclinicians were used by child psychiatrists to make DSM-IV diagnoses. Based on 14 DSM-IV diagnostic categories, the prevalence rate was 9.7% in the British sample of 7- to 14-year-olds and 12.7% in the Taubaté sample. Because the DSM-IV included impairment criteria for more diagnostic categories than did the DSM-III used in the PRCPES, the PRCPES DSM-III rates of 33.9% with CGAS < 71 or 17.9% with CGAS < 61 might provide the most appropriate bases for comparison with the British and Taubaté DAWBA rates.

In addition to other factors that could have contributed to differences in estimated prevalence rates, it is important to consider possible differences in clinicians' tendencies to make particular diagnoses. The U.K.–U.S. comparison showed that psychiatrists from the two countries differed in the diagnoses they made from the same case materials. Considering that the psychiatrists in the British–Taubaté study were either British or were trained by British psychiatrists, it is possible that they tended to draw different diagnostic conclusions from interviews did than the Puerto Rican psychiatrists in the PRCPES. For example, even though the Taubaté and Puerto Rican samples were both from low-income Latin American populations, the prevalence rate for any ADHD diagnosis was 1.8% in Taubaté versus 9.5% in the PRCPES, after application of the most stringent impairment criterion (CGAS < 61).

Analytic Methods

After diagnoses are made for each child in a sample, different methods can be used to analyze the data and to compute prevalence rates. As shown in previous chapters, the items and scales of empirically based instruments can be analyzed both quantitatively in terms of continuous scores and categorically in terms of cutpoints for distinguishing between nondeviant and deviant scores. By contrast, structured diagnostic interviews such as the DISC and DAWBA are designed to assess each criterial feature and each diagnosis as absent versus present. Although it is feasible to score diagnostic criteria quantitatively, the prevalence studies have mainly reported percentages of children who qualify for diagnoses. As a result, the statistical analyses have consisted largely of chi squares, odds ratios, and logistic regressions. If every symptom had been queried for every child, it would be possible to use the sum of symptoms endorsed for each diagnosis as a quantitative measure. However, to save time, structured interviews typically employ "skip" rules, whereby questions are omitted if initial questions about a diagnosis indicate that criteria for making that diagnosis are unlikely to be met. When key questions are skipped for substantial numbers of children, it is not possible to compare responses to a uniform set of diagnostic criteria for all children.

Potentially important analytic variations in how prevalence estimates are made may stem from the selective weighting of prevalence data. Because the samples of children were not completely representative of the target populations and because completion rates for diagnostic interviews were well below 100%, the investigators in most studies have selectively weighted the obtained prevalence data to estimate rates for the entire target population. In the one-stage QCMHS, PRDSM-IVS, and British–Taubaté studies, the investigators applied weights to compensate for the differential selection of particular residential areas and other characteristics of the sampling procedures that limited the representativeness of the target samples. In the two-stage DNS, PRCPES, and ZESCAP, weights were used to compensate for differential Stage 2 proportions and completion rates for children who screened positive versus negative at Stage 1. The MECA investigators did not weight their results because they said it would be "improper to generalize the prevalence rates that were identified in the field trials to the United States or even to demographic subgroups more generally" (Shaffer et al., 1996, p. 874). Although weighting of obtained results may certainly be justified to compensate for the unrepresentativeness of data obtained from samples, the different assumptions and methods used to weight the data reduce the comparability of the prevalence estimates.

Advancing Multicultural Studies of Diagnostic Prevalence Rates

Prevalence studies present major challenges. Even to do a prevalence study within a single culture requires substantial funding, skilled professionals, cadres of trained interviewers, scientific procedures for drawing representative samples, and the cooperation of most of the people who are chosen to participate. Studies of the prevalence of child psychopathology are further complicated by the need to obtain data from parents, teachers, and the children themselves, plus the need to tailor assessment procedures to the ages of the children. The lack of operational definitions for diagnoses requires that standardized assessment procedures be constructed to operationalize diagnoses in large representative samples. When we consider the additional challenges of implementing parallel standardized procedures in multiple cultures, we should not be surprised at the paucity of multicultural diagnostic prevalence studies. The value of new studies could be enhanced by applying uniform procedures to population-based samples rather than to convenience samples or school-based samples of unknown generalizability.

Counting and Measuring

Research on the prevalence of diagnostically defined disorders typically counts the number of individuals who meet criteria for each disorder in a particular sample. However, to advance multicultural prevalence studies, it may be helpful to consider alternatives to counting disorders defined in terms of forced-choice yes/no judgments of each criterial feature and present-versus-absent decisions about each diagnosis. Children vary in the degree to which they manifest various criterial features. Furthermore, both children and adults vary in the degree to which they remember and report manifestations of the criterial features. Consequently, research on prevalence involves *measuring* quantitative variations in responses to diagnostic questions as well as counting the number of individuals who meet diagnostic criteria.

To decide whether particular criterial features are present or absent, diagnosticians and computer algorithms impose yes/no judgments on phenomena that vary quantitatively, both in fact and in interviewees' responses to diagnostic questions. Whether data are analyzed categorically or quantitatively, the measurement processes that yield the data are subject to error. More precise statistical comparisons of the specific criterial features reported in different cultures can be made if quantitative variations in the features are preserved than if they are lost by categorizing each feature as present versus absent. Quantitative aggregation of the features into scores for each diagnostic category can also provide more precise statistical comparisons of the distributions of problems and disorders in multiple cultures. In addition, differences between the distributions of diagnostic scores can be statistically compared for children of each gender and different ages, as assessed by different sources of data. Without necessarily changing the diagnostic categories or cutpoints, quantification of assessment data could increase the precision of multicultural comparisons of diagnostically based disorders.

Diagnostic and Impairment Criteria

An additional way to increase the precision of multicultural comparisons would be to uniformly report data separately for diagnostic criteria and for impairment criteria. The addition of the CGAS to diagnoses and the use of impairment criteria for more diagnoses in DSM-IV than its predecessors have succeeded in reducing the alarmingly high prevalence rates found for DSM diagnoses in many samples. However, requiring that impairment criteria be met raises questions about whether the diagnostic criteria, per se, actually define disorders. One such question is whether informants' reports can really be used to determine whether impairment, such as a child's distress or poor functioning in school, with peers, or in other contexts, is specifically "due to" each symptom that is endorsed in an interview.

Although children who meet diagnostic criteria for disorders are indeed likely to function poorly, some of the criterial symptoms may themselves reflect impairment or the consequences of impairment, rather than "causing" impairment. For example, if a child has poor social skills, no friends, and poor school achievement, these problems could precipitate criterial symptoms of dysthymia, depression, anxiety, social phobia, ADHD, or oppositional defiant disorder. If disorders can be diagnosed only when their criterial symptoms are inferred to *cause* impairment, how can we accurately distinguish between impairment that contributes to or accompanies a particular disorder versus impairment that is specifically *caused by* each symptom of the disorder?

Another kind of question arises when children meet all the diagnostic criteria for a disorder but are not considered to be impaired "due to" each criterial symptom. As pointed out earlier, requiring impairment in order to justify a diagnosis seems inconsistent with medical concepts of disorders, which are diagnosed as present whether or not they cause impairment at the moment when they are diagnosed. Thus, rather than excluding diagnoses if impairment criteria are not met, multicultural studies may be more informative if they document diagnostic criteria and impairment criteria separately.

Uniformity of Assessment Procedures

As shown in Table 7.1, the number of diagnoses assessed in the prevalence studies ranged from 3 in the ANSMHWB to 23 in the DNS and "every psychiatric disorder for which criteria were met" in the PRCPES.

Because inclusion of many diagnoses is likely to produce higher prevalence rates than inclusion of fewer diagnoses, it would be helpful to use the same standardized assessment instruments and procedures to assess children in multiple cultures. Use of the same standardized instruments and procedures would eliminate differences in the number of diagnoses and differences between the data required for making diagnoses as impediments to multicultural comparisons. To reduce the cost and informant burden, prevalence studies could focus on a relatively small set of common and consequential disorders for which prevalence rates can be meaningfully obtained from population samples of practical sizes. Diagnoses such as enuresis might thus be excluded because they do not necessarily involve significant psychopathology. At the other extreme, diagnoses of childhood schizophrenia might be excluded as too rare to warrant detailed assessment in all but the most enormous or high-risk samples.

SUMMARY

This chapter presented diagnostically based prevalence studies that have multicultural implications. Samples have been drawn according to one-stage designs and two-stage designs. In *one-stage designs*, all participants receive diagnostic assessments. In *two-stage designs*, low-cost assessments are used with Stage 1 participants to identify potential cases and a subset of noncases who are then assessed in Stage 2. The prevalence studies that met our criteria for consideration used either the DISC or DAWBA diagnostic interviews. Prevalence rates of DSM diagnoses ranged from 9.7 to 50.6% in cross-sectional prevalence studies and 8.8% at age 11 to 19.6% at age 15 in a longitudinal study of a birth cohort. In the only direct cross-cultural comparison of prevalence rates for diverse diagnoses, the prevalence was 9.7% for a British population-based sample versus 12.7% for a school-based sample in a Brazilian municipality. A comparison of diagnoses made by U.K. and U.S. psychiatrists from the same clinical case information revealed low levels of agreement, indicating cultural differences in diagnostic practices even when psychiatrists received training in the diagnostic systems, spoke the same language, and used the same information.

The following methodological differences among studies were identified: differences in sampling procedures; the ages of the children who were assessed; the use of single informants versus various ways of using multiple informants; the number of diagnoses assessed; the diagnostic criteria; and the analytic methods, especially with respect to how data were weighted in order to estimate prevalence rates.

Based on what has been found so far, multicultural studies of prevalence rates of diagnostically based disorders might be advanced by (1) quantifying the assessment of diagnostic criteria, (2) separating diagnostic and impairment criteria in order to avoid confounding them, and (3) using more uniform procedures for sampling and diagnostic assessment. Although it may be unrealistic to expect new studies to incorporate everything that is needed for precise comparisons of prevalence rates across multiple cultures, the research to date provides a foundation on which to build.

CHAPTER 8

Multicultural Findings
on Correlates and Comorbidity
of Diagnostically Based Disorders

In Chapter 7 we reviewed multicultural findings on the prevalence of disorders defined in terms of standardized diagnostic interviews. In this chapter we present findings on the correlates and comorbidity of disorders defined in terms of standardized diagnostic interviews. As we saw in Chapter 7, rigorous cross-cultural comparisons between prevalence estimates were limited by the paucity of studies in which the same standardized procedures were applied to representative samples from multiple cultures. The paucity of studies in which the same standardized procedures were used also limits comparisons of correlates and comorbidity found for diagnostically based disorders.

Some potentially informative studies have been done with samples that are not fully representative of particular cultures. For example, studies of etiological factors and the effects of interventions have understandably used samples chosen for having high levels of particular problems. Because referral routes, care systems, accessibility, funding contingencies, and attitudes toward problems may differ among cultures, numerous factors can differentially affect the selection of people to be studied. Nevertheless, if standardized assessment procedures reveal similarities between people in different cultures, the correlates and comorbidity that are found to be similar in different cultures warrant considerable confidence, despite possible differences in selective factors. Although our criteria for studies of correlates of diagnoses are consistent with the criteria specified in Chapter 7 for prevalence studies, we did not require the samples reviewed in this chapter to be representative of larger populations.

DEMOGRAPHIC CORRELATES
OF DIAGNOSTICALLY BASED DISORDERS

Table 8.1 summarizes 10 studies that we identified as being consistent with the criteria stated in Chapter 7 and that reported associations of diagnostically based disorders with demographic variables. All studies listed in Table 8.1 used versions of the DISC with general population samples, although not all samples were selected to be representative of the entire population of a particular culture. For example, the Cohen, Cohen, Kasen, et al. (1993), Fergusson, Horwood, and Lynskey (1993), and McGee et al. (1992) studies assessed longitudinal general population samples, whereas the Bird et al. (2001) sample was from the MECA study of children selected by various means in four metropolitan areas of Puerto Rico and the United States, as described in Chapter 7. The studies differed greatly with respect to the number of diagnoses assessed. To provide some comparability across studies, Table 8.1 indicates results for any diagnosis. That is, if a child met criteria for any diagnosis included in the study, the study's authors counted the child as positive in analyses of associations with the demographic variables. Conversely, children who met criteria for none of the diagnoses made in the study were counted as negative.

DEMOGRAPHIC VARIABLES

As Table 8.1 shows, at least two studies reported testing the following demographic variables as possible correlates of diagnoses: gender, age, parents' marital status, SES, and urbanicity (i.e., urban vs. rural residence).

Gender Differences

All 10 studies tested gender effects. Although we might expect gender effects to be fairly consistent across studies, this was not the case. The following significant gender differences were found for "any diagnosis": More boys than girls received diagnoses in four studies that were done in Australia, Puerto Rico, Switzerland, and the United States;

TABLE 8.1. Demographic Correlates of DISC DSM Diagnoses in Different Cultures

Study	Culture	N^c	Ages studied	Age[d]	Gender[e]	Parents' marital[f]	SES[g]	Urbanicity[h]
						Demographic correlates		
Bird et al. (1988, 1989)	Puerto Rico	Stage 1 = 777 Stage 2 = 386	4–16	NS	B	NS	L	NA
Bird et al. (2001)[a]	San Juan, Puerto Rico, and three eastern U.S. areas	1,210	9–17	O	B	NA	NA	NA
Breton et al. (1999)	Quebec, Canada	2,400	6–14	Y	G (ages 12–14)	NA	NA	NS
Canino et al. (2004)	Puerto Rico	1,886	4–17	NS	NS	UM	NS	U
Cohen, Cohen, Kasen, et al. (1993)	Upstate New York	776	10–20	NS	NS	NA	NA	NA

Study	Location	N	Age					
Fergusson et al. (1993)	Christchurch, New Zealand	961	15	NA	G	NA	NA	NA
McGee et al. (1992)	Dunedin, New Zealand	750 750	11 15	O	B (age 11) G (age 15)	NA NA	NA NA	NA NA
Sawyer et al. (2001)[b]	Australia	3,597	6–17	Y	B	UM	L	NA
Steinhausen et al. (1998)	Zurich, Switzerland	Stage 1 = 1,964 Stage 2 = 379	6–17	Y	B	NA	NS	NS
Verhulst et al. (1997)	Netherlands	Stage 1 = 853 Stage 2 = 274	13–18	NA	NS	NA	NA	NA

Note. NA, not assessed; NS, no significant association. Significant effects are shown for associations of demographic variables with total prevalence rate for all diagnoses assessed. All were based on versions of the DISC, in some cases supplemented by other data.

[a]Bird et al. (2001) included only CD and ODD.

[b]Sawyer et al. (2001) included only depressive disorder, CD, and ADHD.

[c]For two-stage studies, *N*s are listed for Stage 1 screening and Stage 2 diagnostic interviews with at least one respondent.

[d]O, Significantly more older children met criteria for any diagnosis; Y, significantly more younger children met criteria for any diagnosis.

[e]B, Significantly more boys met criteria for any diagnosis; G, significantly more girls met criteria for any diagnosis.

[f]UM, Significantly more children of unmarried parents met criteria for any diagnosis (unmarried = never married, divorced, separated).

[g]L, Significantly more lower-SES children met criteria for any diagnosis.

[h]U, Significantly more urban children met criteria for any diagnosis.

more girls than boys received diagnoses in two studies that were done in New Zealand and Quebec; one study in New Zealand found that higher proportions of boys received diagnoses at age 11 but higher proportions of girls received diagnoses at age 15; and the proportion of boys and girls receiving diagnoses did not differ significantly in three studies done in the Netherlands, New York, and Puerto Rico.

The tests of gender effects were, of course, complicated by differences in the ages spanned, the diagnoses that were assessed, the use of impairment criteria, the sources of data (parent, teacher, and/or child), how data were aggregated from different sources, and other factors. When gender differences were analyzed for specific DSM diagnoses at different ages, a fairly consistent finding was that proportionately more girls than boys received depressive diagnoses in adolescence, but not necessarily at younger ages (Breton et al., 1999; Cohen, Cohen, Kasen, et al., 1993; Fergusson et al., 1993). At most ages, proportionately more boys than girls received diagnoses of ADHD (Bird et al., 1988; Breton et al., 1999; Canino et al., 2004; Cohen, Cohen, Kasen, et al., 1993; Fergusson et al., 1993; Sawyer et al., 2001; Verhulst et al., 1997). Additional analyses of the Australian data (Sawyer et al., 2001) revealed interactions between gender and correlates of the ADHD subtypes: Boys with the hyperactive–impulsive and combined types of ADHD were more impaired than girls with these types of ADHD, but boys and girls with the inattentive type of ADHD did not differ in impairment (Graetz, Sawyer, & Baghurst, 2005). Proportionately more boys also received diagnoses of ODD or CD in several studies (Bird et al., 1988; Bird et al., 2001; Breton et al., 1999; Canino et al., 2004; Cohen, Cohen, Kasen, et al., 1993). However, studies in Australia and the Netherlands did not find significantly higher rates of depressive disorders for adolescent girls than boys (Sawyer et al., 2001; Verhulst et al., 1997). Furthermore, studies in Zurich and the Netherlands did not find higher rates of ADHD for boys than girls (Steinhausen et al., 1998; Verhulst et al., 1997). And studies in New Zealand and Zurich did not find higher rates of ODD/CD for boys than girls (Fergusson et al., 1993; McGee et al., 1992; Steinhausen et al., 1998).

Age Differences

In the eight studies that tested age effects, three found that proportionately more younger children received diagnoses, two found that proportionately more older children received diagnoses, and three did not find significant age effects. As with gender effects, the tests of age effects were complicated by many potentially relevant variations among the studies. When age effects were analyzed for specific DSM diagnoses, studies in Puerto Rico and Zurich found depressive disorders to be significantly more prevalent in middle adolescence than at younger ages (Bird et al., 1988; Canino et al., 2004; Steinhausen et al., 1998). However, findings of significantly higher prevalence of depressive disorders among young boys than for other groups in the Quebec and Australian studies argued against concluding that depressive disorders consistently increase with age (Breton et al., 1999; Sawyer et al., 2001).

Diagnoses of ADHD were significantly more prevalent at younger than older ages in some studies (Breton et al., 1999; Cohen, Cohen, Kasen,et al., 1993) but not others (Canino et al., 2004; Steinhausen et al., 1998). When Bird et al. (1988) compared rates at different ages, they found that the rates for ages 4–5 were significantly lower than the rates for ages 6–11 and 12–16, which did not differ significantly from each other. This finding suggests that school attendance increased the proportion of children who met DSM criteria for ADHD, probably because requirements for attention to school tasks make attention problems more salient.

Parental Marital Status, SES, and Urbanicity

Of the three studies that tested associations of parents' marital status with any diagnosis, two found higher prevalence rates for children whose parents were not currently married to each other (Canino et al., 2004; Sawyer et al., 2001). However, one study found no significant association between diagnoses and parents' marital status (Bird et al., 1989).

Of the four studies that tested associations between SES and any diagnosis, one in Puerto Rico and one in Australia found significantly higher prevalence rates for lower, rather than higher, SES levels (Bird, Gould, Yager, Staghezza, & Canino, 1989; Sawyer et al., 2001). Yet a different study in Puerto Rico and a study in Zurich found no significant SES effects (Canino et al., 2004; Steinhausen, 1998).

Studies in Quebec and Zurich that tested associations of urban versus rural residence with any diagnosis found no significant associations (Breton et al., 1999; Steinhausen et al., 1998). However, a study in Puerto Rico reported a significantly higher prevalence rate for any diagnosis among urban children (Canino et al., 2004).

Implications of the Demographic Findings

The 10 studies summarized in Table 8.1 tested demographic correlates of DSM diagnoses made from versions of the DISC for 12,619 children. Two studies were done in New Zealand, two in North America, two in Puerto Rico, one in Puerto Rico and the United States, and one each in Australia, the Netherlands, and Switzerland. For the relatively straightforward demographic variables of gender, age, parents' marital status, SES, and urbanicity, the results were quite inconsistent across studies. Inconsistency is to be expected when the studies varied in so many ways, in addition to differences that might be associated with culture. However, all the samples were from "Western" cultures with similar religious, economic, educational, and political systems where European languages were spoken.

One way to determine whether methodological differences between studies accounted for much of the variation in the results shown in Table 8.1 might be to compare the results for studies in a single culture. This can be done by comparing results for the two Puerto Rican samples with each other (Bird et al., 1988, 1989; Canino et al., 2004) and for the two New Zealand samples with each other (Fergusson et al., 1993; McGee et al., 1992). It might also make sense to compare the results for the Australian sample with the results for the U.S. sample (Cohen, Cohen, Kasen, et al., 1993; Sawyer et al., 2001), because reports of children's problems have been found to be very highly correlated between Australian and U.S. samples (Crijnen et al. 1997; Rescorla et al., 2006a, 2006b, in press; Verhulst et al., 2003). However, even when research teams were led by the same people, and they tested the same variables over similar ages in Puerto Rican probability samples, the findings in Table 8.1 differed for gender, parents' marital status, and SES (Bird et al., 1988, 1989; Canino et al., 2004). Although both Puerto Rican studies found nonsignificant effects of age, only the Canino et al. (2004) study tested effects of urbanicity.

Comparisons between the two New Zealand studies are limited by the assessment of only 15-year-olds by Fergusson et al. (1993) and 11- and 15-year-olds by McGee et al. (1992), plus a lack of tests of the effects of marital status, SES, and urbanicity. For 15-year-olds, the two studies agreed in finding a higher prevalence for any diagnosis among girls than boys, but comparisons with other cultures are precluded by the lack of studies reporting data specifically for 15-year-olds. Comparisons between the Australian and U.S. samples are limited by major differences in design, sampling procedures, age ranges, and the diagnoses assessed (Cohen, Cohen, Kasen, et al., 1993; Sawyer et al., 2001). It should therefore not be surprising that the Australian and U.S. studies reported different gender and age effects.

In Chapter 7 we described use of the DAWBA to make DSM-IV diagnoses in general population samples from Britain and the municipality of Taubaté, Brazil. Although not directly comparable to the DISC studies summarized in Table 8.1, associations of DSM-IV diagnoses with age and gender were reported for the 1,251 Taubaté 7- to 14-year-olds assessed with the DAWBA (Fleitlich-Bilyk & Goodman, 2004). No significant associations were found between age or gender and the presence of any diagnosis from the 14 diagnostic categories analyzed. However, significantly more 11- to 14-year-olds than 7- to 10-year-olds received diagnoses of "any depressive disorder," and significantly more boys than girls received diagnoses of "any ADHD disorder" and "any oppositional–conduct disorder."

MENTAL HEALTH SERVICE CORRELATES

Several studies listed in Table 8.1 reported data on receipt of mental health services. However, only the two Puerto Rican studies reported the percentage of children with and without DSM diagnoses who had received services during a specified period preceding the diagnostic interviews (Bird et al., 1993; Canino et al., 2004). These two studies were done on different islandwide probability samples, both with high completion rates. For 222 9- to 16-year-olds, Bird et al. (1993) reported that 13.5% of those who obtained DSM-III diagnoses on the DISC had received mental health services in the preceding 6 months, compared to 6.8% of those who did not obtain DSM-III diagnoses. No statistical test of this difference was reported.

For 1,879 4- to 17-year-olds, Canino et al. (2004) reported that 25.7% of those who obtained DSM-IV diagnoses had received services in the preceding year. Of children who obtained CGAS scores indicating impairment (i.e., CGAS < 69), 39.5% of those without DSM-IV diagnoses had received services, whereas 49.6% with CGAS scores < 69 and DSM-IV diagnoses had received services. Of children who obtained neither DSM-IV diagnoses nor CGAS scores < 69, 9.7% had received services. DSM-IV diagnoses (including diagnosis-specific impairment) and CGAS scores < 69 were each significantly associated with receipt of services. However, CGAS scores < 69 were more strongly associated with receipt of services (OR = 3.9) than were DSM-IV diagnoses (OR = 1.8). Both Puerto Rican studies thus showed that children who obtain DISC-based DSM diagnoses are more likely to have received services than those who do not receive diagnoses. The Puerto Rican studies also showed that other factors, such as impairment not assessed by the DISC, are important as well.

LONGITUDINAL CORRELATES OF DIAGNOSTICALLY BASED DISORDERS

The correlates of diagnostically based disorders reviewed thus far have been cross-sectional. Two of the studies listed in Table 8.1 reported longitudinal analyses of associations between DSM diagnoses made from versions of the DISC and subsequent diagnoses obtained by the same children. Using the upstate New York sample assessed for the Cohen, Cohen, Kasen, et al. (1993) study listed in Table 8.1, Cohen, Cohen, and Brook (1993) analyzed associations between six DSM-III-R diagnoses that were made from mother and child interviews when the 734 children were 9–18 years old and diagnoses that were made 2½ years later. For agreement between Time 1 and Time 2 diagnoses of ADHD, CD, overanxious disorder, ODD, and alcohol abuse, modest 2½-year stabilities were indicated by kappas ranging from .20 to .44 (mean = .34 for kappas computed separately for mild, moderate, and severe levels of each diagnosis). The association between Time 1 and Time 2 diagnoses of major depressive disorder was so weak that it was described as "not persistent" (p. 871), and no kappa was reported.

In the Dunedin study listed in Table 8.1, McGee et al. (1992) reported DSM-III diagnoses made from parents' questionnaire reports plus DISC interviews of 750 adolescents at ages 11 and 15. Analyses of 10 diagnostic categories showed that 42% of adolescents who received any diagnosis at age 11 received at least one diagnosis at age 15, although not necessarily the same diagnosis. Reflecting an increase in the overall prevalence from 8.8% for any diagnosis at age 11 to 19.6% for any diagnosis at age 15, 81% of the adolescents receiving any diagnosis at age 15 had received no diagnosis at age 11. Although the samples were too small to test predictive relations between specific diagnoses, McGee et al. (1992) computed ORs for predictive relations from age 11 internalizing (anxiety, depression) and externalizing (CD, ODD) disorders to age 15 internalizing and externalizing disorders, separately for each gender. For boys, age 11 internalizing disorders unexpectedly predicted age 15 externalizing disorders but not internalizing disorders. For girls, age 11 internalizing disorders significantly predicted age 15 internalizing disorders, but age 15 externalizing disorders were not predicted by age 11 disorders of any kind. For boys, age 11 externalizing disorders predicted only age 15 externalizing disorders. Thus, for boys, age 15 externalizing disorders were preceded by *both* internalizing and externalizing disorders. Conversely, for girls, age 15 externalizing disorders were preceded by *neither* internalizing nor externalizing disorders. However, for girls only, age 15 internalizing disorders were preceded by age 11 internalizing disorders.

Based on a subsequent reassessment of the Dunedin sample at age 18, Feehan, McGee, and Williams (1993) reported predictive relations from age 15 to age 18 diagnoses for 890 adolescents who were interviewed at both ages. The age 15 diagnoses were based on the DSM-III version of the DISC, whereas the age 18 diagnoses were based on a DSM-III-R version of the adult DIS that was modified to make it consistent with the DISC that had been used at age 15. Feehan et al. (1993)

found that age 15 diagnoses of ADHD, simple phobia, and ODD did not significantly predict any age 18 diagnoses. Age 15 diagnoses of CD, depressive disorders, and anxiety disorders other than simple phobia did predict the presence of diagnoses at age 18, but not necessarily the same diagnoses.

COMORBIDITY AMONG DIAGNOSTICALLY BASED DISORDERS

In the preceding sections we considered various correlates of diagnoses made from interviews that were intended to operationalize the diagnoses. In this section we consider diagnoses made from the interviews as correlates of other diagnoses made from the same interviews. Associations among diagnoses began to attract attention when many children were found to obtain multiple diagnoses from interviews for operationalizing DSM-III (Costello et al., 1982). The apparent co-occurrence of multiple disorders in the same individual is called *comorbidity*. Although it may not be surprising that some people have more than one disorder, the rates of comorbidity among DSM-III diagnoses of children were amazingly high. For example, two studies reported 96% comorbidity between ODD and CD, and a third study reported 84% comorbidity between ODD and CD (Faraone, Biederman, Keenan, & Tsuang, 1991; Spitzer, Davies, & Barkley, 1990; Walker et al., 1991).

The findings of very high comorbidity among DSM-III disorders unleashed a flood of publications on comorbidity. The comorbidity among diagnoses prompted changes in DSM criteria, including the addition of rules whereby certain diagnoses preempted others. For example, DSM-III-R specified that ODD should not be diagnosed if the criteria for CD were met. ODD should also not be diagnosed if the criterial behaviors for ODD "occur exclusively during the course of a psychotic disorder, Dysthymia, or a Major Depressive, Hypomanic, or Manic Episode" (American Psychiatric Association, 1987, p. 58). Nevertheless, many children who meet criteria for one DSM diagnosis are still found to meet criteria for additional diagnoses.

If we could be certain that each diagnosis truly indicates a different disorder, findings that certain disorders tend to occur together might be very informative. For example, the frequent co-occurrence of certain disorders might indicate that they have particular risk or etiological factors in common. The frequent co-occurrence of certain disorders might also indicate that one disorder causes or increases the risk for the other disorder. On the other hand, if many children meet criteria for a particular combination of disorders, the criteria should be reexamined to determine whether apparent comorbidity is an artifact of overlapping or closely related criteria. In any event, to accurately determine the degree to which particular disorders really tend to co-occur, we need to assess samples of children that are not biased by factors that could influence comorbidity findings, as discussed in the following sections.

Berkson's Bias

A particularly important type of bias occurs in the tabulation of co-occurring disorders among people who are referred for treatment of one or more of the disorders under study. Known as *Berkson's bias* (Berkson, 1946), this pertains to the tendency of people referred for services to have higher rates of comorbidity than nonreferred or general population samples. Berkson's bias results from the fact that people with more than one disorder are more likely to seek help or to be referred for help than people who have only one disorder. This fact is based on another fact: that the probability of referral for people with multiple disorders is a function of the combined probabilities of referral for each disorder taken separately.

As an example, if X is the probability of referral for people who have Disorder 1, and Y is the probability of referral for people who have Disorder 2, then the probability of referral for people having both 1 and 2 is $(X + Y) - XY$. (The probability of truly having both Disorder 1 and 2 is XY, which must be subtracted from $X + Y$ to avoid counting comorbid disorders twice.) The higher probability of referral for people who have both Disorder 1 and Disorder 2 than for people who have only one of the disorders inflates the observed comorbidity rate above the rate that would be found in general population samples, where fewer people would have both Disorder 1 and Disorder 2 (Caron & Rutter, 1991). Furthermore, increased distress resulting from multiple disorders may also increase the probability of referral beyond what is predicted by combining the independent probabilities of referral for each disorder. Lilienfeld (2003) has called this additional inflation factor in comorbidity among referred people the "straw that breaks the camel's back" (p. 286).

Numerous studies have reported comorbidity in clinical samples. For example, Youngstrom, Findling, and Calabrese (2003) reported comorbidity among youths seen at a clinic specializing in mood and disruptive behavior disorders. Although the findings for the Youngstrom et al. clinic sample may be informative, they cannot tell us the typical level of comorbidity among disorders, because youths with multiple disorders (i.e., comorbid disorders) were more likely to be referred to the clinic than youths with only one disorder. Research has demonstrated Berkson's bias in terms of higher comorbidity rates among a variety of children's problems in clinical than in nonclinical samples (Biederman, Newcorn, & Sprich, 1991; McConaughy & Achenbach, 1994).

Biases Caused by Unidirectional Computation of Comorbidity Rates

If we want to know the comorbidity of CD with ADHD, it might seem logical to determine the percentage of individuals diagnosed as having ADHD who are also diagnosed as having CD. For example, suppose that we administer the DISC to 1,000 youths and find that 100 of them qualify for a diagnosis of ADHD. We also find that 50 of the youths with ADHD diagnoses qualify for a diagnosis of CD. Can we conclude that the comorbidity between diagnoses of ADHD and CD is 50/100 = 50%? This is a typical way to compute comorbidity. However, we would be right to conclude that there is 50% comorbidty between ADHD and CD *only if* exactly 100 of the 1,000 youths obtained diagnoses of CD. Why is this? Suppose that 150 of the 1,000 youths obtained diagnoses of CD, but only 50 of the 150 youths with CD obtained diagnoses of ADHD. If we started with the 150 CD diagnoses and found that only 50 were comorbid with diagnoses of ADHD, we might conclude that comorbidity between CD and ADHD is 33%, instead of the 50% rate obtained when we started with diagnoses of ADHD. However, because only 33% of the youths with diagnoses of CD obtained diagnoses of ADHD, we would be wrong to conclude that ADHD is 50% comorbid with CD among youths who obtain diagnoses of CD.

What should we do about the discrepant comorbidity rates obtained for a pair of disorders having different base rates (e.g., ADHD having a base rate of 100/1,000 = 10%, and CD having a base rate of 150/1,000 = 15%)? To resolve the discrepancy, McConaughy and Achenbach (1994) proposed that comorbidities be computed *bidirectionally*. This is easily done by computing the mean of the comorbidity rates computed for Disorder 1 with Disorder 2 and Disorder 2 with Disorder 1. In our hypothetical example, the 50% comorbidity rate for ADHD with CD is averaged with the 33% rate for CD with ADHD to obtain a bidirectional comorbidity of 41.5% between ADHD and CD.

CRITERIA FOR STUDIES OF COMORBIDITY

In reviewing findings on comorbidity, we sought to avoid Berkson's bias as well as biases caused by unidirectional computation of comorbidity. We did this by giving priority to studies that assessed samples of general populations and that reported data that enabled us to compute bidirectional comorbidity. Unlike our criteria for studies of the prevalence and correlates of diagnoses, we did not require a minimum sample size of 300. Although all the studies that qualified according to the other criteria did report some data for at least 300 children, the fact that comorbidity could only be computed for children who obtained diagnoses in certain target categories meant that only the subgroups who obtained diagnoses were relevant for estimating comorbidity.

FINDINGS ON COMORBIDITY
AMONG DIAGNOSTICALLY BASED DISORDERS

We first consider comorbidity that was computed in terms of bidirectional percentages. We then consider comorbidity that was computed in terms of ORs.

Comorbidities in Terms of Bidirectional Percentages

Table 8.2 displays the total percentage of cases receiving multiple diagnoses, plus bidirectional comorbidities that were found for major diagnostic categories in general population samples. The data reported by Bird et al. (1988) and Bird et al. (1993) were from the same Puerto Rican Child Psychiatry Epidemiological Study (PRCPES). However, Bird et al. (1988) computed comorbidities for the entire sample of 4- to 16-year-olds who obtained any diagnoses, whereas Bird et al. (1993) computed comorbidities for the 9- to 16-year-olds who obtained any diagnoses according to either the DISC-C or DISC-P. By looking at the first line in Table 8.2, you can see in the column headed "*N* of cases" that Bird et al. (1988) reported on 215 "cases," that is, 4- to 16-year-olds who obtained DSM diagnoses. In the column headed "Total % comorbid," you can see that 46% of the 215 cases obtained multiple diagnoses. By looking at the second row in Table 8.2, you can see that Bird et al. (1993) reported on 159 cases (many of which were included in the 215 cases reported on by Bird et al., 1988).

Because Bird et al. (1988, 1993) and Steinhausen et al. (1998) reported unidirectional percentages of comorbidity, we averaged the two unidirectional percentages for each pair of diagnostic categories in order to obtain the bidirectional percentage for that pair of categories. For example, Bird et al. (1988) reported that 17.0% of the children who obtained ADHD diagnoses also obtained affective diagnoses, and that 30.7% of the children who obtained affective diagnoses also obtained

TABLE 8.2. Percentage of Cases with Comorbid Diagnoses Computed Bidirectionally

Study	Culture	N of cases	Ages studied	Total % comorbid[a]	ADHD × Aff %	ADHD × Anx %	ADHD × CD/ODD %	Aff × Anx %	Aff × CD/ODD %	Anx × CD/ODD %
Bird et al. (1988)	Puerto Rico	215	4–16	46	24	22	49	24	38	37
Bird et al. (1993)	Puerto Rico	159	9–16	63	37	36	64	34	50	59
Steinhausen et al. (1998)	Zurich	125	6–17	40	NA	NA	NA	56	58[b]	72[b]

Note. NA, not assessed; Aff, affective disorders; Anx, anxiety disorders.
[a]Total % comorbid reflects cases that received more than one diagnosis.
[b]Steinhausen et al. (1998) combined ADHD with CD/ODD for computation of comorbidity with affective and anxiety disorders.

ADHD diagnoses. To compute the bidirectional comorbidity, we averaged $17.0 + 30.7 = 47.7/2 = 23.85$ and rounded to 24% in the column headed ADHD $\times$ Aff % in Table 8.2. Because Steinhausen et al. combined ADHD diagnoses with CD and ODD diagnoses into a category of disruptive disorders, the results for ADHD are merged with the results for CD/ODD in the columns headed CD/ODD.

As Table 8.2 shows, the total percentage of cases with multiple diagnoses ranged from 40% of the 125 6- to 17-year-olds in the Steinhausen et al. (1998) study to 63% of the 159 9- to 16-year-olds in the Bird et al. (1993) study. For affective $\times$ anxiety diagnoses, which are the only paired diagnoses that are comparable between the two Bird studies and the Steinhausen study, the comorbidity ranged from 26 to 56%. Across all paired categories, the comorbidity ranged from 22% for ADHD $\times$ affective diagnoses among Puerto Rican 4- to 16-year-olds to 72% for anxiety $\times$ CD/ODD/ADHD diagnoses among Zurich 6- to 17-year-olds. Numerous factors in addition to culture could affect the actual rates of comorbidity. However, the overall findings indicate that many of the children in general population samples who qualify for a particular diagnosis also qualify for other diagnoses.

Comorbidities in Terms of ORs

In addition to the few studies that have reported comparable comorbidities in terms of percentages, others have reported ORs for comorbidity between particular pairs of diagnoses. Although ORs are useful statistics, their magnitude can be strongly affected by the proportion of individuals who receive each of the dichotomous classifications. For example, a very large OR can be obtained in a sample where 1% of individuals are classified as "yes" and 99% are classified as "no" on one variable, and 1% are classified as "yes" and 99% are classified as "no" on the other variable. The possible ORs would be much smaller if 50% of the individuals were classified as "yes" and "no" on the first variable and 50% were also classified as "yes" and "no" on the second variable. Because the size of ORs can vary so much as a function of the percentage of individuals classified in each way, the absolute magnitude of any OR is less informative than whether the confidence interval (CI) around the OR includes 1.00. If the CI does include 1.00, it means that the OR does not deviate from chance, because the odds of the "yes–yes" combination for the two variables equal the odds of the "yes–no" combination (i.e., the odds of the two combinations are 1.00 to 1.00).

The lack of comparability between ORs computed on different data precludes averaging ORs unless mathematical transformations are applied for meta-analytic purposes (Lipsey & Wilson, 2001). It is also difficult to draw generalizable conclusions about the precise magnitude of comorbidities across the different studies that have reported ORs. However, for various general population samples, substantial ORs have been reported for comorbidity between various DSM diagnoses made from the DISC, the DAWBA, and the CAPA (Costello, Mustillo, Erkanli, Keeler, & Angold, 2003; Fergusson et al., 1993; Fleitlich-Bilyk & Goodman, 2004; Ford et al., 2003). In addition, Angold, Costello, and Erkanli (1999) tabulated ORs from several studies that reported comorbidities among the same four DSM diagnostic categories for which we displayed comorbidity rates in Table 8.2.

The studies reviewed by Angold et al. used a variety of procedures to make DSM diagnoses, including the DISC-based diagnoses reported in studies that we reviewed in the present chapter (Bird et al., 1993; Cohen, Cohen, & Brook, 1993; Cohen, Cohen, Kasen, et al., 1993; Fergusson et al., 1993). However, the data used by Angold et al. for these studies were not necessarily from the publications that we reviewed. Furthermore, several of the studies included in the Angold et al. tabulations would not have met our criteria, because they were unpublished, the samples were too small or not representative of general populations, or they did not use diagnostic interviews for which data have been reported for more than one culture. Moreover, many of the ORs were from repeated assessments of the same samples. The exact results must therefore be viewed with considerable caution. The ORs cannot be assumed to be generalizable to any particular populations.

Most ORs reported by Angold et al. showed significant comorbidity between each pairing of ADHD, CD/ODD, depression, and anxiety diagnoses. Angold et al. also computed the median of the ORs for each pairing of the four diagnostic categories. However, Angold et al. did not report the number of cases or corrections for effects that may have been significant by chance. Consequently, the specific ORs are not apt to be generalizable. The largest median OR was 10.7 for comorbidity of ADHD with CD/ODD, followed by median ORs of 8.2 for depression with anxiety, 6.6 for CD/ODD with depression, and 5.5 for ADHD with depression. The 95% CI for the OR of 10.7 overlapped with the CIs for the other ORs. The overlapping CIs meant that the ORs of 10.7, 8.2, 6.6, and 5.5 did not differ significantly from each other. The lowest median ORs were 3.1 for CD/ODD with anxiety and 3.0 for ADHD with anxiety, indicating substantial comorbidity even for these combinations of very different kinds of disorders. The CI for CD/ODD with anxiety overlapped the CIs for ADHD with depression, ADHD with anxiety, and CD/ODD with depression, meaning that the ORs for these four pairings did not differ significantly from each other. The CI for ADHD with anxiety also overlapped the CI for ADHD with depression.

Far more precise data for many more independent and representative samples are needed to draw conclusions about the typical degree of comorbidity between different combinations of diagnoses. Nevertheless, the Angold et al. findings are certainly consistent with conclusions that comorbidity among the major DSM categories of child diagnoses is very high. The broad confidence intervals around the Angold et al. ORs and the large differences among the percentages shown in Table 8.2 for each kind of comorbidity indicate that comorbidity estimates are also highly variable among studies.

SUMMARY

This chapter presented findings on correlates and comorbidity of disorders defined in terms of diagnostic interviews. Ten studies were identified as providing usable data on correlates of diagnostically based disorders in general population samples of at least 300 children. Because the studies differed greatly with respect to the specific diagnoses and the criteria that were used to make them, we compared correlates found for children classified as having any diagnosis in a particular study versus children classified as having no diagnosis. At least two of the 10 studies tested associations of diagnoses with the following demographic variables: gender, age, parents' marital status, SES, and urbanicity. The findings varied too much to support firm conclusions about whether any of the demographic variables are consistently associated with elevated rates of DSM diagnoses. Where sufficient data were reported for specific diagnostic categories, a fairly consistent finding across cultures was that proportionately more adolescent girls received depressive diagnoses, whereas proportionately more boys received diagnoses of ADHD and CD/ODD. There were also tendencies for depressive disorders to be most prevalent in middle adolescence and for ADHD to be most prevalent during the primary school years. However, differences among the age ranges studied and other methodological variations precluded generalizable conclusions about associations with age, even for samples from similar cultures.

Receipt of mental health services during specified periods preceding the diagnostic interviews was analyzed as a correlate of diagnoses only in two Puerto Rican studies. Both found higher rates of mental health service usage by children who received diagnoses than by children who did not, as expected. However, in the Puerto Rican study that assessed impairment in addition to diagnoses, service usage was more strongly associated with CGAS impairment scores < 69 than with DSM diagnoses.

Two longitudinal studies have reported significant associations between some childhood diagnoses and diagnoses 2½–3 years later. However, the associations were often between different categories of diagnoses at Time 1 versus Time 2, such as between Time 1 internalizing diagnoses and Time 2 externalizing diagnoses.

Since it was discovered in the 1980s that children who meet criteria for one DSM diagnosis often meet criteria for additional DSM diagnoses, many publications have addressed the issue of comorbidity. However, to determine the degree to which particular disorders really tend to co-occur, comorbidity must be assessed without distortion by factors such as Berkson's bias or unidirectional computation of comorbidity. Based on the very few studies that have reported adequate data, it can be concluded that comorbidity among DSM diagnoses of childhood disorders is high. Unfortunately, the estimates from different studies differ too much to support conclusions about the typical rates of comorbidity between even the most common diagnoses.

CHAPTER 9

Comparisons of Empirically Based and Diagnostically Based Findings

In Chapters 2 and 3 we presented the empirically based and diagnostically based approaches to psychopathology. We then presented samples of multicultural findings obtained with the empirically based approach in Chapters 4 through 6 and with the diagnostically based approach in Chapters 7 and 8. In this chapter, we highlight and compare the main findings from the two approaches.

MAIN FINDINGS FROM THE EMPIRICALLY BASED APPROACH

The primary sources of multicultural findings from the empirically based approach have been the ASEBA, Conners, and SDQ rating forms completed by parents, teachers, and youths.

Psychometric Findings

For the empirically based scales presented in Chapter 2, the alpha coefficients averaged .90 for the ASEBA scales, .87 for the Conners scales, and .75 for the SDQ scales. The test–retest rs averaged .90 for the ASEBA scales, .73 for the Conners scales, and .69 for the SDQ scales. The lower mean alpha for the SDQ may result from the fact that the SDQ scales have fewer items than most of the ASEBA and Conners scales. The lower test–retest rs for the Conners and SDQ may reflect longer test–test intervals than were used for the ASEBA scales.

Cross-informant rs averaged .78 between mothers' and fathers' CBCL/6–18 ratings and .62 between TRF ratings by pairs of teachers. Cross-informant rs were not available for these combinations of raters on the Conners or SDQ. Between parent and teacher ratings, the mean r was .31 for ASEBA scales, .32 for Conners scales, and .42 for SDQ scales. Between parent and youth ratings, the mean r was .51 for ASEBA scales and .45 for SDQ scales. Between teacher and youth ratings, the mean r was .21 for ASEBA scales and .30 for SDQ scales. Cross-informant rs were not available for youths' self-ratings on the Conners scales.

Validity Findings

Chapter 2 presented evidence for the content validity of ASEBA problem items in terms of the ways in which the items were formulated and selected. International experts' identification of particular ASEBA problem items as being very consistent with particular DSM-IV diagnostic categories has supported the content validity of those items in relation to DSM-IV. The criterion-related validity of the ASEBA items and scales has been supported by strong associations of scale scores with referral status after controlling for demographic variables in several cultures, according to both quantitative and categorical analyses.

The construct validity of ASEBA scales has been supported by significant associations with many other variables. These include DSM diagnoses, scores on scales of the Conners, BASC, and SDQ instruments, genetic and biochemical factors, developmental course, and long-term outcomes. The construct validity of the ASEBA syndromes has also been supported by findings of configural invariance in CFA of problem scores from many cultures, as detailed in Chapter 6 (Ivanova et al., 2006a, 2006b, 2006c).

Because the main use of the Conners scales is for assessment of ADHD, inclusion of paraphrased versions of the 18 symptom criteria for DSM-IV ADHD implies content validity for assessment of ADHD, as defined by DSM-IV. Criterion-related validity has been supported by findings that scores on the Conners scales discriminated significantly between children who were diagnosed as having ADHD versus those who were not.

In addition to significant associations with ADHD diagnoses, which are the main foci of the Conners scales, Chapter 2 summarized findings on construct validity in terms of significant associations between Conners scores and scores from other assessment instruments. The other instruments included the CBCL, TRF, and Revised Behavior Problem Checklist. Significant associations have also been reported with genetic factors and with long-term outcomes.

As reported in Chapter 2, the SDQ's content validity can be evaluated mainly in terms of its correlations with scales of the Rutter parent and teacher questionnaires, on which the SDQ is based. According to the SDQ's author (Goodman, 1997), rs averaged .84 with scores on scales of the Rutter parent questionnaire and .90 with scores on scales of the Rutter teacher questionnaire. These correlations thus indicate very similar meaning for the content of the SDQ and Rutter scales, according to parent and teacher ratings. Criterion-related validity has been indicated by significant differences between SDQ Total Difficulties scores obtained by children referred to three London mental health clinics and children participating in a pilot study for a national survey, although age, gender, ethnicity, and SES were evidently not analyzed nor controlled.

Evidence for the construct validity of SDQ scales has been reported in terms of significant associations with ICD-10 and DSM-IV diagnoses made from the DAWBA. Significant correlations have also been reported between SDQ scale scores and scores from CBCL and YSR scales.

Multicultural Findings on Distributions of Problem Scores

As we presented in Chapter 4, distributions of CBCL, TRF, and YSR problem scores have been statistically compared for many cultures. The most comprehensive comparisons have included CBCLs from 31 cultures, TRFs from 21 cultures, and YSRs from 24 cultures (Rescorla et al., 2006a, 2006b; Rescorla et al., in press). ESs for culture on the Total Problems scores were medium for the CBCL, TRF, and YSR. Total Problems scores for most cultures were within one standard deviation of the omnicultural mean (the mean of the means for all cultures). Even for cultures whose mean Total Problems scores were below or above one standard deviation of the omnicultural mean, the distributions of scores had substantial overlaps with the distributions from the other cultures. In other words, despite tendencies for Total Problems scores in some cultures to be lower or higher than in most other cultures, large proportions of children from all the cultures obtained scores within the same range. In multicultural comparisons of scores on syndromes, DSM-oriented, Internalizing, and Externalizing scales, ESs for culture were generally small to medium, with much overlap between the distributions of scores from the different cultures. Statistical interactions of culture with gender and age were negligible, indicating that gender and age differences were similar in most of the cultures analyzed.

The obtained problem scores may well have been affected by cultural factors as well as by age, gender, and vicissitudes of translation and sampling. However, the statistical analyses showed that far more of the variance in scores was accounted for by individual differences within each culture than by differences between cultures. And studies in several cultures have shown significantly elevated problem scale scores for children who were referred for mental health services and/or who met criteria for psychiatric diagnoses. Thus, despite some differences between cultures in mean scale scores, high problem scores are apt to indicate a need for help rather than merely typifying a particular culture. Of course, the meaning of a particular child's scores obtained from ratings by a particular informant should be interpreted in relation to appropriate norms and to scores obtained from other informants who know the child.

Findings for 48-item versions of the CPRS from two Sudanese cities and one Indian city were compared with findings for Canadian and American children, respectively. Sudanese problem scores for four of the five CPRS scales were significantly lower than scores reported in a previous study of Canadian children, whereas Indian scores were within one standard deviation of mean scores reported in a previous study of American children (Al-Awad & Sonuga-Barke, 2002; Rosenberg & Jani, 1995).

In the same Sudanese sample for which CPRS scores were obtained, problem scores on a 39-item version of the CTRS were found to be significantly lower than Canadian scores on four of the six scales. Using four scales scored from an earlier version of the 39-item CTRS, Luk et al. (1988) compared scores from England, Hong Kong, New Zealand, and the United States. Although not tested statistically, the problem scores were highest for the New Zealand children and lowest for the American children. Several studies have reported prevalence rates in different cultures for deviant scores on 10-item versions of the CTRS, but without statistical tests of the differences between cultures.

SDQ scores have been reported for general population samples in the United Kingdom, Finland, Germany, and other countries. Statistical comparisons of SDQ ratings by teachers yielded significantly higher Hyperactivity/Inattention scores for 7- to 8-year-olds in Portugal than in Italy or Spain (Marzocchi et al., 2004).

Multicultural Findings on Correlates of Empirically Based Scale Scores

The findings presented in Chapters 4 and 5 included many correlates of empirically based scales, as summarized next.

Gender Differences

With considerable consistency in many cultures, girls obtained higher scores than boys on Internalizing problems but lower scores than boys on Externalizing problems. The girls' higher scores on Internalizing problems became more consistent with age across cultures, whereas their lower scores on Externalizing problems became less consistent with age. Although parents and teachers rated boys significantly higher on attention problems in most cultures, boys' self-ratings of attention problems did not differ significantly from girls' self-ratings.

Age Differences

Age effects varied across parent ratings, teacher ratings, and self-ratings. In parent ratings, Internalizing scores generally increased with age, whereas Externalizing scores generally decreased with age. In teacher ratings, Internalizing scores generally increased with age, but Externalizing scores did not generally decrease with age. In self-ratings, 14- to 16-year-olds tended to report more problems than 11- to 13-year-olds on most scales.

SES Differences

In addition to the associations of empirically based scale scores with age and gender that were presented in Chapter 4, Chapter 5 presented multicultural findings on SES differences. When various measures of SES were used in very diverse cultures, higher problem scores and lower competence scores were consistently found for children from lower-SES families than for children from higher-SES families. ESs ranged from 1 to 5% for problem scores and were somewhat larger for competence scores.

Parents' Marital Status

Only a few studies have reported associations with marital status, but the results have consistently indicated lower problem scores for children from intact families than for children from divorced, single-parent, or reconstituted families. Although intact families tend to be financially more secure than single-parent families, multilevel analyses have shown that family and neighborhood SES both have independent effects on problem scores, over and above the effects of parents' marital status, per se (Kalff, Kroes, Vies, Bosma, et al., 2001; Kalff, Kroes, Vies, Hendriksen, 2001).

Diagnoses

Studies in several cultures have found that children who obtain high scores on empirically based problem scales are more likely to meet criteria for diagnoses such as ADHD that correspond to the problem scales than are children who obtain low problem scores. Significantly higher problem scores have also been found for children referred for mental health services than for nonreferred children in several cultures.

Long-Term Outcomes

Longitudinal studies in Australia, the Netherlands, and the United States have obtained similar predictive rs between initial scores on empirically based scales and subsequent scores on the same or similar scales. The Dutch and American studies also found similar predictive relations for signs of disturbance, such as referral for mental health services, suicidal behavior, substance abuse, and police contacts. Furthermore, the Dutch longitudinal study found that adult DSM diagnoses were significantly predicted by child and adolescent scores on empirically based scales.

Genetic Factors

Numerous behavior genetic studies in several cultures have reported various levels of genetic, shared environmental, and nonshared environmental effects on empirically based problem scale scores. These studies have included analyses of genetic and environmental effects associated with ratings by different informants, such as mothers, fathers, and teachers. Substantial genetic effects have been found for measures of attention problems and anxious/depressed problems. Although the Aggressive Behavior and Delinquent (Rule-Breaking) Behavior syndromes are both included in the broad Externalizing grouping, larger genetic effects have typically been found for Aggressive Behavior than for Delinquent Behavior scores. Important age differences have been found for genetic effects on some problem scales, such as substantial declines with age in genetic effects on Anxious/Depressed syndrome scores.

Immigrant Children

Scores obtained on empirically based problem scales by immigrant children have shown significant differences from the scores obtained by nonimmigrant children in the host cultures. The particular differences have varied according to whether the rating forms were completed by parents, teachers, or the children themselves. Problem scores have been associated with acculturation status and with various family characteristics, stress, and first- versus second-generation immigration status in the host country. The data obtained with the same instruments on general population samples in dozens of cultures offer many possibilities for comparing problems reported for immigrant children with problems reported for peers in both the immigrant children's cultures of origin and in the host cultures.

Multicultural Findings
on Empirically Based Patterns of Problems

In Chapter 6 we reviewed patterns of problems found in factor analyses of data from many cultures. Following studies that found varying degrees of support for the 1983 and 1991 ASEBA syndrome models in several cultures, a more comprehensive approach was taken by applying uniform CFA procedures to test the 2001 ASEBA syndrome model in CBCL data from 30 cultures, TRF data from 20 cultures, and YSR data from 23 cultures (Ivanova, 2006a, 2006b, 2006c). With a few small deviations, the 2001 eight-syndrome model was supported for all three instruments.

Factor analyses of the Conners CTRS in a few cultures have yielded support for some of the factors in the 1969 and 1978 CTRS models. CFA have found varying degrees of support for the SDQ scales in several cultures. Finnish and U.S. findings supported 3-factor models for the SDQ consisting of internalizing, externalizing, and prosocial factors (Dickey & Blumberg, 2004; Koskelainen et al., 2001). The internalizing and externalizing factors are analogous to the groupings found in second-order factor analyses of ASEBA syndromes. Although the results of some analyses that were constrained to fit the five SDQ scales were fairly consistent with those scales, CFA research in more cultures is needed to determine whether there is multicultural support for patterns of SDQ problem items that are more differentiated than the broad internalizing and externalizing groupings.

MAIN FINDINGS
FROM THE DIAGNOSTICALLY BASED APPROACH

Multicultural findings from the diagnostically based approach rest mainly on diagnoses made from the DISC. However, we know of no published studies that reported direct statistical comparisons between DISC findings for more than two diagnoses in different cultures. To our knowledge, the only published study that statistically compared the prevalence of more than two diagnoses for children in different cultures was a comparison of DAWBA diagnoses obtained in Taubaté, Brazil with diagnoses obtained in a U.K. national sample (Fleitlich-Bilyk & Goodman, 2004). Other than this one bicultural comparison, our summary of diagnostically based findings is based on studies done in single cultures that were similar enough to other single-culture studies to afford at least rough comparisons between their findings.

Psychometric Findings

When interviews such as the DISC are developed to operationalize diagnoses, the interviews state the diagnostic criteria as questions whose answers determine whether the diagnostic criteria are met. The DISC questions are thus not viewed as comprising scales for measuring quantitative constructs or latent variables but as criteria for making yes/no decisions about whether individuals have particular disorders. Consequently, properties of scales, such as internal consistency, are not typically reported for interviews such as the DISC. Nevertheless, test–retest reliability and cross-informant agreement are as important to know for diagnostic interviews as for other assessment procedures.

As we reported in Chapter 3, the mean test–retest kappa obtained in the MECA study of the DISC was .52 for parent interviews and .33 for youth interviews (Schwab-Stone et al., 1996). These low kappas for test–retest reliability were consistent with kappas ranging from .42 to .52 in other studies of Quebec, Puerto Rican, and multiethnic U.S. samples (Bravo et al., 2001; Breton et al., 1998; Canino et al., 1987; Roberts et al., 1996). For DSM-based rating scales, test–retest rs have averaged from .60 to .86 (Conners, 2001; DuPaul et al., 1998; Gadow et al., 2002). For the DSM-oriented scales of the CBCL/6–18, TRF, and YSR, the mean test–retest reliabilities have been .88, .85, and .79, respectively (Achenbach & Rescorla, 2001).

The mean cross-informant kappa was .12 between diagnoses made from DISC interviews with parents and with their 9- to 18-year-old children in the MECA study (Jensen et al., 1999). Without specifying measures of agreement, several other studies have reported that there was little overlap between diagnoses made from parent and child DISC interviews (Breton et al., 1999; Shaffer et al., 1996; Verhulst et al., 1997). Cross-informant rs for DSM-based rating scales have averaged .42 for parent versus teacher ratings and .30 for parent versus youth ratings (Conners, 2001; DuPaul et al., 1998; Gadow et al., 2002). For the

DSM-oriented ASEBA scales, the mean cross-informant rs have been .29 for parent versus teacher, .45 for parent versus youth, and .21 for teacher versus youth.

Validity Findings

Two studies that obtained diagnoses from parent and youth DISC interviews and diagnoses from extensive clinical evaluations reported mean kappas of .12 and .09 between the DISC and clinical diagnoses (Jensen & Weisz, 2002; Lewczyk et al., 2003). We found one study that reported associations between DAWBA diagnoses and clinical diagnoses. In this study Goodman, Ford, Richards, et al. (2000) obtained a mean Kendall *tau b* correlation of .56 between three broad categories of diagnoses made for 39 children by psychiatrists from DAWBA data and diagnoses made by a child psychiatrist who read clinical case notes for the children and rated the diagnoses as absent, possible, or definite. The diagnoses could be made in terms of either ICD-10 or DSM-III criteria. A meta-analysis yielded a mean kappa of .15 between diagnoses of children made from standardized diagnostic interviews and from clinical evaluations (Rettew et al., 2006).

Point-biserial rs between DSM-based rating scales and DSM diagnoses have averaged from .25 to .31 (DuPaul et al., 1998; Gadow et al., 2002). However, the authors of these scales reported much higher rs between their DSM-based rating scales and empirically based scales, including scales scored from the YSR and CTRS. Between the CBCL/6–18 DSM-oriented scales and DSM-IV diagnoses, point-biserial rs have averaged .46 (Achenbach & Rescorla, 2001).

Multicultural Findings on the Prevalence of Diagnostically Based Disorders

As detailed in Chapter 7, the data for multicultural comparisons of diagnostically based disorders come largely from studies that used various versions of the DISC in single cultures. The prevalence rates of DSM diagnoses in general population samples ranged from 8.8% for 11-year-olds in a Dunedin, New Zealand, longitudinal sample to 50.6% for 9- to 17-year-olds in the MECA study of three metropolitan areas in the United States and one in Puerto Rico. In the only direct multicultural comparison of diverse DSM diagnoses made with the same interview, Fleitlich-Bilyk and Goodman (2004) reported a prevalence rate of 9.7% for British 7- to 14-year-olds versus 12.7% for 7- to 14-year-olds attending mainstream schools in Taubaté, Brazil. The addition of various impairment criteria reduced the prevalence rates in several studies, although the prevalence rates continued to differ markedly among the studies. The large methodological differences among the studies preclude firm conclusions about the contribution of cultural factors to differences in the prevalence rates of DSM diagnoses.

Multicultural Findings on Correlates of Diagnostically Based Disorders

The most feasible multicultural comparisons of correlates were for demographic characteristics associated with "any diagnosis" versus "no diagnosis." However, the findings varied too much to support firm conclusions about whether gender, age, parents' marital status, SES, or urbanicity were consistently associated with prevalence rates for "any diagnosis." Two epidemiological studies, both in Puerto Rico, reported positive associations between receipt of any diagnosis and previous receipt of mental health services.

In the few studies that reported sufficient data for specific diagnostic categories, a fairly consistent finding was that depressive diagnoses tended to be most prevalent among adolescent girls, whereas ADHD and CD/ODD diagnoses tended to be most prevalent among boys. There were also tendencies for depressive diagnoses to be most prevalent in middle adolescence and ADHD to be most prevalent during the primary school years, but methodological variations precluded firm conclusions about age differences in diagnoses.

Multicultural Findings on Comorbidity among Diagnostically Based Disorders

There is an enormous literature on comorbidity in clinical samples. However, Berkson's bias and other factors often cause comorbidity estimates made from clinical samples to be inflated above those made from more representative samples. Consequently, representative general population samples are needed to determine the typical rate of co-occurrence among particular disorders. Furthermore, to obtain accurate estimates of the frequency with which two disorders co-occur, it is necessary to compute *bidirectional* comorbidity, which is the mean of the percentage of co-occurrence of Disorder A with Disorder B and the co-occurrence of Disorder B with Disorder A (McConaughy & Achenbach, 1994).

Among the large general population samples that were assessed with standardized diagnostic interviews, only studies in Puerto Rico and Zurich reported data from which bidirectional comorbidity could be computed (Bird et al., 1988, 1993; Steinhausen et al., 1998). In these studies, from 40 to 63% of the children received multiple diagnoses. For the few pairs of diagnostic categories for which bidirectional comorbidity could be computed, comorbidities ranged from 22% for ADHD × affective diagnoses among Puerto Rican 4- to 16-year-olds to 72% for anxiety × "disruptive" (ADHD, CD, ODD) diagnoses among Zurich 6- to 17-year-olds. Several studies have reported significant ORs between various combinations of diagnoses, but the findings cannot be aggregated across studies into credible estimates of typical comorbidity rates.

COMPARISONS OF FINDINGS FROM THE EMPIRICALLY BASED AND DIAGNOSTICALLY BASED APPROACHES

In the following sections we compare those findings from the empirically based and diagnostically based approaches that may be particularly instructive for advancing assessment and understanding of psychopathology.

Psychometric Comparisons

We first address two fundamental psychometric properties: internal consistency and test–retest reliability.

Internal Consistency

With respect to psychometric findings, the mean alphas of .90 and .87 for the ASEBA and Conners scales, respectively, indicate that the items of the scales consistently measure particular constructs. Because standardized diagnostic interviews such as the DISC are intended to operationalize diagnoses by translating the diagnostic criteria into yes/no questions, the internal consistency of the questions may not be considered relevant. Also, the diagnostic interviews typically omit some questions when answers to initial screening questions for a diagnosis fail to reach a preselected threshold. Consequently, the interviews do not assess all the same criteria for every child. However, acceptable alphas have been obtained for DSM-oriented scales on which respondents rate every symptom (Achenbach & Rescorla, 2001; DuPaul et al., 1998; Gadow et al., 2002). This finding indicates that the symptoms specified for at least some DSM diagnoses can consistently measure a particular construct when assessed via rating scales.

Test–Retest Reliability

Test–retest reliability is equally relevant to empirically based and diagnostically based assessment. To be useful, assessment procedures should produce similar findings regarding psychopathology when readministered over intervals brief enough to preclude major changes in the psychopathology. Empirically based rating scales have yielded a mean test–retest r of .90 for ASEBA scales, .73 for Conners scales, and .69 for the SDQ.

The test–retest kappas for diagnoses made from DISC interviews have been considerably lower, ranging from about .33 to .52. The findings that test–retest kappas for diagnoses are typically smaller than the rs for empirically based scales are not mere artifacts of differences between the formulas for kappa versus r. As pointed out by the inventor of kappa (Cohen, 1960), the magnitude of kappa closely approximates the magnitude of r computed for binary data, such as yes/no diagnoses.

Whether agreement is measured by kappa or by other statistics, the prevailing conceptual model for diagnoses dictates that test–retest reliability be defined in terms of agreement between yes/no diagnoses made at two assessments. To illuminate the poor test–retest reliability of diagnoses, Jensen et al. (1995) investigated DISC interviews administered at 2- to 3-week intervals in the MECA general population sample. Most of the test-retest unreliability was explained by *test–retest attenuation*, which is the tendency for interviewees to report fewer problems at the second interview than at the first. This tendency is often found for rating forms as well as for diagnostic interviews and for adults as well as for children (e.g., Achenbach & Rescorla, 2001; Evans, 1975; Miller, Hampe, & Noble, 1972; Helzer, Spitznagel, & McEvoy, 1987; Robins, 1985; Vandiver & Sher, 1991).

Because a reduction of only one reported symptom can change a diagnostic decision from yes to no, test–retest attenuation has a much more dramatic effect on the reliability of yes/no diagnoses than on the reliability of quantitative scale scores. For example, suppose that, in Time 1 interviews with 200 children, 100 of the children qualified for diagnoses of ODD by reporting four criterial symptoms, which is the number of criterial symptoms required to meet the threshold for the diagnosis. The initial prevalence of ODD would thus be $100/200 = 50\%$. If 50 of the 100 children reported one less symptom in Time 2 interviews, the prevalence rate would drop to 25% and the kappa between the Time 1 and Time 2 interviews would be .50. Because test-retest attenuation may involve decreases of more than one symptom per diagnosis, declines in symptoms even for children whose Time 1 symptoms exceeded the diagnostic threshold could cause diagnostic conclusions to change from Time 1 to Time 2 for these children as well. Although Jensen et al. (1995) found that most changes from Time 1 to Time 2 were decreases in reported symptoms, they did find a few cases in which more symptoms were reported at Time 2 than Time 1. This "augmentation" effect may further reduce test–retest reliability in yes/no diagnoses by causing some children to change from no diagnosis at Time 1 to a diagnosis at Time 2. We return to the issue of test–retest attenuation later in this chapter.

Cross-Informant Agreement

The impact of a difference of only one reported symptom on diagnostic conclusions might help to explain the extremely low agreement between diagnoses made from DISC interviews with parents versus their children. In the MECA study, for example, the mean cross-informant kappa was .12 for agreement between diagnoses made from parent versus child interviews (Jensen et al., 1999). Other studies have also reported that there was little overlap between diagnoses made from parent and child DISC interviews (Breton et al., 1999; Shaffer et al., 1996; Verhulst et al., 1997). Although Table 2.4 reported correlations in the .40s and .50s between quantified parent and youth reports of the youths' problems, the requirement for yes/no diagnostic conclusions may keep agreement much lower. Disagreement about even a single symptom can cause 100% disagreement between "yes" for a diagnosis based on one informant's report and "no" for that diagnosis based on the other informant's report. The lack of published data on agreement between diagnoses made from interviews with pairs of adult informants who see children in similar contexts, such as mothers and fathers, leaves open the question of whether agreement between such diagnoses would be as good as indicated by the correlations of .73–.80 reported in Table 2.4 for empirically based scales.

Validity Comparisons

The content validity of ASEBA scales has been supported by the ways in which their items were formulated and selected and by international experts' identification of items that are very consistent with DSM diagnostic categories. For the Conners ADHD items and for the DISC items, content validity is assumed on the grounds that the items are paraphrased from the DSM criteria.

Questions of criterion-related validity and construct validity are more complex. The criterion-related validity of the ASEBA syndromes has been supported by strong associations with clinical referral un-confounded with demographic differences, which were controlled. The criterion-related validity of the Conners scales has been supported by significant discrimination between children who were diagnosed as having ADHD versus those who were not, after controlling for demographic differences. The criterion-related validity of SDQ scales has been supported by a study that reported significant discrimination between referred and nonreferred children, although the study did not report associations with demographic differences or controls for these differences (Goodman, 1999).

For standardized diagnostic interviews such as the DISC, it might seem that criterion-related validity should be evaluated in terms of associations with diagnoses made by other means. However, meta-analyses of associations between diagnoses made from standardized interviews and from clinical evaluations have shown that agreement between them is typically quite low not only for children but also for adults (Rettew et al., 2006).

Because the standardized interviews were developed to operation-alize diagnoses, it might be argued that diagnoses made from these interviews are so much better than clinical diagnoses that the low agreement with clinical diagnoses is explained by the poor quality of the clinical diagnoses. Yet, if clinical diagnoses are not acceptable as validity criteria for the standardized interviews, then how can we judge the validity of the interviews? As Cronbach and Meehl (1955) explained long ago, the construct validity of assessment procedures should be evaluated in terms of networks of associations with other measures of the same construct and/or related constructs.

One basic way to test the validity of assessment procedures for which there is no clear external criterion is by testing the agreement between different procedures that are intended to measure the same constructs. For example, validity data for intelligence tests such as the Stanford–Binet Intelligence Scales, Fifth Edition (SB5; Roid, 2003) typically include correlations with other intelligence tests, such as Wechsler (2003) Intelligence Scales, that have been administered to the same children at about the same time. Because the tests differ in structure and content, they are not expected to correlate perfectly. However, correlations of SB5 Verbal IQ, Performance IQ, and Full Scale IQ scores with scores on the corresponding Wechsler scales range from .66 to .85 (Roid, 2003). These correlations are high enough to indicate that both tests measure similar constructs. Analogously, as we reported in Chapter 2, correlations of .71–.89 between corresponding ASEBA and Conners scales support the validity of both the ASEBA and Conners scales for assessing similar taxonomic constructs for children's problems.

Because the DISC, DAWBA, and other standardized diagnostic interviews are designed to operationalize many of the same diagnoses, a basic way to test their construct validity is to compute agreement between diagnoses made for the same children by the different interviews. We found only one published report of agreement between diagnoses made from different standardized interviews administered to the same children and/or their parents. In the one study, DSM-III-R diagnoses were initially made from separate DISC interviews with 100 9- to 12-year-olds and with their mothers, drawn from an epidemiological sample in upstate New York (Cohen, O'Connor, Lewis, Velez, & Malachowski, 1987). Clinicians then administered the K-SADS separately to the children and their mothers 3–4 months later, an interval over which the diagnoses were "not expected to change" (p. 663). Kappas were computed in various ways to test agreement between diagnoses made from the DISC and K-SADS, with the child and mother data combined. Averaged over different methods for computing agreement for the most common diagnoses, the mean kappa was .03 for agreement between "definite" diagnoses—that is, diagnoses "made when the symptoms were considered by the clinician to have reached a standard of clinical significance" (p. 663). The mean kappa was .14 for agreement between "possible" diagnoses—that is, diagnoses "made whenever the presence of symptoms matching diagnostic criteria were noted" (p. 663). Whether computed for definite or possible diagnoses, agreement between diagnoses made from the DISC and K-SADS was thus very low.

Although studies such as those reviewed in Chapter 8 have reported associations between the standardized diagnostic interviews and other variables, inconsistencies among the studies preclude inferences about the construct validity of the diagnostic interviews. Furthermore, the low test–retest reliability of diagnoses made from the interviews limits the strength of associations that diagnoses can attain with other data. This limitation is due to the fact that, given poor agreement between diagnoses obtained with the same interview administered twice to the same people, the diagnoses are not likely to agree better with data obtained by different procedures.

As discussed earlier, Jensen et al. (1995) found that test–retest attenuation accounted for much of the unreliability in DISC diagnoses. In the Jensen et al. sample, intraclass correlations (ICCs) between the number of symptoms reported for each Time 1 and Time 2 DISC diagnostic category exceeded the kappas for all but one diagnostic category. This finding indicated that test–retest attenuation reduced Time 1 versus Time 2 agreement for yes/no diagnoses more than it reduced Time 1 versus Time 2 agreement for the number of symptoms reported for each diagnosis in the same interviews. In addition, both the test–retest and cross-informant correlations that we reviewed in Chapters 2 and 3 were considerably higher for quantified DSM-based and DSM-oriented scales than for yes/no diagnoses. These findings suggest that diagnostic reliability could be improved by quantifying diagnostic data rather than requiring diagnoses to be based exclusively on yes/no decisions about each diagnostic criterion. More reliable diagnoses would, in turn, improve the possibilities for agreement with validity criteria.

Comparisons of Distributions and Prevalence Rates

Many studies have tested differences between empirically based scale scores obtained by children in numerous cultures. The most comprehensive statistical tests have compared scores on the CBCL in 31 cultures, on the TRF in 21 cultures, and on the YSR in 24 cultures (Rescorla et al., 2006a, 2006b, in press). These tests yielded small to medium ESs for multicultural differences in problem scores. Patterns of gender and age effects on scale scores were quite consistent across most cultures.

Prevalence rates have been compared for 14 DAWBA-based DSM-IV diagnoses in two cultures (Fleitlich-Bilyk & Goodman, 2004) and for two DISC-based DSM-III-R diagnoses in two cultures (Bird et al., 2001). The bicultural DAWBA comparison yielded prevalence rates of 9.7% for any of the 14 DSM-IV diagnoses in the United Kingdom versus 12.7% in Taubaté, Brazil. The bicultural DISC comparison yielded prevalence rates of 4.1% for CD and 3.0% for ODD in Puerto Rico versus 5.4% and 8.0%, respectively, for a non-Hispanic white U.S. mainland sample. The Taubaté rate for any diagnosis was significantly higher than the U.K. rate, and the U.S. mainland rate for ODD was significantly higher than the Puerto Rican rate. The prevalence rates for any DISC-based diagnosis in other studies ranged from 8.8 to 50.6%, but the many methodological differences (detailed in Chapter 7) preclude rigorous cross-cultural comparisons and inferences about true differences in prevalence rates among the seven cultures from which DISC-based prevalence rates were reported.

It may seem that comparing distributions of scores on empirically based scales versus prevalence rates for diagnoses is like comparing apples and oranges—they differ in too many ways to afford direct comparisons. However, the scores on empirically based scales and the diagnoses obtained from interviews are both based on informants' reports of children's behavioral and emotional problems. Both approaches assess many similar problems. Furthermore, prevalence rates for "cases" can be obtained from empirically based scales by tabulating the number of children who obtain problem scores above particular cutpoints. Conversely, quantitative scores for diagnoses can be computed by tabulating the number of symptoms endorsed by each informant. (As discussed later, this approach requires dispensing with "skip-out" procedures that omit interview questions when it appears that criteria will not be met for a diagnosis.) In any event, it is possible to obtain comparable data from both approaches. To date, however, the diagnostically based approach has not been applied uniformly enough in a sufficient number of cultures to support firm conclusions about multicultural similarities and differences in the prevalence of disorders defined according to diagnostic criteria. The more uniform applications of empirically based assessment procedures, on the other hand, have facilitated direct statistical comparisons of problems reported by parents, teachers, and youths in many cultures.

Comparisons of Correlates

Tendencies for girls to obtain higher Internalizing and lower Externalizing scores than boys on empirically based scales have been quite consistent in parent, teacher, and self-ratings across many cultures. Boys have tended to score higher than girls on attention problems in parent and teacher ratings, but not in self-ratings in most cultures. Certain age trends in empirically based scale scores have also been consistently found in many cultures. Although studied in fewer cultures, children from higher-SES and intact families have consistently obtained lower problem scores than other children. Longitudinal studies have found similar predictive relations from empirically based scale scores to later outcomes in three cultures. Numerous studies in several cultures have quantified genetic and environmental effects on empirically based scale scores. Differences in empirically based scale scores have been found between immigrant children, children of host cultures, and children residing in the immigrant children's home culture. Various characteristics of immigration status and immigrant children's families have been identified as correlates of scores on empirically based problem scales.

Although most diagnostically based studies have reported findings for "any diagnosis," the findings were inconsistent with respect to demographic correlates of any diagnosis. In the few studies that reported sufficient data for specific diagnostic categories, depressive diagnoses tended to be most prevalent among adolescent girls, whereas ADHD and CD/ODD diagnoses tended to be most prevalent among boys. These tendencies are consistent with the findings of higher Internalizing scores for girls and higher Externalizing and attention problems scores for boys on empirically based scales.

Comparisons of Patterns and Comorbidity

CFA has been used to test the generalizability of empirically based ASEBA syndrome patterns. When uniform CFA methods were applied to large samples assessed with parallel parent, teacher, and self-report instruments, similar patterns of co-occurring problems were found in many cultures (Ivanova et al., 2006a, 2006b, 2006c). Support has also been found for broad internalizing and externalizing patterns of problems in SDQ ratings of children in two cultures (Dickey & Blumberg, 2004; Koskelainen et al., 2001).

The problems that comprise particular diagnoses are chosen by the experts who formulate the diagnostic criteria. Because the criterial problems are thus taken for granted as a priori constituents of the diagnoses, few efforts have been made to test the patterning of the specific problems reported in diagnostic interviews in different cultures. However, comorbidities between different diagnoses have been reported in several studies. In the general population studies that provided sufficient data for computing bidirectional comorbidities, from 40 to 63% of children received multiple diagnoses. For specific combinations of diagnoses, comorbidities ranged from 22% for ADHD × affective diagnoses to 72% for anxiety × "disruptive" diagnoses. The high rates of comorbidity suggest systematic associations among problems that the experts assigned to different diagnoses. However, the paucity of studies reporting comorbidity in sufficiently comparable ways precludes firm conclusions about the co-occurrence of particular diagnoses and the problems they include.

For some kinds of problems, considerable congruence exists between an empirically based syndrome (e.g., ASEBA Attention Problems) and a particular DSM diagnosis (e.g., attention deficit/hyperactivity disorder). However, for other kinds of problems, the empirically based approach and the DSM approach are less congruent. For example, the ASEBA eight-syndrome model identifies separate Aggressive Behavior and Rule-Breaking Behavior syndromes. Although these syndromes are significantly correlated (e.g., $r = .67$ in the U.S. CBCL normative sample), the syndromes emerged as separate factors in EFA and CFA. Furthermore, as summarized in Chapters 4 and 5, these two syndromes have quite different age, longitudinal, and genetic patterns. In contrast, the DSM-IV combines aggressive and unaggressive forms of antisocial behavior into a heterogeneous set of 15 criteria for the diagnosis of CD. To receive a diagnosis of CD, a child must be deemed to manifest ≥ 3 of these 15 symptoms. Because there are many possible combinations of 3 symptoms out of 15, children meeting criteria for CD may have very different patterns of symptoms. Some may have ≥ 3 aggressive symptoms, whereas others may have ≥ 3 unaggressive symptoms, and still others may have various mixtures of aggressive and unaggressive symptoms.

Despite the DSM's failure to distinguish between aggressive and unaggressive symptoms as criteria for CD, factor analyses of DSM-IV CD symptoms assessed with the DISC for 1,669 Australian 6- to 17-year-olds yielded separate aggressive and rule-breaking patterns (Tackett, Krueger, Sawyer, & Graetz, 2003). The numbers of aggressive CD symptoms reported for the Australian children were strongly associated with Aggressive Behavior syndrome scores on CBCLs completed by the children's parents, whereas the numbers of unaggressive CD symptoms were strongly associated with CBCL Delinquent (Rule-Breaking) Behavior syndrome scores.

The ASEBA and the DSM also differ in how they handle problems of anxiety and depression. Factor analyses of ASEBA items have repeatedly indicated that problems of anxiety and depression co-occur to such a degree that they form a syndrome designated as Anxious/Depressed, consistent with the construct of negative affectivity (Clark, Watson, & Mineka, 1994). In contrast, the DSM-IV has separate diagnostic categories for anxiety disorders and depressive disorders, although many children and adolescents are identified as comorbid for anxiety and depression. In addition, studies of adults have also indicated that chronic dispositions to both anxiety and depression have a similar genetic basis (Kendler, Neale, Kessler, Heath, & Eaves, 1992; Kendler & Roy, 1995).

Comparisons of Organizational Structure

The empirically based approach as instantiated by the ASEBA and the diagnostically based approach as instantiated by the DSM differ with respect to their organizational structure. Although both approaches have numerous problem items and various groupings of these problem items, the approaches differ both in how their organizational structure was derived and in the nature of the organizational structure, as outlined next.

Organizational Structure of ASEBA Items and Scales

The ASEBA employs statistical methods, such as factor analysis, to identify patterns of co-occurring problems. Each empirically based syndrome reflects a particular pattern of co-occurring problems. Patterns of associations among scores on different syndromes can also be identified by performing second-order factor analyses of correlations among syndrome scores. Such analyses have identified the groupings of syndromes designated as Internalizing and Externalizing. And because most problems reported for children are associated with each other to at least a small degree when analyzed in large representative samples, the sum of scores on all problems serves as a global measure of psychopathology.

The ASEBA eight-syndrome model constitutes one level in a hierarchical assessment pyramid. At the base of the pyramid, children are assessed in terms of specific behavioral and emotional problems that are rated on three-step scales. The eight syndromes derived from EFA and CFA of the problem items form the next higher level of the pyramid. Above the syndrome level, Internalizing and Externalizing groupings derived from second-order factor analyses form the next level. And the Total Problems score forms the apex of the pyramid, as illustrated in Figure 9.1.

Pyramids of problems ranging from individual problem items to syndromes, Internalizing and Externalizing groupings of syndromes, and Total Problems scores are analogous to models of children's abilities, as follows: Individual problem items are analogous to individual ability test items; problem items and test items are analogously aggregated into scales and subtests, respectively; related scales are then aggregated into broader groupings, such as Internalizing and Externalizing groupings of syndromes and Verbal and Nonverbal groupings of ability subtests. All the problem items are combined to provide a global measure of psychopathology, just as all the ability items are combined to provide a global measure of intelligence.

A child's ASEBA syndrome scores are displayed on a profile. This profile is analogous to profiles for displaying subtest scores from ability tests such as the Wechsler (2003) tests. Although a child's profile may be quite specific to that child, certain profile patterns may also be found to characterize multiple children. Profile patterns that characterize substantial numbers of children can be identified through statistical methods such as cluster analysis and latent profile analysis.

The eight-syndrome model is supported by empirical data from many cultures and has generated hypotheses about differences in the nature and course of different patterns of problems. Because the problem items can be aggregated in additional ways, they can also be scored according to diagnostically based, top-down methods, such as the DSM-oriented scales derived from judgments by international experts. Furthermore, items can be aggregated using a combination of top-down and bottom-up approaches. For example, specific items can be grouped into scales based on constructs other than those reflected in the DSM-oriented scales. The validity of such scales can then be empirically tested. Scales using ASEBA items for assessing posttraumatic

Total Problems

Broad Groupings

Syndromes

Examples of Problem Items[a]

Anxious/ Depressed	Withdrawn/ Depressed	Somatic Complaints	Social Problems	Thought Problems	Attention Problems	Rule-Breaking Behavior	Aggressive Behavior
Cries	Enjoys little	Aches, pains	Clumsy	Can't get mind off thoughts	Acts young	Bad companions	Argues
Fears	Lacks energy	Eye problems	Gets teased	Hears things	Can't concentrate	Breaks rules	Attacks people
Feels unloved	Rather be alone	Feels dizzy	Jealous	Repeats acts	Can't sit still	Lacks guilt	Disobedient
Feels too guilty	Refuses to talk	Headaches	Lonely	Sees things	Confused	Lies, cheats	Fights
Talks or thinks of suicide	Sad	Nausea	Not liked	Strange behavior	Daydreams	Sets fires	Loud
Worries	Secretive	Overtired	Prefers younger kids	Strange ideas	Fails to finish	Steals	Mean
	Shy, timid	Stomach-aches	Too dependent		Impulsive	Swearing	Screams
	Withdrawn	Tired			Inattentive	Truant	Temper
		Vomiting			Stares	Vandalism	Threatens

FIGURE 9.1. Pyramid of empirically based assessment levels. Copyright T. M. Achenbach. Reprinted by permission.
[a] Abbreviated versions of CBCL/6–18, TRF, and YSR items.

stress disorder (PTSD; Wolfe & Birt, 1997), obsessive–compulsive disorder (OCD; Hudziak et al., 2004), and sluggish cognitive tempo (SCT; Bauermeister et al., 2005) have been tested with data from cultures outside the United States.

Organizational Structure of DSM Symptoms and Diagnoses

The DSM also consists of groupings of problem items, namely its diagnoses with their respective symptom criteria. However, the organizational structure of the DSM and the method used to derive this organizational structure differ from those of the ASEBA. As embodied in the DSM-III, each diagnostic category of childhood disorders started "with a clinical concept for which there is some degree of face validity. . . . Initial criteria were generally developed by asking the clinicians to describe what they consider to be the most characteristic features of the disorder" (Spitzer & Cantwell, 1980, p. 360). The conceptual model is one in which each category represents a disorder whose nature is known to the experts who formulate the category. In effect, the diagnostic criteria for a particular diagnostic category define a particular taxonomic construct.

The process of generating diagnostic categories and criteria for childhood disorders has become progressively more complex from DSM-III to DSM-III-R and DSM-IV. However, the products of this process are still diagnostic categories that are defined in terms of yes/no decision rules based on yes/no judgments of whether a child meets each of the criteria for a diagnosis. Standardized diagnostic interviews operationalize the verbally stated criteria for each diagnostic category by stating them in terms of questions whose answers are coded as yes/no judgments of whether each criterion is met. The ICD paradigm is similar, although less research on children has been published for the ICD than for the DSM.

The DSM was not designed to form an explicitly hierarchical structure. However, inspection of DSM categories suggests that some sections of the DSM have a roughly hierarchical organization. For example, within the "Disorders Usually First Diagnosed in Infancy, Childhood, or Adolescence" section of the DSM-IV, a major subdivision is "Attention Deficit and Disruptive Behavior Disorders." This subdivision contains five diagnoses, two of which have subtypes: ADHD (with three nested subtypes), AHDH/NOS, CD (with three nested subtypes), ODD, and disruptive behavior disorder NOS (*NOS* stands for "not otherwise specified"). Nested within each diagnosis is a set of diagnostic criteria. Most of the diagnostic criteria are behavioral or emotional problems considered symptomatic of the disorder.

Many DSM symptom criteria are analogous to problem items on empirically based scales. For example, the CD criteria *Often bullies, threatens, or intimidates others* and *Often initiates physical fights* are similar to CBCL items *16. Cruelty, bullying, or meanness to others*; *37. Gets in many fights*; and *57. Physically attacks people.* Similarly, many DSM-IV ADHD criteria are similar to CBCL items. For example, the DSM symptom *Is often easily distracted by extraneous stimuli* is similar to CBCL item *78. Inattentive or easily distracted.* Thus, empirically based scales and DSM diagnoses both contain sets of discrete items that describe behavioral and emotional problems. The approaches differ, however, in their methods for grouping the items. In the empirically based approach, statistical analyses are used to identify syndromes that form part of a hierarchical pyramid. In the DSM approach, by contrast, experts define diagnostic categories in terms of particular symptoms and other criteria. Some DSM diagnoses are grouped together into subdivisions of the DSM-IV, such as "Attention-Deficit and Disruptive Behavior Disorders." However, neither the assignments of symptom items to diagnoses nor the assignments of diagnoses to subdivisions were based on statistical co-occurrence.

SUMMARY

In this chapter we compared findings obtained with the empirically based and diagnostically based approaches, including psychometric and validity findings for assessment instruments; multicultural findings on the distributions of problem scores and the prevalence of diagnoses; correlates of empirically based scale scores and diagnoses; and findings on empirically based patterns of problems as well as on comorbidity among diagnoses.

An important difference between the psychometric findings for the two approaches was the much lower test–retest reliability of diagnoses than of empirically based scales. This finding may be due in part to the effects of yes/no assessment of diagnoses on test–retest attenuation and on regression toward the mean, which is discussed in Chapter 10.

As instantiated by the ASEBA, the organization of empirically based items and scales can be represented in terms of a pyramid in which behavioral and emotional problem items form the base and the Total Problems scale forms the apex. The level above the items includes eight syndromes. At the next level an Internalizing grouping comprises three of the syndromes, and an Externalizing grouping, two of the syndromes. Items were assigned to syndromes and the syndromes were assigned to the Internalizing and Externalizing groupings on the basis of statistical findings. The diagnostically based approach, as instantiated by the DSM, is organized according to discrete diagnostic categories, some of which have subtypes. Each diagnosis is defined by a set of criteria, most of which are behavioral and emotional problems. Some diagnoses, such as CD, are nested within subdivisions of disorders, such as disruptive behavior disorders. The assignment of symptoms to diagnoses and diagnostic subtypes, as well as the assignment of diagnostic categories to broader subdivisions, is based on expert judgment rather than statistical findings.

CHAPTER 10

Meeting Challenges Posed by Multicultural Research on Children's Problems

To advance our multicultural understanding of children's problems, we need to address challenges that are evident from the findings to date. In this chapter we address methodological and conceptual challenges that confront empirically based and diagnostically based assessment. We also outline strategies for meeting these challenges.

METHODOLOGICAL CHALLENGES

In the following sections, we discuss several challenges that confront both empirically based and diagnostically based approaches to assessment. Regardless of how child psychopathology is assessed, obtaining and effectively using multisource data present major methodological challenges. Test–retest attenuation and regression toward the mean also present challenges that need to be met by all approaches to assessment of child psychopathology. Assessing uniform sets of problems, obtaining accurate prevalence rates, and taking account of base-rate differences associated with age and gender present additional challenges for all approaches to assessment. Lastly, both empirically based and diagnostically based approaches need to deal with the fact that children often manifest many kinds of problems and meet the criteria for multiple diagnoses.

Collecting and Using Multisource Data

It is now widely accepted that important decisions about child psychopathology require information from multiple informants, such as mothers, fathers, teachers, and the children themselves. Different methods may be needed to obtain information from different informants and about different aspects of children's functioning. Consequently, this challenge can be thought of in terms of multiple sources, which include both multiple informants and multiple methods, such as questionnaires, rating forms, interviews, tests, laboratory procedures, and observations. Whether the goals are viewed from empirically based or diagnostically based perspectives, proper assessment of psychopathology for both clinical and research purposes requires data from multiple sources.

As summarized in Chapter 2, correlations between parent, teacher, and self-ratings are typically quite modest. Correlations between ratings by pairs of informants who interact with the child in the same general setting (e.g., pairs of parents) are higher but seldom exceed the .60s. Agreement between parents and their children on DSM diagnoses is typically quite low, as summarized in Chapter 3. Low agreement between informants thus poses a major challenge for both empirically based and diagnostically based approaches to assessment.

When data from different sources suggest different conclusions, it is tempting to respond by asking "Which source should I believe?" Such a response implies that discrepancies must be resolved by determining which source is right and which is wrong. However, dichotomous decisions (i.e., right/wrong) ignore the possibility that each source may provide valuable though different information. Even information that seems contradictory may reveal important aspects of a child's functioning and how he or she is viewed by different people. Consequently, we may understand a child better if we take account of contradictory information from different sources than if we believe only one source.

Making better use of information from multiple sources is a major challenge for all approaches to psychopathology. To meet this challenge, it is helpful to distinguish between the different kinds of data that are needed for different phases of assessment. For multicultural research and for the initial stages of clinical assessment, better pictures of children's everyday functioning may be obtained from parent, teacher, and self-reports than from more specialized procedures. Of course, custom-tailored procedures administered by highly trained clinicians may be needed for the advanced phases of clinical evaluations. However, standardized instruments can be used to obtain parallel parent, teacher, and self-reports in most service and research contexts.

Data from parallel instruments can be compared and interpreted in various ways. Figure 10.1 portrays a typical location for standardized parent, teacher, and self-report data in clinical evaluations of individual children. Research assessment may often use only the standardized procedures at the top of Figure 10.1.

Integrating Multi-Informant Data

One way to integrate multi-informant data is to compare the scores a child obtains from ratings by each type of informant on each scale. To systematically compare information from parents, teachers, and youths, it is necessary to preserve those reports as separate data sources. For research purposes, children can then be grouped according to the scales on which multiple informants report numerous problems. When data from each kind of informant are compared, it is also possible to

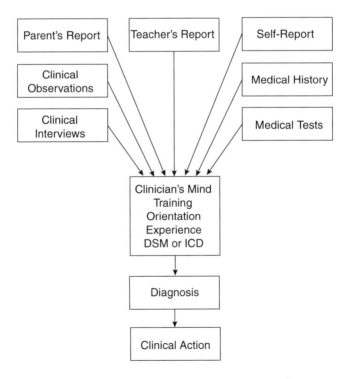

FIGURE 10.1. Schematic model for clinical assessment of child psychopathology. Reproduced by permission of L. Dumenci (2005).

determine whether particular kinds of informants tend to report more or fewer problems than do other kinds of informants. For example, multicultural findings reviewed in Chapter 4 showed that parents and teachers tend to report fewer problems for youths than youths report for themselves. For certain research purposes, it may be better to aggregate information from different informants, such as by summing the standard scores obtained from multiple informants on each scale. For other purposes, information from different informants can be compared to determine whether a child is deviant on particular scales according to most or all informants.

Identifying areas where informants disagree can be as important as finding areas where they agree. When all informants agree about the nature and severity of a child's problems, decisions may be relatively easy regarding the need for treatment, the problems to be treated, and the optimal treatment. However, when informants do not agree, clinicians may decide to give priority to the reports of one informant rather than another, depending on the situation. One strategy might be for clinicians to give priority to parents' reports for externalizing kinds of problems, to self-reports for internalizing kinds of problems, and to teachers' reports for attentional problems.

Another approach to integrating multi-informant data for a given child is to use algorithms derived from multi-informant data for large samples of children. For example, the Psychometric Latent Agreement Model (PLAM; Dumenci, 2006) uses ratings of multiple items by multiple informants to estimate the probability with which a child's scores match each of several latent (inferred) classes. The latent classes can be defined either in terms of diagnoses or in terms of deviance on quantitative scales. When the PLAM is used to estimate the probability that a child's scores match a particular diagnostic class, such as the class of children who have ADHD, it yields one probability for the child's membership in that class and a second probability for the child's membership in the class of children who do not have ADHD.

An important additional benefit of the PLAM is that it also estimates the probability for whether the child can be classified as a true case or noncase of ADHD and the probability that the data for the child do not exceed chance levels of resemblance to the classes of children with ADHD and without ADHD. In other words, the PLAM identifies children whose scores do not justify clear-cut assignments to the classes of cases versus noncases. Because it is unrealistic to expect all children to be accurately classified as cases versus noncases of each kind of disorder, it is very helpful to explicitly identify children for whom decisions should be deferred until more data are obtained.

Dealing with Test–Retest Attenuation

The tendency for people to report fewer problems at a second assessment than at an initial assessment affects the results of interviews, tests, questionnaires, and rating forms in both quantitative and yes/no formats. However, test–retest attenuation has different consequences for quantitative than for yes/no formats, as explained in the following sections.

Quantitative Formats

When individual items are scored quantitatively and their scores are aggregated to form quantitative scales, the test–retest attenuation effect is evident as a decline in scale scores from the first to the second assessment. The effect of this decline is typically quite small in terms of the percentage of variance accounted for (e.g., Achenbach & Rescorla, 2001). Furthermore, when deviance is assessed in terms of a quantitative continuum, a decline in scores that contributes only a portion of variation along the continuum need not materially affect conclusions about whether children need help. Even if clinical cutpoints are specified on a continuum of scores, it is clear that a child who scored slightly above the cutpoint at the initial assessment and slightly below the cutpoint at the next assessment has not changed from needing help to not needing help. For both clinical and research purposes, users can readily see that the small decline in scores does not indicate an important change in the level of problems.

When quantitative scores are evaluated in relation to norms, the norms are typically based on an initial administration of an assessment procedure. Even if an assessment procedure is susceptible to test–retest attenuation, judgments about the deviance of a child's scores in relation to norms should be based on the initial assessment of that child. In other words, norms provide a valuable standard metric by which to judge the degree of deviance (or lack of deviance) that a child's score indicates in comparison to scores obtained by the normative sample. If the norms are based on the initial assessments of children in the normative sample, then the scores obtained at the initial assessment of new children are the ones that should be compared to the scores of the normative sample.

Test–retest attenuation may vary with the length of the retest interval and with other factors, such as whether interventions are implemented. Consequently, steps must be taken to avoid mistaking test–retest attenuation for improvement in the condition that is being assessed. For example, in tests of the efficacy of Intervention A, it is important to include control (or comparison) groups that receive no intervention or a different intervention, such as Intervention B. The groups that do not receive Intervention A should receive the same pre- and postintervention assessments as the Intervention A group. Because test–retest attenuation presumably has the same effects on changes from pre- to postintervention scores for all groups, significantly more favorable changes in pre- to postintervention scores for the Intervention A group than for other groups provide evidence for the efficacy of Intervention A.

Yes/No Formats

For quantitative scale scores that are judged by comparison with norms and/or by comparison with scores for groups receiving the same assessment sequences, the challenges of test–retest attenuation are easily met. However, test–retest attenuation presents greater challenges for yes/no reports of diagnostic criteria and for yes/no decisions about diagnoses (Jensen et al.,1995). If even one less criterion for a diagnosis is met at a second interview than at an initial interview, the diagnosis may change from "yes" to "no." Dichotomous scoring may also reduce agreements between different informants (Jensen et al., 1999), between different diagnostic interviews (Cohen et al., 1987), between standardized diagnostic interviews and clinical diagnoses (Rettew et al., 2006), and between diagnoses assigned to the same children by different editions of diagnostic criteria (Lahey et al., 1990).

It seems likely that quantification of diagnostic criteria could reduce many of these problems. By allowing criteria to be rated even on simple three-step scales regarding the severity and/or frequency of symptoms, the benefits of quantification could be obtained for the assessment of each criterial symptom. Summing or otherwise aggregating the ratings for all the criterial symptoms would enable users to obtain scores for diagnoses. These scores could, in turn, be used in making the ultimate diagnostic decisions.

If standardized diagnostic interviews are used to compare outcomes for children receiving different intervention conditions, the challenge of test–retest attenuation can be met by comparing the results of parallel pre- and postintervention assessments for children receiving each intervention, as we illustrated for quantitative scales. However, because diagnoses are not norm-referenced, the conceptual problem of whether children truly have certain disorders is not so easily solved. The assumption that meeting yes/no diagnostic criteria provides yes/no answers as to the presence of disorders poses similar problems for dealing with contradictory data from different sources and for regression toward the mean, as discussed next.

Dealing with Regression toward the Mean

Another type of effect that can lead to changes in results from one assessment occasion to another is *regression toward the mean*. Unlike test–retest attenuation, regression toward the mean is a statistical phenomenon whereby individuals who initially obtain scores that are either far below or far above the mean for their group will subsequently tend to obtain scores that are closer to the mean of their group. Not confined to reports of problems, regression toward the mean is also found in scores for tests of abilities and other nonproblematic characteristics, observational measures, and even measures of physical characteristics such as height and weight.

Regression toward the mean reflects the fact that, whenever individuals are assessed, chance factors (including errors of measurement) contribute to the scores obtained by every individual. For those individuals who obtain the most extreme scores (both high and low), the chance factors are likely to have contributed toward making those scores more extreme than if the chance factors had not been present or had influenced the scores in the opposite way. When the same individuals are assessed again, those who initially obtained the most extreme scores will now obtain scores that tend to be, on the average, somewhat closer to the mean of the entire group of individuals who were assessed on both occasions.

The tendency for extreme scorers to obtain less extreme scores at a subsequent assessment occurs because the chance factors that initially helped to push some individuals' scores toward the extremes are not likely to affect those individuals' scores in precisely the same way at a subsequent assessment. Instead, being chance, the chance factors are as likely to influence those individuals' scores in the opposite direction or in no direction at all as in the initial direction. Although most individuals who initially scored far above the mean will again tend to obtain scores above the mean, their scores will tend to be, on the average, lower than their initial scores. Conversely, most individuals who initially scored far below the mean will again tend to score below the mean, but their scores will tend to be, on the average, higher than their initial scores.

Implications for Evaluating Outcomes

Regression toward the mean has important implications for evaluating outcomes. Because extreme scorers tend to obtain less extreme scores at a subsequent assessment, we cannot draw conclusions about the efficacy of an intervention unless we also do parallel pre- and postintervention assessments of control (or comparison) groups of extreme scorers who receive different intervention conditions. Regression toward the mean must thus be controlled for in the same way as test–retest attenuation when evaluating the efficacy of interventions.

Quantitative scoring of both problems and competencies makes it relatively easy to document and analyze regression toward the mean. However, regression effects also need to be recognized in assessing and reassessing individuals on the basis of yes/no reports of diagnostic criteria and yes/no diagnostic decisions. Because of regression toward the mean, people who initially report the most symptoms will tend to report fewer symptoms at the next assessment, even if their true condition has not changed. As a result, regression toward the mean may cause some people who meet criteria for a diagnosis at an initial assessment to slip below the diagnostic threshold at a subsequent assessment. Conversely, people who initially report the fewest symptoms may tend to report somewhat more symptoms at the next assessment.

Assessing Uniform Sets of Problems

To compare findings on children's problems across cultures, it is necessary to assess the same problems in each culture. However, using a uniform item set may result in missing problems that might be specific to a given culture. Thus, a basic challenge facing both empirically based and diagnostically based approaches to multicultural child psychopathology involves the choice of problems to be assessed. An instrument must include enough items to obtain a differentiated and comprehensive picture of children's behavioral and emotional functioning without being too long to be practical.

One reason that more multicultural comparisons have used empirically based than diagnostically based approaches is that empirically based instruments provide uniform item sets that can be administered in multiple cultures. Multicultural studies using empirically based instruments may also be more numerous because large samples of children can be assessed at far lower cost with empirically based instruments than with diagnostic interviews.

Empirically based instruments vary in length, from 20 problem items for the SDQ to 120 problem items for the CBCL and TRF. No instrument can assess every problem that could possibly be manifested by every child in every culture. However, problems that are thought to be specific to a particular culture can be added to the standard set of items. In addition, problems that are specific to a particular child can be assessed by asking respondents to enter and rate problems that are not in the standard set. For example, the CBCL and TRF provide extra spaces for respondents to add problems and to rate these problems. If many respondents in a culture add the same problem, this problem is deemed sufficiently important in that culture to warrant further investigation.

Comparing cultures on uniform sets of problems is more complicated when using diagnostically based assessment, owing to the many hundreds of symptoms and diagnoses specified by the DSM-IV and the ICD-10. As noted in Chapters 7 and 8, comparisons of findings from diagnostically based studies have been complicated by great variations in the numbers of diagnoses that have been assessed. Among the prevalence studies using the DISC, the number of diagnoses has ranged from three in the Australian ANSMHWB (Sawyer et al., 2001) to 23 in the Dutch DNS (Verhulst et al., 1997) and "every psychiatric disorder for which criteria were met" in the Puerto Rican PRCPES (Bird et al., 1988). Furthermore, even when similar diagnoses have been assessed in different studies, they have been aggregated in different ways for analysis. For example, the Zurich ZESCAP (Steinhausen et al., 1998) combined ADHD with CD and ODD into a category of disruptive disorders for computation of comorbidity with nondisruptive disorders. By contrast, the Puerto Rican PRCPES (Bird et al., 1988, 1993) computed comorbidity separately for ADHD and CD/ODD.

Although costs and logistics inevitably affect the number of diagnoses assessed, multicultural comparisons require that a common set of diagnoses be assessed in each culture. The best way to fulfill this requirement is for studies to use a standard set of diagnoses and to aggregate them in the same way for analysis. As with the empirically based approach, investigators can add diagnoses that may be especially relevant to each culture.

An additional complication in using the diagnostically based approach is that diagnostic interviews generally have "skip-out" procedures. For example, because the DISC includes nearly 3,000 questions (Shaffer et al., 2000), interviewers can omit questions for a diagnosis if earlier questions make it clear that the criteria for that diagnosis will not be met. If some criteria are omitted for some children, it is impossible to compare all children on the same criteria and to test various ways of using the data, such as by summing all symptoms or experimenting with different cutpoints. One way to avoid this problem is to have respondents initially complete forms for rating each criterial symptom relevant to the diagnoses to be assessed for the child's age. Because most respondents can rate about 10 items per minute, they can provide data on large numbers of criterial symptoms much more quickly than in interviews. The ratings could then be used to determine which diagnostic criteria that are not easily rated should be queried in a standardized interview. The interview could include a standard set of questions for all respondents, plus questions designed to clarify responses to criterial symptoms that are endorsed on the rating forms.

Other complications arise from the changes in diagnostic criteria from DSM-III to DSM-III-R and DSM-IV (American Psychiatric Association, 1980, 1987, 1994). There have also been substantial differences between versions of the DISC that were based on the same edition of the DSM. The fact that DSM-V is scheduled for 2012, 18 years after the publication of DSM-IV in 1994, should allow sufficient time to conduct prevalence and comorbidity studies using a uniform version of the DISC based on the DSM-IV.

Obtaining Accurate Estimates of Prevalence Rates

As reported in Chapter 4, distributions of problem scale scores have been compared from CBCLs completed by parents in 31 cultures. Similar comparisons were reported in Chapter 4 for TRFs completed by teachers in 21 cultures and YSRs completed by youths in 24 cultures. These comparisons made it possible to identify cultures with relatively low, intermediate, and high scores on empirically based and DSM-oriented scales, according to parent, teacher, and self-reports. Other studies have reported bicultural comparisons of scores for specific problems (e.g., Achenbach, Bird, et al., 1990; Achenbach, Hensley, Phares, & Grayson, 1990; Lambert, Knight, Taylor, & Achenbach, 1996; Weisz et al., 1989).

Because the item and scale scores were quantitative, it was possible to perform quantitative statistical analyses of the differences between cultures. Statistically significant differences reflect multicultural variations in the magnitudes of problem scores, rather than the prevalence of problems or disorders, per se. However, the results can be converted to prevalence rates for each problem by counting ratings of 0 as indicating the absence of the problem and ratings of 1 and 2 as indicating the presence of the problem, as was done for some bicultural comparisons (e.g., Stanger, Fombonne, & Achenbach, 1994). As an alternative, to compare the prevalence of relatively severe problems, we can count each problem as present only if it was rated 2, and we can count the problem as absent if it was rated 0 or 1.

Analogously, scale scores can be converted to prevalence rates by counting the number of children who obtained scores above a particular cutpoint, such as the clinical or borderline clinical cutpoints that have been established to discriminate between children who are most likely to need professional help and children who are less likely to need professional help. Although the clinical and borderline clinical cutpoints were established on the basis of normative distributions of scale scores, cutpoints can also be established on the basis of other considerations. For example, cutpoints can be based on scores that are found to discriminate between particular criterion groups defined by the presence of known pathogens, tissue damage, genetic factors, criteria such as DSM diagnoses, etc.

Unlike the empirically based approach, the diagnostically based approach defines disorders as being present or absent according to a priori criteria. Consequently, operationalization of diagnoses in terms of standardized interviews directly yields prevalence rates for the samples of children for whom the interviews are used. However, as reported in Chapter 7, there is a paucity of directly comparable prevalence data for diagnoses made from standardized interviews in different cultures. Reasons for the paucity of comparable prevalence data include differences among the interviews that were used; differences between the diagnostic categories that were assessed even when the same interview was used; one-stage versus two-stage sampling designs; use of data from parents versus children; differences in how data from different sources were used to draw diagnostic conclusions; and different ways of aggregating diagnoses for statistical analysis. Thus, although the diagnoses made from the standardized interviews can be directly tabulated to provide prevalence rates, the findings published to date do not afford firm conclusions about variations in the prevalence of diagnostically defined disorders found for children in different cultures.

For both empirically based and diagnostically based approaches, data collected from probability samples of children in the general population are likely to yield the most useful and accurate estimates of prevalence. In addition, the higher the completion rate in a sample, the more likely it is that the results are not biased by unknown selection factors. Our review in Chapter 4 of multicultural comparisons of scores on empirically based instruments revealed that completion rates varied widely. Furthermore, low completion rates tended to be associated with lower problem scores, although there were exceptions to this general trend. In addition, completion rates tended to be low when forms were sent to respondents by mail. It is expensive to conduct general population studies with large samples and to use data collection procedures likely to yield high completion rates. However, such studies are likely to yield the most reliable and informative data on prevalence rates for children's problems.

As reviewed in Chapter 7, some diagnostically based prevalence studies have used probability samples and have achieved completion rates as high as 90.1% (Canino et al., 2004). However, other studies have used samples that were less likely to be representative and/or have failed to achieve high completion rates. Although two-stage prevalence studies have been viewed as more efficient and cost effective than one-stage studies, two-stage studies have suffered from serious attrition between Stage 1 and Stage 2. This attrition reduces the representativeness of the data obtained, even when the initial target sample was well chosen (e.g., Bird et al., 1988; Steinhausen et al., 1998; Verhulst et al., 1997). Furthermore, the relatively low costs of Stage 1 screening may be offset by the costs of subsequently locating and assessing all individuals chosen for the Stage 2 sample.

Dealing with Base-Rate Differences in Problems Associated with Age and Gender

Base rates of emotional and behavioral problems vary considerably with age and gender. For example, 4-year-old boys are more likely to manifest hyperactive, impulsive, and inattentive behavior than 16-year-old girls. Conversely, 16-year-old girls are more likely to report feelings of depression than 4-year-old boys. Because the empirically based approach stems from psychometric concepts, a core element of this approach is that an individual's scores should be compared with those obtained by a normative sample of peers. Research using empirically based scales has revealed consistent age and gender differences in scores on empirically based scales in most cultures, as reviewed in Chapter 4. For example, boys typically had higher raw scores than girls on attention problems and aggressive behavior, whereas older children typically had higher scores than younger children on depression and withdrawal. Because of these base-rate differences, deviance should be evaluated by comparing a child's scores with scores obtained by peers of the same age and gender.

The diagnostically based approach to assessment stems from medical practice, in which diseases are often assumed to be present or absent. For some diseases, such as measles, a known pathogen typically produces a particular disease. If the pathogen is not present, the disease is absent. However, even some physical illnesses are defined in terms of deviance on quantitative measures (e.g., high blood pressure), rather than as categorical conditions that are either present or absent. For emotional and behavioral disorders such as depression and ADHD, research has not yet identified specific pathogens or physical abnormalities. Instead, symptoms of disorders such as ADHD are widely distributed among members of the population. For example, 7-year-old boys vary widely in the number of problems characteristic of ADHD they manifest, with many manifesting few such problems and a smaller percentage manifesting many such problems. The variations are even greater when children of different ages and genders are compared.

Although some problems, such as hallucinations, delusions, and compulsive fire setting, may not need to be judged in relation to norms, many of the criterial symptoms of disorders such as ADHD, ODD, CD, and separation anxiety disorder are apt to vary significantly by gender and age. The DSM implicitly acknowledges base-rate differences in problems in some of its criteria. For example, the criteria for some disorders, such as ADHD, are only deemed to be met if "inconsistent with developmental level" (American Psychiatric Association, 2000, p. 92). However, the DSM provides no basis for judging whether symptoms are inconsistent with an individual's developmental level. Additionally, for some disorders a "child" variant of a presenting symptom is allowed, such as irritability instead of depressed mood for major depressive disorder. Yet the DSM does not provide norms or correlates for irritability in children of different ages and genders, making it difficult to determine when reports of irritability indicate a depressive disorder.

Normative data on the distributions of symptoms by gender, age, informant, and culture could be used to adjust diagnostic criteria in relation to the base rates of the symptoms in different groups. For example, it might be found that so many 4-year-old boys manifest six of the nine ADHD hyperactive/impulsive symptoms that this criterion does not indicate deviance for 4-year-old boys. Similarly, it might be found that so few 16-year-old girls manifest even four of the hyperactive/impulsive symptoms that a lower threshold for deviance might be needed for this group. Were the DSM normed by age and gender, particular symptoms and aggregates of symptoms could also be tested for their ability to discriminate between normal and clinical criterion groups of each gender and age, as assessed by different informants, in order to evaluate how well they function for various groups and to make norm-referenced adjustments to criteria, if needed.

Dealing with Patterning and Comorbidity of Problems

Whether viewed at the level of specific problems or of diagnostic categories, it is clear that there are many associations among children's problems. That is, many children manifest multiple kinds of problems and qualify for multiple diagnoses.

Statistical analyses of children's problems take account of co-occurrence among problems by identifying patterns of co-occurrence that may themselves be used as taxonomic constructs. A methodological challenge for research on child psychopathology is to find patterns of co-occurring problems that are particularly useful for assessing individual children, for training people to work with children, and for research and theory on the cause, course, prevention, treatment, and outcome of particular patterns of problems. For multicultural purposes, it is especially important that the patterns be supported across many cultures. As reported in Chapter 6, an eight-syndrome model has been supported by data from 31 cultures, and, as reported in Chapter 5, numerous correlates of these syndromes have been found in multiple cultures.

Findings that many children qualify for multiple diagnoses have been interpreted as reflecting the co-occurrence of different disorders; that is, comorbidity. However, as reported in Chapter 8, very few of the many studies of comorbidity have reported comorbidity between diagnoses in general population samples in ways that permit multicultural comparisons. Our comparisons of findings from these few studies indicated that comorbidity among certain diagnoses is undoubtedly high. However, variations between the studies and their results preclude firm conclusions about the precise patterns and rates of comorbidity. In addition, the difficulty of analyzing bidirectional comorbidity among more than two disorders at a time presents a challenge for identifying higher-order patterns such as those that are readily identified via cluster analysis, latent profile analysis, and second-order factor analysis of syndrome scores. The methodological challenges posed by comorbidity among diagnoses arise partly from unresolved conceptual issues regarding the degree to which current versions of diagnoses truly represent categorically different disorders. These and other unresolved conceptual issues are addressed in the following section.

CONCEPTUAL CHALLENGES

Next we discuss some major conceptual challenges that confront assessment of childhood psychopathology. First, we examine the notion of construct validity as it pertains to relations between assessment procedures and what they are intended to assess. Thereafter, we consider issues of taxonomic validity in relation to diagnostically and empirically based approaches.

Examining Construct Validity

In Chapter 2 we cited a dictionary definition of a *construct* as "an object of thought constituted by the ordering or systematic uniting of experiential elements" (Gove, 1971, p. 489). We drew an analogy between constructs and the statistical concept of a *latent variable,* which is a variable whose value is inferred from associations among multiple manifest (observed or measured) variables. We also cited a classic paper by Cronbach and Meehl (1955) titled "Construct Validity in Psychological Tests." A major point made by Cronbach and Meehl was that many tests are intended to measure attributes for which there is no operationally defined validity criterion. For such tests to be considered valid, various kinds of evidence must be obtained to substantiate a set of lawful relations (i.e., a *nomological network*) among observations and statements regarding the construct and the test that purports to measure it. Although a nomological network may comprise a theory that gives meaning to a construct, Cronbach and Meehl stated that "in the early stages of the development of a construct or even at more advanced stages when our orientation is thoroughly practical, little or no theory in the usual sense of the word need be involved" (p. 292). They also stated that "constructs may vary in nature from those very close to 'pure description' (involving little more than extrapolation of relations among observation-variables) to highly theoretical constructs" (p. 300).

Since Cronbach and Meehl (1955) laid the conceptual foundations for construct validity, others have sought to differentiate among various aspects of it (e.g., Benson, 1998; Messick, 1995; Nunnally & Bernstein, 1994). In doing so, they have focused on determining the validity with which a particular instrument assesses a construct (or latent variable) for which there is no single external validity criterion. Where there is no single external validity criterion, associations between the instrument's scores and various other data thought to tap the construct are used to evaluate the validity of the instrument for measuring the construct.

The Construct Validity of Intelligence Tests

Intelligence tests provide classic examples of the process of establishing construct validity. When Alfred Binet and Théophile Simon (1905/1916) were asked to find ways to identify French children whose cognitive development was sufficiently delayed to warrant special education, they invented a test that was validated on the basis of the following findings:

1. Children whose teachers judged them to be very bright all did well on the test.
2. Children whose school performance lagged 3 or more years behind that of their agemates all obtained mental ages (MAs) on the test below their chronological ages (CAs). (An MA is the level of cognitive performance typically achieved by normal children of a particular CA.)

3. Most children performing normally in school obtained MAs corresponding to their CAs.
4. Children could rarely pass items located above their ceiling levels—i.e., the MA levels at which they had failed all items.

After Binet and Simon published their test in France, translated versions were adopted in many countries. One kind of support for the construct validity of the American version of the test was Frederick Kuhlmann's (1912) finding that MA scores correlated well with the mean of several teachers' ratings of the abilities of children with mental retardation, even though the teachers' ratings correlated poorly with each other. Construct validity was also supported by findings that children who obtained high scores on Lewis Terman's (1916) Stanford–Binet test subsequently achieved high levels of success in school and in adult life, as documented by a longitudinal study that eventually spanned 50 years (Sears, 1977).

When new tests were developed, such as the Wechsler (1939) intelligence scales, their construct validity was supported by their substantial correlations with the Binet tests. As we noted earlier, corresponding scales scored from 21st-century versions of the Wechsler and Stanford–Binet tests correlate from .66 to .85 (Roid, 2003). Such high correlations indicate that both kinds of tests are measuring similar constructs, even though there is no single "gold standard" criterion for those constructs. In addition to substantial correlations between different tests of intelligence, the construct validity of the tests has been supported by their significant predictive correlations with academic performance and other measures of intellectual achievement under many conditions. The construct validity of particular scales of the tests has also been supported by CFAs, which confirm the hypothesized patterning of test items (Roid, 2003; Wechsler, 2003).

Developing Valid Taxonomic Constructs for Child Psychopathology

At our current stage of knowledge about child psychopathology, it is helpful to work toward valid taxonomic constructs. In other words, we need to identify constructs that validly represent important differences in kinds and degrees of psychopathology. Although it is expected that taxonomic constructs will eventually provide a basis for theories about the nature and cause of specific kinds of psychopathology, neither the diagnostically based nor empirically based approaches to taxonomy of child psychopathology are derived from well-supported theories about causes of psychopathology. First we consider diagnostically based taxonomic constructs because they stem from the tradition of deriving diagnostic criteria from clinicians' concepts of disorders, in contrast to deriving empirically based taxonomic constructs from psychometric findings.

Diagnostically Based Taxonomic Constructs

The diagnostically based approach rests on clinicians' concepts of disorders (Spitzer & Cantwell, 1980). Based on their own experience and knowledge, clinicians provide categories and criteria for the DSM and ICD. However, they do not specify operations for assessing behavioral and emotional problems. The lack of operational definitions in the DSM and ICD prompted the development of standardized interviews to operationalize the diagnostic criteria. Because the standardized interviews are intended to assess diagnostic constructs, substantial associations between diagnoses made from the interviews and diagnoses made by other means would support the construct validity of the interviews for assessing and discriminating between diagnostic constructs. However, meta-analyses have yielded kappas averaging only .15 between diagnoses of children made from standardized interviews and diagnoses made from clinical evaluations (Rettew et al., 2006). The kappas were too low to validate diagnoses made from standardized interviews in terms of clinical diagnoses of children, even when the clinical diagnoses were made by teams of clinicians using data from multiple sources (e.g., Jensen & Weisz, 2002; Lewczyk et al., 2003).

If we think of clinicians' diagnoses as being analogous to teachers' ratings of children's intelligence, perhaps the low agreement with interview-based diagnoses is analogous to the low agreement between individual teachers' ratings and the early Binet–Simon intelligence test. Although even the low agreement with individual teachers' ratings provided one type of support for the construct validity of early intelligence tests, other kinds of evidence for the construct validity of the tests, including higher correlations with ratings averaged from multiple teachers than with individual teachers' ratings (Kuhlmann, 1912), soon showed that the tests were more valid measures of intelligence than were individual teachers' ratings.

At this writing, there is evidence that diagnoses made from standardized interviews are significantly associated with some other variables. However, as reviewed in Chapter 8, the findings are not consistent enough to argue that the standardized interviews have greater construct validity than diagnoses of children made by clinical teams (e.g., Jensen & Weisz, 2002; Lewczyk et al., 2003). Furthermore, what is apparently the only published study of agreement between diagnoses made for the same children from different standardized interviews (the

DISC vs. the K-SADS) yielded mean kappas of only .03 for agreement between "definite" diagnoses and .14 for agreement between "possible" diagnoses (Cohen et al., 1987). Finding high agreement between diagnoses made from two or more standardized interviews would support the construct validity of the interviews, just as high correlations between intelligence tests indicate that the different tests measure similar constructs.

An important taxonomic function of diagnostic constructs is to differentiate between disorders. However, the high rates of comorbidity found between diagnoses and the variations in comorbidity from one study to another suggest a lack of clear separation between the disorders represented by different diagnoses. Nevertheless, DSM and ICD diagnoses will continue to be used for numerous important purposes. These purposes include communicating about psychopathology, training mental health professionals, determining whether and what treatment is needed, and obtaining reimbursement for services.

Empirically Based Taxonomic Constructs

Unlike diagnostically based taxonomic constructs, empirically based taxonomic constructs consist of patterns of co-occurring problems identified via statistical analyses of data for large samples of children. In other words, the procedures for deriving empirically based constructs are designed to determine which problems tend to co-occur and then to operationalize the identified patterns in terms of quantified scales. Individual children can be scored on the scales and their scale scores can be compared with scores for normative samples of peers to assess degrees of deviance and nondeviance. Because the taxonomic constructs are based on statistical findings and because individuals are assessed in terms of quantitative scale scores, it is not assumed that each construct represents a categorically separate disorder. Nor is it assumed that deviance on multiple scales necessarily indicates the presence of multiple disorders. Instead, the statistically identified patterns of problems and the patterns of scale scores obtained by individual children may be shaped by diverse causal factors that contribute to the co-occurrence of particular problems. The patterns may be caused by the co-occurrence of disorders that are categorically distinct as well as by other factors.

The validity of scales for assessing several empirically based taxonomic constructs has been supported by findings analogous to findings that have supported the construct validity of intelligence tests. Like the high correlations between corresponding scales of the Stanford–Binet and Wechsler intelligence tests, high correlations have been found between corresponding scales of the ASEBA and Conners instruments. For parents' ratings, correlations have ranged from .71 to .80, with a mean of .77. For teachers' ratings, correlations have ranged from .77 to .89, with a mean of .84 (Achenbach & Rescorla, 2001).

Analogous to the CFA evidence for the construct validity of intelligence test scales, the CFA findings reported in Chapter 6 support the configural invariance of ASEBA syndromes in ratings of children's problems, although the CFA findings include far more cultures than do the findings for intelligence tests (Ivanova et al., 2006a, 2006b, 2006c). As reviewed in Chapters 2 and 5, significant associations have been found between scores on the empirically based taxonomic scales and many other variables, including genetic, biochemical, developmental, and outcome variables. Although not specifically designed to assess DSM diagnostic constructs, scores on the empirically based taxonomic scales have also been significantly associated with DSM diagnoses in diverse samples. On the other hand, some kinds of disorders, such as severe infantile autism, may not be effectively captured by the empirically based approach. Nevertheless, for disorders that may be effectively captured by both approaches, a major challenge is to develop taxonomic constructs for representing distinctive patterns of psychopathology in ways that are acceptable to mental health providers working from both the empirically based and diagnostically based perspectives in multiple cultures.

Dealing with the Lack of a "Gold Standard" for Psychopathology

Because no physical pathogens or physical abnormalities have yet been found to underlie most behavioral and emotional disorders of children, there is no definitive medical test to determine whether such disorders are present. In other words, we currently lack a "gold standard" for these behavioral and emotional disorders. Consequently, deciding whether a disorder such as ADHD, depression, conduct disorder, or autism is present requires weighing evidence derived from various assessment procedures. All assessment procedures are subject to error. However, the degree of error cannot be precisely determined without a gold standard against which the assessment procedures can be tested.

When researchers lack a gold standard, they often test the validity of assessment procedures by comparing their results to the results of other procedures for assessing the same constructs. Good agreement among multiple procedures for assessing a particular construct is one kind of evidence for the construct validity of the procedures. New assessment procedures are often developed because of perceived deficiencies in old assessment procedures. Ironically, however, the presumably deficient procedures are often used as validation criteria for new procedures. For example, the DISC was developed because of perceived deficiencies in existing diagnostic procedures, such as clinical evaluations. However, one way to test the validity of the DISC is to compare its diagnoses with diagnoses obtained from clinical evaluations (Rettew et al., 2006).

Meta-analyses have revealed poor agreement between diagnoses made from standardized diagnostic interviews and diagnoses made from clinical evaluations of children. The lack of a gold standard and the poor agreement between diagnoses made from standardized interviews and clinical evaluations also present challenges for adult diagnoses, for which meta-analyses have yielded a mean kappa of only .29 (Rettew et al., 2006). The poor agreement found for adult diagnoses has been interpreted by some as indicating that standardized interviews administered by "lay" (i.e., nonclinician) interviewers are less valid than "systematic clinical assessment" (Brugha, Bebbington, & Jenkins, 1999, p. 1015). When Brugha et al. attempted to "calibrate" lay interviews using the Clinical Interview Schedule–Revised (CIS-R) with clinician-administered Schedules for Clinical Assessment in Neuropsychiatry (SCAN) interviews (Taub et al., 2005), they obtained disappointing results. With SCAN diagnoses serving as gold standards, Taub et al. sought to modify diagnostic findings from less costly CIS-R interviews to agree better with gold standard SCAN diagnoses. Despite sophisticated statistical analyses of their large sample ($N = 612$), however, Taub et al. concluded that lay interviews would have to be greatly improved in order to increase their agreement with clinical interviews before calibration efforts could succeed.

In contrast to the view that lay interviews are at fault, others have argued that "clinical interviews, especially those administered in community settings, might have serious problems of both reliability and validity" (Wittchen, Üstün, & Kessler, 1999, p. 1022). Wittchen et al. cited a variety of evidence indicating that structured lay interviews actually yielded more reliable and valid data than semistructured clinical interviews in community samples.

Another option for validating diagnostic interviews is to compare the results obtained from two different diagnostic interviews, such as the DISC and the K-SADS. Surprisingly few findings of this sort have been published. The few comparisons of diagnoses made from two different diagnostic interviews have yielded quite poor agreement. However, better agreement has been obtained between diagnostic interviews and scores on empirically based instruments, as reviewed in Chapter 5.

Despite decades of sophisticated and costly studies of large and diverse samples, the challenges of finding appropriate gold standards for diagnostically based instruments have not yet been mastered, even for adult diagnoses. As exemplified by the debate between Brugha et al. (1999) and Wittchen et al. (1999), diagnostic interview methodology has received a great deal of attention. However, in the methodological efforts to improve the reliability and validity of diagnostic interviews, less attention has been paid to conceptualizations of the diagnoses that the interviews are supposed to assess. If specific physical etiologies are discovered for particular forms of psychopathology, tests of those etiologies will become key components of the operational definitions for the relevant diagnoses. Finding such physical etiologies is a major goal of research in molecular genetics and neuroimaging. Yet, until physical etiologies are pinpointed, diagnostic constructs depend on data that are practical to obtain for clinical and research purposes. Many assessment procedures can be used to collect such data, but all procedures arc inevitably subject to error. It is therefore essential to quantify error and to minimize its effects on assessment decisions. Quantification and norm referencing are two ways to do this.

SUMMARY

To advance our understanding of children's problems, certain challenges must be met. Among the methodological challenges are the need to obtain multisource data; effective use of multisource data for making decisions; dealing with test–retest attenuation and regression toward the mean; attaining uniformity in problems assessed across cultures; obtaining accurate estimates of prevalence rates; dealing with base-rate differences associated with age and gender; and documenting the patterning and comorbidity of children's problems.

Important conceptual challenges are posed by issues of construct validity and their implications for the validity of taxonomic constructs for child psychopathology. A fundamental conceptual challenge is the current lack of a "gold standard" for most disorders. The low agreement between clinical diagnoses and diagnoses made from standardized interviews raises questions about how to test the validity of both kinds of diagnoses. A variety of evidence supports the construct and criterion-related validity of empirically based scales in relation to diverse criteria. A major challenge for the future is to formulate constructs for psychopathology that can be validly assessed and effectively used to link clinical services with research in multiple cultures.

CHAPTER 11

Contributions of Multicultural Research to Understanding, Assessing, Preventing, and Treating Child Psychopathology

Chapter 1 posed the question, "Why should we do multicultural research on children's problems?" The findings presented in Chapters 2–9 demonstrate many kinds of knowledge that can be gained from multicultural research on children's problems. An especially compelling reason for doing multicultural research is that findings of similarities and differences among diverse cultures can advance our understanding more than findings that may only reflect idiosyncrasies of a particular culture. This is because findings from a particular culture may be affected by culture-specific factors, such as that culture's language, the possibilities for recruiting participants, the degree to which people are willing to provide relevant information, and characteristics of mental health, medical, educational, and other systems.

The benefits of multicultural research are like those of meta-analyses of diverse studies. Because each study in a meta-analysis differs from each other study in various ways, findings that are general across diverse studies deserve more confidence than findings from one study or a few very similar studies. Likewise, findings that are general across diverse cultures deserve more confidence regarding principles of human functioning than findings from one culture or a few very similar cultures. On the other hand, findings that differ sharply from one culture to another may reveal important variables that are espe-

273

cially intertwined with culture. This can, in turn, provide leads about culture-specific processes that affect development and psychopathology. In other words, viewing multicultural research from meta-analytic perspectives can advance our understanding by distinguishing between factors that are culture specific and those that are general across diverse cultures.

BEYOND "WE" VERSUS "THEY"

In Chapter 1 we pointed out that people often simplify the complexity of cultural differences by imposing categories of "we" versus "they." We also discussed other categories that people impose on cultural variations. As Hermans and Kempen (1998) have argued, conceptualization of cultural variations in terms of categories falsely represents "cultures as internally homogeneous and externally distinctive" (p. 1119). Research that applies similar standardized assessment procedures to people in diverse cultures can help us move beyond views of cultures as internally homogeneous and externally distinctive and toward broader understanding of issues that cut across all cultures.

The significant within-culture gender, age, and SES differences in scores on empirically based instruments reported in Chapters 4 and 5 indicate that cultures are not "internally homogeneous" with respect to children's behavioral and emotional problems. Conversely, findings presented in Chapters 4, 5, and 6 indicate considerable multicultural consistency in ratings of children's behavioral and emotional problems. The findings include (1) good fit for the eight-syndrome model in many cultures; (2) similar scale scores in many cultures; (3) similar associations of scale scores with age and gender in nearly all cultures and with SES and parents' marital status in cultures where these associations were tested; (4) consistency in heritability estimates and longitudinal patterns for empirically based scale scores in several cultures; and (5) consistent associations of scale scores with diagnoses and with referral for services in several cultures.

NEW WAYS TO UNDERSTAND CHILD PSYCHOPATHOLOGY

Although much remains to be done, multicultural research on many thousands of children has yielded a great deal of knowledge on which to base new ways of understanding child psychopathology. Until recently, most theories and practices were based mainly on children in a few very similar cultures. These theories and practices were assumed to apply to children in general. However, various forms of globalization confront us with both needs and opportunities to extend the study of child psychopathology to many more cultures. Studies of children in diverse cultures broaden the range of questions that can be addressed and the generalizability of the findings. Adapting standardized assessment procedures to the practical realities of different cultures can help to demystify both what is being assessed and differences between cultures.

Because assessment of child psychopathology depends heavily on reports by people who know the children and by the children themselves, the characteristics to be assessed must be formulated in ways that enable people from different cultures to provide similarly meaningful information. This requires assessment instruments that can be administered in cost-effective ways under diverse conditions. For research purposes, the instruments should be used to assess samples of children who are appropriately representative of particular groups. Determining the prevalence of problems among children in a particular culture requires samples that are representative of the general population of children in that culture.

Standardized data on the prevalence and patterning of numerous problems have been obtained in many cultures, as detailed in Chapters 4 and 6. As summarized in Chapter 5, correlates of problems have been compared in fewer cultures, but the standardization of empirically based assessment procedures across many cultures makes it possible to test correlates in additional cultures. Various theoretical approaches have been applied to child psychopathology and adaptive functioning. However, standardized data on the prevalence, patterning, and correlates of problems in many cultures now provide a far more comprehensive basis for understanding and dealing with the developmental course of psychopathology. In other words, the large multicultural database, obtained with methods that are easily applied to research and services, provides a solid foundation for advancing knowledge of child psychopathology. This knowledge can, in turn, foster new ways to assess, prevent, and treat child psychopathology, as outlined next.

Assessing Child Psychopathology

Since the publication of DSM-III (American Psychiatric Association, 1980), the diagnostically based approach to assessment has shared with the empirically based approach a focus on explicitly specified problems. Although the diagnostically based approach designates the problems as "symptoms," the symptoms specified for diagnoses such as ADHD, ODD, CD, anxiety disorders, and depressive disorders have many clear counterparts among the problem items of empirically based assessment instruments. Furthermore, reports of whether a child manifests the criterial symptoms of a particular diagnosis are crucial for determining whether the child qualifies for the diagnosis. Other criteria, such as the age when the symptoms first appeared, impairment caused by the symptoms, and whether the symptoms are due to some other disorder are often so difficult to assess with certainty that they may have little practical effect on diagnostic decisions. Consequently, for both research and clinical purposes, the diagnostically based approach relies heavily on parent, teacher, and self-reports of children's behavioral and emotional problems, just as the empirically based approach does.

The two approaches assess some different problem items and aggregate the items into different constructs. Yet they may share enough common ground to provide a basis for multicultural research that includes problem items and constructs from both approaches. To improve both reliability and agreement with other assessment procedures, it may be more productive to assess diagnostically based problem items quantitatively rather than in yes/no terms. It would also be more productive to experiment with different ways of aggregating the diagnostically based problem items rather than requiring that they be aggregated solely according to preexisting fixed rules for making yes/no diagnostic decisions. Quantifying the assessment of problem items would not preclude also categorizing judgments of the problems as yes versus no. For example, if respondents rated the problem items as 0, 1, or 2, the data could be categorized as *0 = No* versus *1 or 2 = Yes*. They could also be categorized as *0 or 1 = No* versus *2 = Yes*. Analogously, experimenting with different ways of aggregating items would not preclude also applying existing diagnostic rules to decisions about whether a child has a disorder.

The items could be experimentally aggregated via such statistical procedures as factor analysis, cluster analysis, latent class analysis, and latent profile analysis. After the items are aggregated, different rules can be tested for deciding which children should be classified as having, versus not having, particular disorders. For example, if factor analysis is used to aggregate items, various cutpoints can be tested on the distribution of scores computed by aggregating ratings of items found to load highly on a particular factor. If cluster analysis is used to aggregate items, the similarity between a child's pattern of item ratings and various cluster types can be computed via measures of association, such as intraclass correlation and Euclidean distance. If latent class analysis is used, children can be assigned to the classes for which their patterns of item scores have the highest probability of membership.

By assessing large samples of children from multiple cultures in terms of diagnostically based problem items and by experimenting with quantitative scoring and different ways of aggregating the items, researchers can compare the prevalence and patterning of the problem items across cultures. They can also test whether the findings are consistent with existing diagnostic categories and criteria.

Preventing Child Psychopathology

Systematic research that employs the same standardized assessment procedures in different cultures can potentially identify risk factors for psychopathology that are common to multiple cultures. As illustrated by findings reviewed in Chapter 5, longitudinal studies in the Netherlands and the United States have revealed similar predictive relations between developmentally early variables and later psychopathology. In addition, cross-sectional findings have revealed tendencies for problem scores to be higher among children from lower-SES than higher-SES families in a variety of cultures. Longitudinal research on developmental changes in problem levels has also revealed that the prevalence of elevated problem scores tends to increase with development among children from lower-SES but not higher-SES families (Wadsworth & Achenbach, 2005). For some kinds of problems, increases in the prevalence of elevated scores among lower-SES children reflected a greater incidence of new "cases" than among higher-SES children. For other kinds of problems, increases in the proportions of elevated scores reflected a greater accumulation of elevated scores among lower-SES than higher-SES children. In other words, once these problems reached elevated levels, they were less likely to be ameliorated (i.e., to drop to the normal range) among lower-SES than higher-SES children at subsequent ages.

Although not measurable in precisely the same way in all cultures, SES is typically a proxy for multiple social, economic, and educational variables. Measures of SES that are appropriate for a culture may be useful markers for risks that could be targeted for efforts to prevent certain kinds of problems. For some children in some cultures, economic deprivation may contribute to higher problem levels. However, low SES is associated with higher problem levels even in cultures such as Sweden (Larsson & Frisk, 1999), where excellent public support services and protections against poverty mean that economic deprivation is unlikely to play a major role.

To prevent problems that are associated with SES, we should look closely at such factors as attitudes, stressors, microenvironments, aspirations, role models, and adaptational competencies that may be related to SES. We should also consider risk factors for low-SES children that may be related to risk factors for minority and immigrant children. In some cultures, immigrant and minority families tend to be of lower SES than indigenous families. However, associations of higher problem scores with lower SES have been found even in cultures that had few minority and immigrant children when the studies were done, such as Iceland (Hannesdottir & Einarsdottir, 1995), Jamaica (Lambert et al., 1994), Lithuania (Zukauskiene et al., 2003), and Sweden (Larsson & Frisk, 1999), as well as in cultures with many minority and immigrant children, such as Australia (Sawyer et al., 2001) and the United States (Achenbach & Rescorla, 2001; Bourdon, 2005).

It is possible that combinations of low SES with immigrant and minority status may increase risks for certain kinds of problems. Yet analyses of SES effects on U.S. parent and teacher ratings, with ethnicity partialed out, still showed significantly higher problem scores for lower-SES than for higher-SES children (Achenbach & Rescorla, 2001). After SES was partialed out, associations between ethnicity and problem scores were negligible. This finding indicates that, even in cultures where many children are immigrants and minorities, SES has significant associations with problem scores independent of immigration and minority status.

Associations between the marital status of parents and problems reported for their children have been published for a few cultures. Lower problem scores have been found for children from intact families than nonintact families in cultures as different as the United States and China (Bourdon et al., 2005; Liu, Kurita, Guo, et al., 1999). Proportionately more lower-SES children than higher-SES children live in nonintact families, which often include only one parent figure. Because SES and marital status may be mutually associated, and both may also be associated with immigration status, questions arise about whether each of these variables represents different risk factors or whether elevated risks for problems are primarily associated with only one of them. Because lower-SES families tend to live in more deprived neighborhoods than higher-SES families, questions also arise about whether neighborhood characteristics are associated with children's problems, over and above family SES and parents' marital status.

To identify relations among risk factors at the level of family characteristics and at other levels, such as neighborhood characteristics, we need multilevel modeling of data. As reviewed in Chapter 5, a study in the Dutch city of Maastricht found that neighborhood SES indeed had an effect on CBCL problem scores for 5- to 7-year-olds, over and above the effects of family SES and parents' marital status (Kalff, Kroes, Vles, Bosma, et al., 2001; Kalff, Kroes, Vles, Henricksen, et al., 2001). Specifically, children from low-SES nonintact families had higher problem scores if they lived in low-SES neighborhoods than if they lived in higher-SES neighborhoods.

A study in the Dutch city of Rotterdam showed that neighborhood socioeconomic disadvantage (NSD) was associated with high problem scores on both the CBCL and YSR for 10- to 12-year-olds, after controlling for parental SES (Schneiders et al., 2003). Furthermore, NSD predicted increases in problem scores over a 2-year follow-up period. The findings from Maastricht and Rotterdam thus indicate that characteristics of low-SES neighborhoods, in addition to family characteristics associated with low SES, may contribute to children's problems. Although additional factors are apt to be associated with particular kinds of problems, one fruitful prevention strategy may be to concentrate resources for strengthening protective factors in schools and other neighborhood institutions that serve predominantly low-SES families. The multicultural consistency of associations between low SES and high problem scores even in cultures lacking significant poverty and immigration indicates that characteristics associated with low SES may be especially good targets for preventive efforts in many cultures.

In addition to SES differences, other variations in family characteristics may potentially affect children's problems and adaptive functioning. Certain childrearing practices, for example, may elevate risks for particular kinds of problems. Other childrearing practices may strengthen children's adaptive functioning in ways that protect against particular kinds of problems. By using the same standardized procedures to assess children's problems in different cultures and by also assessing childrearing practices in the different cultures, researchers can determine whether particular problems are consistently associated with certain childrearing practices in the different cultures.

As an example, Landsford et al. (2005) tested associations between reports of corporal punishment and scores on the CBCL and YSR in samples from China, India, Italy, Kenya, the Philippines, and Thailand. Across all six cultures, mothers who used the most corporal punishment rated their children highest on the CBCL Aggressive and Anxious/Depressed syndromes. However, individual mothers' reported use of corporal punishment had the strongest effects on CBCL problem scores in cultures where other mothers reported little use of corporal punishment. Equally interesting, children who reported that parents in their cultures frequently used corporal punishment rated themselves high on the YSR Aggressive Behavior syndrome, regardless of how much corporal punishment their own mothers were reported to use. There were thus some consistencies in relations between reports of corporal punishment and children's problems that could guide multicultural prevention programs. There were also important interactions between culture and other variables that need to be considered when implementing such programs.

Treating Child Psychopathology

When feasible, it is usually better to prevent problems than to try to eliminate them after they emerge. Treatment of children's mental health problems is costly and time consuming. Furthermore, appropriate treatment requires well-qualified practitioners, plus significant commitments by the children, their parents, and often their schools. Even in affluent cultures, estimates of need for help far exceed the availability of appropriate services (U.S. Public Health Service, 2000). Less affluent cultures have fewer child mental health professionals, and they are typically concentrated in a very few locations within the cultures.

Both to improve the accessibility of existing services and to guide the development of new services, we need to consider multicultural perspectives. In cultures that have substantial service infrastructures, improving the accessibility of services requires adapting referral, assessment, and treatment procedures to the unmet needs of immigrant, minority, and low-SES families and children. In cultures that lack substantial service infrastructures, new services may be based on methods and training from cultures that already have substantial infrastructures.

In cultures that have substantial infrastructures, there has been growing recognition that mental health services may not always be intrinsically beneficial. Instead, some services may fail to ameliorate problems or may even cause harm. Recognition of these facts has inspired the development of *EBT*, which refers to "empirically based treatment," also known as "evidence-based treatment." EBT is treatment whose efficacy is supported by research. The clearest kind of research support is typically provided by randomized clinical trials in which outcomes are compared for participants who have been randomly assigned to different treatment conditions. Meta-analyses of many well-controlled studies have yielded evidence that several kinds of treatment can substantially reduce some childhood problems (Weisz, 2004). These findings provide empirically based guidance for developing new services and for improving existing services. However, EBT has not yet been widely implemented in clinical practice, and research has not found much evidence for the effectiveness of child mental health services as they are typically rendered (Weisz & Addis, 2006). Consequently, much remains to be learned about how to identify children who will benefit from each kind of service and how to ensure that children actually receive the most effective service for their particular needs.

To translate EBT into more effective mental health services, we need stronger links between assessment of children, on the one hand, and the choice of treatment, on the other (Mash & Hunsley, 2005). In EBT studies, children are typically recruited according to a priori categories of problems for which particular EBTs are designed, such as anxiety disorders and obsessive–compulsive disorders. Although EBT may well be effective in controlled studies of children who are recruited in this way, many children who need help may not be easily identified according to the a priori categories used in EBT research. Instead, children may have problems that fit multiple categories or none of the categories. Furthermore, multi-informant assessment may yield major differences between children's views of their own problems and the views of mothers, fathers, teachers, and clinicians, each of whom may, in turn, hold different views (Achenbach, McConaughy, et al., 1987; Yeh & Weisz, 2001). Consequently, EBT needs to be more closely meshed with *EBA*, that is, "empirically based" or "evidence-based" assessment (Achenbach, 2005; Mash & Hunsley, 2005). The need for EBAs in addition to EBTs may be especially pertinent to economically undeveloped cultures, as well as for minority, immigrant, and low-SES children and their families in all cultures.

Although multi-informant data can enhance the assessment of all children, such data are especially helpful for avoiding premature closure on mental health labels and diagnoses. As reviewed in Chapters 4–6, EBA methods have yielded similar results in many cultural groups. These findings suggest that EBA can provide a foundation for extending treatment to immigrant, minority, and low-SES children in cultures that already have substantial infrastructures, as well to children in cultures that do not.

SUMMARY

Etic comparisons across many cultures are analogous to meta-analyes of diverse studies. Findings that are consistent across diverse cultures deserve more confidence regarding general principles of psychopathology than findings from individual cultures. Conversely, findings that are specific to only one or a few distinct cultures may suggest culture-specific processes that need to be investigated.

Multicultural research opens new vistas on child psychopathology that extend beyond theories and practices rooted in a few cultures.

Because assessment of child psychopathology depends heavily on reports by people who know the children and by the children themselves, the assessment process should enable people from different cultures to provide similarly meaningful information. Standardized assessment procedures have produced a multicultural database that can foster new ways to assess, prevent, and treat children's behavioral, emotional, and social problems. Current versions of diagnostically based assessment and empirically based assessment both focus on explicitly specified problems. Ways were outlined to use both approaches in multicultural research and practice.

Multicultural findings on relations between risk factors and psychopathology suggest targets for prevention that are relevant to many cultural contexts. Because not all problems can be prevented and because need for help exceeds the supply of effective services in most cultures, it is useful to consider multicultural perspectives on improving access to EBT. Even in affluent cultures, EBT is typically least available to immigrant, minority, and low-SES families. To improve accessibility in cultures that have substantial mental health infrastructures and in those that do not, an essential step is to identify children who will benefit from particular treatments. Making this identification requires closing the gap between EBT and EBA in order to pinpoint specific needs and evaluate treatment outcomes.

References

Achenbach, T. M. (1965, March). *A factor-analytic study of juvenile psychiatric symptoms.* Paper presented at the meeting of the Society for Research in Child Development, Minneapolis, MN.

Achenbach, T. M. (1966). The classification of children's psychiatric symptoms: A factor-analytic study. *Psychological Monographs, 80* (No. 615).

Achenbach, T. M. (1991a). *Manual for the Child Behavior Checklist/4–18 and 1991 Profile.* Burlington: University of Vermont, Department of Psychiatry.

Achenbach, T. M. (1991b). *Manual for the Teacher's Report Form and 1991 Profile.* Burlington: University of Vermont, Department of Psychiatry.

Achenbach, T. M. (1991c). *Manual for the Youth Self-Report and 1991 Profile.* Burlington: University of Vermont, Department of Psychiatry.

Achenbach, T. M. (1997). *Manual for the Young Adult Self-Report and Young Adult Behavior Checklist.* Burlington: University of Vermont, Department of Psychiatry.

Achenbach, T. M. (2005). Advancing assessment of children and adolescents: Commentary on evidence-based assessment of child and adolescent disorders. *Journal of Clinical Child and Adolescent Psychology, 34,* 541–547.

Achenbach, T. M., Bird, H. R., Canino, G. J., Phares, V., Gould, M., & Rubio-Stipec, M. (1990). Epidemiological comparisons of Puerto Rican and U.S. mainland children: Parent, teacher, and self reports. *Journal of the American Academy of Child and Adolescent Psychiatry, 29,* 84–93.

Achenbach, T. M., Dumenci, L., Erol, N., & Roussos, A. C. (2000). *Rejoinder: Despite the limitations of their data and analyses, the Hartman et al. results support the CBCL/TRF syndrome structure.* Unpublished manuscript.

Achenbach, T. M., Dumenci, L., & Rescorla, L. A. (2001). *Ratings of relations between DSM-IV diagnostic categories and items of the CBCL/6–18, TRF, and YSR.* Burlington: University of Vermont, Research Center for Children, Youth, and Families. Available at www.ASEBA.org

Achenbach, T. M., Dumenci, L., & Rescorla, L. A. (2002). Is American student behavior getting worse? Teacher ratings over an 18-year period. *School Psychology Review, 31,* 428–442.

Achenbach, T. M., Dumenci, L., & Rescorla, L. A. (2003a). Are American children's problems still getting worse? A 23-year comparison. *Journal of Abnormal Child Psychology, 31,* 1–11.

Achenbach, T. M., Dumenci, L., & Rescorla, L. A. (2003b). *Ratings of relations between DSM-IV diagnostic categories and items of the Adult Self-Report (ASR) and Adult Behavior Checklist (ABCL).* Burlington: University of Vermont, Research Center for Children, Youth, and Families. Available at www.ASEBA.org

Achenbach, T. M., & Edelbrock, C. (1978). The classification of child psychopathology: A review and analysis of empirical efforts. *Psychological Bulletin, 85,* 1275–1301.

Achenbach, T. M., & Edelbrock, C. (1981). Behavioral problems and competencies reported by parents of normal and disturbed children aged four to sixteen. *Monographs of the Society for Research in Child Development, 46*(1, Serial No. 188).

Achenbach, T. M., & Edelbrock, C. (1983). *Manual for the Child Behavior Checklist and Revised Child Behavior Profile.* Burlington: University of Vermont, Department of Psychiatry.

Achenbach, T. M., & Edelbrock, C. (1986). *Manual for the Teacher's Report Form and Teacher Version of the Child Behavior Profile.* Burlington: University of Vermont, Department of Psychiatry.

Achenbach, T. M., & Edelbrock, C. (1987). *Manual for the Youth Self-Report and Profile.* Burlington: University of Vermont, Department of Psychiatry.

Achenbach, T. M., Hensley, V. R., Phares, V., & Grayson, D. (1990). Problems and competencies reported by parents of Australian and American children. *Journal of Child Psychology and Psychiatry, 31,* 265–286.

Achenbach, T. M., Howell, C. T., McConaughy, S. H., & Stanger, C. (1995a). Six-year predictors of problems in a national sample of children and youth: I. Cross-informant syndromes. *Journal of the American Academy of Child and Adolescent Psychiatry, 34,* 336–347.

Achenbach, T. M., Howell, C. T., McConaughy, S. H., & Stanger, C. (1995b). Six-year predictors of problems in a national sample of children and youth: II. Signs of disturbance. *Journal of the American Academy of Child and Adolescent Psychiatry, 34,* 488–498.

Achenbach, T. M., Howell, C. T., McConaughy, S. H., & Stanger, C. (1995c). Six-year predictors of problems in a national sample: III. Transitions to young adult syndromes. *Journal of the American Academy of Child and Adolescent Psychiatry, 34,* 658–669.

Achenbach, T. M., Howell, C. T., McConaughy, S. H., & Stanger, C. (1998). Six-year predictors of problems in a national sample: IV. Young adult signs of disturbance. *Journal of the American Academy of Child and Adolescent Psychiatry, 37,* 718–727.

Achenbach, T. M., Howell, C. T., Quay, H. C., & Conners, C. K. (1991). National survey of problems and competencies among 4- to 16-year-olds:

Parents' reports for normative and clinical samples. *Monographs of the Society for Research in Child Development, 56*(3, Serial No. 225).

Achenbach, T. M., Krukowski, R. A., Dumenci, L., & Ivanova, M. Y. (2005). Assessment of adult psychopathology: Meta-analyses and implications of cross-informant correlations. *Psychological Bulletin, 131,* 361–382.

Achenbach, T. M., & Lewis, M. (1971). A proposed model for clinical research and its application to encopresis and enuresis. *Journal of the American Academy of Child Psychiatry, 10,* 535–554.

Achenbach, T. M., McConaughy, S. H., & Howell, C. T. (1987). Child/adolescent behavioral and emotional problems: Implications of cross-informant correlations for situational specificity. *Psychological Bulletin, 101,* 213–232.

Achenbach, T. M., Newhouse, P. A., & Rescorla, L. A. (2004). *Manual for the ASEBA Older Adult Forms and Profiles.* Burlington: University of Vermont, Research Center for Children, Youth, and Families.

Achenbach, T. M., & Rescorla, L. A. (2000). *Manual for the ASEBA Preschool Forms and Profiles.* Burlington: University of Vermont, Research Center for Children, Youth, and Families.

Achenbach, T. M., & Rescorla, L. A. (2001). *Manual for the ASEBA School-Age Forms and Profiles.* Burlington: University of Vermont, Research Center for Children, Youth, and Families.

Achenbach, T. M., & Rescorla, L. A. (2003). *Manual for the ASEBA Adult Forms and Profiles.* Burlington: University of Vermont, Research Center for Children, Youth, and Families.

Achenbach, T. M., & Rescorla, L. A. (in press). *Multicultural supplement to the manual for the ASEBA school-age forms and profiles.* Burlington: University of Vermont, Research Center for Children, Youth, and Families.

Achenbach, T. M., Verhulst, F. C., Baron, G. D., & Akkerhuis, G. W. (1987). Epidemiological comparisons of American and Dutch children: I. Behavioral/emotional problems and competencies reported by parents for ages 4 to 16. *Journal of the American Academy of Child and Adolescent Psychiatry, 26,* 317–325.

Achenbach, T. M., Verhulst, F. C., Baron, G. D., & Althaus, M. (1987). A comparison of syndromes derived from the Child Behavior Checklist for American and Dutch boys aged 6–11 and 12–16. *Journal of Child Psychology and Psychiatry, 28,* 437–453.

Achenbach, T. M., Verhulst, F. C., Edelbrock, C., Baron, G. D., & Akkerhuis, G. W. (1987). Epidemiological comparisons of American and Dutch children: II. Behavioral/emotional problems reported by teachers for ages 6 to 11. *Journal of the American Academy of Child and Adolescent Psychiatry, 26,* 326–332.

Al-Awad, A. M. E., & Sonuga-Barke, E. J. S. (2002). The application of the Conners' Rating Scales to a Sudanese sample: An analysis of parents' and teachers' ratings of childhood behaviour problems. *Psychology and Psychotherapy: Theory, Research and Practice, 75,* 177–187.

Albrecht, G., Veerman, J. W., Damen, H., & Kroes, G. (2001). The Child Behavior Checklist for group care workers: A study regarding the factor structure. *Journal of Abnormal Child Psychology, 29,* 83–89.

Ambrosini, P. J. (2000). Historical development and present status of the Schedule for Affective Disorders and Schizophrenia for School-Age Children (K-SADS). *Journal of the American Academy of Child and Adolescent Psychiatry, 39*, 49–58.

American Psychiatric Association. (1952; 1968; 1980; 1987; 1994, 2000). *Diagnostic and statistical manual of mental disorders* (1st ed., 2nd ed., 3rd ed., 3rd ed., rev., 4th ed.; 4th ed., text rev.). Washington, DC: Author.

Angold, A., & Costello, E. J. (2000). The Child and Adolescent Psychiatric Assessment (CAPA). *Journal of the American Academy of Child and Adolescent Psychiatry, 39*, 39–48.

Angold, A., Costello, E. J., & Erkanli, A. (1999). Comorbidity. *Journal of Child Psychology and Psychiatry, 40*, 57–87.

Arnett, J. J. (2002). The psychology of globalization. *American Psychologist, 57*, 774–783.

Arsenault, L., Moffitt, T. E., Caspi, A., Taylor, A., Rijsdijk, F. V., Jaffee, S. R., et al. (2003). Strong genetic effects on cross-situational antisocial behaviour among 5-year-old children according to mothers, teachers, examiner–observers, and twins' self-reports. *Journal of Child Psychology and Psychiatry, 44*, 832–848.

Bartels, M., van den Oord, E. J. C. G., Hudziak, J. J., Rietveld, M. J. H., van Beijsterveldt, C. E. M., & Boomsma, D. I. (2004). Genetic and environmental mechanisms underlying stability and change in problem behaviors at ages 3, 7, 10, and 12. *Developmental Psychology, 40*, 852–867.

Bauermeister, J. J., Matos, M., Reina, G., Salas, C. C. Martinez, J. V., Cumba, E., et al. (2005). Comparison of the DSM-IV combined and inattentive type of ADHD in a school-based sample of Latino/Hispanic children. *Journal of Child Psychology and Psychiatry, 46*, 166–179.

Becker, A., Hagenberg, N., Roessner, V., Woerner, W., & Rothenberger, A. (2004). Evaluation of the self-reported SDQ in a clinical setting: Do self-reports tell us more than ratings by adult informants? *European Child and Adolescent Psychiatry, 13*(Suppl. 2), 17–24.

Becker, A., Woerner, W., Hasselhorn, M., Banaschewski, T., & Rothenberger, A. (2004). Validation of the parent and teacher SDQ in a clinical sample. *European Child and Adolescent Psychiatry, 13*(Suppl. 2), 11–16.

Bengi-Arslan, L., Verhulst, F. C., van der Ende, J., & Erol, N. (1997). Understanding childhood (problems) behaviors from a cultural perspective: Comparison of problem behaviors and competencies in Turkish immigrant, Turkish and Dutch children. *Social Psychiatry and Psychiatric Epidemiology, 32*, 477–484.

Benson, J. (1998). Developing a strong program of construct validation: A test anxiety example. *Educational Measurement: Issues and Practice, 17*, 10–17.

Bentler, P. M. (1990). Comparative fit indices in structural models. *Psychological Bulletin, 107*, 238–246.

Berg, I., Fombonne, E., McGuire, R., & Verhulst, F. C. (1997). A cross-cultural comparison of French and Dutch disturbed children using the Child Behaviour Checklist (CBCL). *European Child and Adolescent Psychiatry, 6*, 7–11.

Berkson, J. (1946). Limitations of the application of fourfold table analysis to hospital data. *Biometrics Bulletin, 2*, 47–53.

Bérubé, R. L., & Achenbach, T. M. (2006). *Bibliography of published studies using the Achenbach System of Empirically Based Assessment (ASEBA): 2006 edition.* Burlington: University of Vermont, Research Center for Children, Youth, and Families.

Biederman, J., Newcorn, J., & Sprich, S. (1991). Comorbidity of attention deficit hyperactivity disorder with conduct, depressive, anxiety, and other disorders. *American Journal of Psychiatry, 148,* 564–577.

Bilenberg, N. (1999). The Child Behavior Checklist (CBCL) and related material: Standardization and validation in Danish population and clinically based samples. *Acta Psychiatrica Scandinavica, Supplementum, 100*(398), 1–52.

Binet, A., & Simon, T. (1916). New methods for the diagnosis of the intellectual level of subnormals. *The development of intelligence in children* (pp. 31–90). Baltimore: Williams & Wilkins. (Original work published in French in *L'Année Psychologique*, 1905)

Bird, H. R. (1996). Epidemiology of childhood disorders in cross-cultural context. *Journal of Child Psychology and Psychiatry, 37,* 35–49.

Bird, H. R., Canino, G. J., Davies, M., Zhang, H., Ramirez, R., & Lahey, B. B. (2001). Prevalence and correlates of antisocial behaviors among three ethnic groups. *Journal of Abnormal Child Psychology, 29,* 465–478.

Bird, H. R., Canino, G., Rubio-Stipec, M., Gould, M. S., Ribera, J., Sesman, M., et al. (1988). Estimates of the prevalence of childhood maladjustment in a community survey in Puerto Rico: The use of combined measures. *Archives of General Psychiatry, 45,* 1120–1126.

Bird, H. R., Gould, M. S., Rubio-Stipec, M., Staghezza, B. M., & Canino, G. (1991). Screening for childhood psychopathology in the community using the Child Behavior Checklist. *Journal of the American Academy of Child and Adolescent Psychiatry, 30,* 116–123.

Bird, H. R., Gould, M. S., & Staghezza, B. M. (1993). Patterns of diagnostic comorbidity in a community sample of children aged 9 through 16 years. *Journal of the American Academy of Child and Adolescent Psychiatry, 32,* 361–368.

Bird, H. R., Gould, M. S., Yager, T., Staghezza, B., & Canino, G. (1989). Risk factors for maladjustment in Puerto Rican children. *Journal of the American Academy of Child and Adolescent Psychiatry, 28,* 847–850.

Birmaher, B., Stanley, M., Greenhill, L., Twomey, J., Gavrilescu, A., & Rabinovich, H. (1990). Platelet imipramine binding in children and adolescents with impulsive behavior. *Journal of the American Academy of Child and Adolescent Psychiatry, 29,* 914–918.

Bongers, I. L., Koot, H. M., van der Ende, J., & Verhulst, F. C. (2003). The normative development of child and adolescent problem behavior. *Journal of Abnormal Psychology, 112,* 179–192.

Bongers, I. L., Koot, H. M., van der Ende, J., & Verhulst, F. C. (2004). Developmental trajectories of externalizing behaviors in childhood and adolescence. *Child Development, 75,* 1523–1537.

Boomsma, D. I., van Beijsterveldt, C. E. M., & Hudziak, J. J. (2005). Genetic and environmental influences on anxious/depression during childhood: A study from the Netherlands Twin Register. *Genes, Brain, and Behavior, 10,* 1–16.

Borgatta, E. F., & Fanshel, D. (1965). *Behavioral characteristics of children known to psychiatric outpatient clinics.* New York: Child Welfare League of America.

Bourdon, K. H., Goodman, R., Rae, D. S., Simpson, G., & Koretz, D. S. (2005). The Strengths and Difficulties Questionnaire: U.S. normative data and psychometric properties. *Journal of the American Academy of Child and Adolescent Psychiatry, 44,* 557–564.

Bravo, M., Ribera, J., Rubio-Stipec, M., Canino, G., Shrout, P., Ramírez, R., et al. (2001). Test–retest reliability of the Spanish version of the Diagnostic Interview Schedule for Children (DISC-IV). *Journal of Abnormal Child Psychology, 29,* 433–444.

Breton, J.-J., Bergeron, L., Valla, J.-P., Berthiaume, C., Gaudet, N., Lambert, J., et al. (1999). Quebec child mental health survey: Prevalence of DSM-III-R mental health disorders. *Journal of Child Psychology and Psychiatry, 40,* 375–384.

Breton, J.-J., Bergeron, L., Valla, J.-P., Berthiaume, C., & St-Georges, M. (1998). Diagnostic Interview Schedule for children (DISC-2.25) in Quebec: Reliability findings in light of the MECA study. *Journal of the American Academy of Child and Adolescent Psychiatry, 37,* 1167–1174.

Breton, J.-J., Bergeron, L., Valla, J.-P., Lepine, S., Houde, L., & Gaudet, N. (1995). Do children aged 9 through 11 years understand the DISC Version 2.5 questions? *Journal of the American Academy of Child and Adolescent Psychiatry, 34,* 946–954.

Brown, S.-L., & van Praag, H. M. (1991). *The role of serotonin in psychiatric disorders.* New York: Brunner/Mazel.

Browne, N. W., & Cudeck, R. (1993). Alternative ways of assessing model fit. In K. A. Bollen & J. S. Long (Eds.), *Testing structural equation models* (pp. 136–162). Newbury Park, CA: Sage.

Brugha, T. S., Bebbington, P. E., & Jenkins, R. (1999). A difference that matters: Comparisons of structured and semi-structured psychiatric diagnostic interviews in the general population. *Psychological Medicine, 29,* 1013–1020.

Canino, G. J., Bird, H. R., Rubio-Stipec, M., Woodbury, M. A., Ribera, J. C., Huertas, S. E., et al. (1987). Reliability of child diagnosis in a Hispanic sample. *Journal of the American Academy of Child and Adolescent Psychiatry, 26,* 560–565.

Canino, G. J., Shrout, P. E., Rubio-Stipec, M., Bird, H. R., Bravo, M., Ramirez, R., et al. (2004). The DSM-IV rates of child and adolescent disorders in Puerto Rico. *Archives of General Psychiatry, 61,* 85–93.

Caron, C., & Rutter, M. (1991). Comorbidity in child psychopathology: Concepts, issues and research strategies. *Journal of Child Psychology and Psychiatry, 32,* 1063–1080.

Clark, L. A., Watson, D., & Mineka, S. (1994). Temperament, personality, and the mood and anxiety disorders. *Journal of Abnormal Psychology, 103,* 103–116.

Cohen, J. (1960). A coefficient of agreement for nominal scales. *Educational and Psychological Measurement, 20,* 37–46.

Cohen, J. (1988). *Statistical power analysis for the behavioral sciences* (2nd ed.). New York: Academic Press.

Cohen, M. (1988). The Revised Conners Parent Rating Scale: Factor structure replication with a diversified clinical sample. *Journal of Abnormal Child Psychology, 16*, 187–196.

Cohen, P., Cohen, J., & Brook, J. (1993). An epidemiological study of disorders in late childhood and adolescence: II. Persistence of disorders. *Journal of Child Psychology and Psychiatry, 34*, 869–877.

Cohen, P., Cohen, J., Kasen, S., Velez, C. N., Harmark, C., Johnson, J., et al. (1993). An epidemiological study of disorders in late childhood and adolescence: I. Age- and gender-specific prevalence. *Journal of Child Psychology and Psychiatry, 34*, 851–867.

Cohen, P., O'Connor, P., Lewis, S., Velez, C. N., & Malachowski, B. (1987). Comparison of DISC and K-SADS-P interviews of an epidemiological sample of children. *Journal of the American Academy of Child and Adolescent Psychiatry, 26*, 662–667.

Conners, C. K. (1969). A teacher rating scale for use in drug studies with children. *American Journal of Psychiatry, 126*, 884–888.

Conners, C. K. (1970). Symptom patterns in hyperkinetic, neurotic and normal children. *Child Development, 4*, 667–682.

Conners, C. K. (1973). Rating scales for use in drug studies with children. In *Psychopharmacology Bulletin: Pharmacotherapy with children* (Vol. 9, pp. 24–29). Washington, DC: U.S. Government Printing Office.

Conners, C. K. (1978). *Parent questionnaire.* Washington, DC: Children's Hospital National Medical Center.

Conners, C. K. (1989). *Conners Rating Scales manual.* North Tonawanda, NY: Multi-Health Systems.

Conners, C. K. (1990). *Conners Rating Scales Manual.* North Tonawanda, NY: Multi-Health Systems.

Conners, C. K. (1994). Conners Rating Scales. In M. E. Maruish (Ed.), *The use of psychological testing for treatment planning and outcome assessment* (pp. 550–578). Mahwah, NJ: Erlbaum.

Conners, C. K. (1997, 2001). *Conners Rating Scales–Revised technical manual.* North Tonawanda, NY: Multi-Health Systems.

Conners, C. K., Erhardt, D., & Sparrow, E. (1999). *Conners Adult ADHD Rating Scales.* Toronto: Multi-Health Systems Inc.

Conners, C. K., Sitarenios, G., Parker, J. D. A., & Epstein, J. N. (1998a). Revision and restandardization of the Conners Teacher Rating Scale (CTRS-R): Factor structure, reliability, and criterion validity. *Journal of Abnormal Child Psychology, 26*, 279–291.

Conners, C. K., Sitarenios, G., Parker, J. D. A., & Epstein, J. N. (1998b). The Revised Conners Parent Rating Scale (CPRS-R): Factor structure, reliability, and criterion validity. *Journal of Abnormal Child Psychology, 26*, 257–268.

Costello, A., Edelbrock, C., Kalas, R., Kessler, M., & Klaric, S. A. (1982). *Diagnostic Interview Schedule for Children* (DISC) (Contract No. RFP-DB-81-0027). Bethesda, MD: National Institute of Mental Health.

Costello, E. J., Mustillo, S., Erkanli, A., Keeler, G., & Angold, A. (2003). Prevalence and development of psychiatric disorders in childhood and adolescence. *Archives of General Psychiatry, 60,* 837–844.

Cox, A., Rutter, M., Yule, B., & Quinton, D. (1977). Bias resulting from missing information: Some epidemiological findings. *British Journal of Preventive and Social Medicine, 31,* 131–136.

Crijnen, A. A. M., Achenbach, T. M., & Verhulst, F. C. (1997). Comparisons of problems reported by parents of children in 12 cultures: Total Problems, Externalizing, and Internalizing. *Journal of the American Academy of Child and Adolescent Psychiatry, 36,* 1269–1277.

Crijnen, A. A. M., Achenbach, T. M., & Verhulst, F. C. (1999). Comparisons of problems reported by parents of children in twelve cultures: The CBCL/4–18 syndrome constructs. *American Journal of Psychiatry, 156,* 569–574.

Crijnen, A. A. M., Bengi-Arslan, L., & Verhulst, F. C. (2000). Teacher-reported problem behaviour in Turkish immigrant and Dutch children: A cross-cultural comparison. *Acta Psychiatrica Scandinavica, 102,* 439–444.

Cronbach, L. J. (1951). Coefficient alpha and the internal structure of tests. *Psychometrika, 16,* 297–334.

Cronbach, L. J., & Meehl, P. E. (1955). Construct validity in psychological tests. *Psychological Bulletin, 52,* 281–302.

De Groot, A., Koot, H. M., & Verhulst, F. C. (1994). Cross-cultural generalizability of the Child Behavior Checklist cross-informant syndromes. *Psychological Assessment, 6,* 225–230.

De Groot, A., Koot, H. M., & Verhulst, F. C. (1996). Cross-cultural generalizability of the Youth Self-Report and Teacher's Report Form cross-informant syndromes. *Journal of Abnormal Child Psychology, 24,* 651–664.

Dedrick, R. F., Greenbaum, P. E., Friedman, R. M., Wetherington, C. M., & Knoff, H. M. (1997). Testing the structure of the Child Behavior Checklist/4–18 using confirmatory factor analyses. *Educational and Psychological Measurement, 57,* 306–313.

Dickey, W. C., & Blumberg, S. J. (2004). Revisiting the factor structure of the Strengths and Difficulties Questionnaire: United States, 2001. *Journal of the American Academy of Child and Adolescent Psychiatry, 43,* 1159–1167.

DeVito, T. J., Drost, D. J., Pavlosky, W., Neufeld, R. W. J., Rajakumar, N., McKinlay, D., et al. (2005). Brain magnetic resonance spectroscopy in Tourette's disorder. *Journal of the American Academy of Child and Adolescent Psychiatry, 44,* 1301–1308.

Dumenci, L. (2006). *The Psychometric Latent Agreement Model (PLAM) for discrete traits measured by multiple items.* Manuscript submitted for publication.

Dumenci, L., Erol, N., Achenbach, T. M., & Simsek, Z. (2004). Measurement structure of the Turkish translation of the Child Behavior Checklist using confirmatory factor analytic approaches to validation of syndromal constructs. *Journal of Abnormal Child Psychology, 32,* 337–342.

Dumenci, L., McConaughy, S. H., & Achenbach, T. M. (2004). A hierarchical three-factor model of inattention–hyperactivity–impulsivity derived from the attention problems syndrome of the Teacher's Report Form. *School Psychology Review, 33,* 287–301.

Dumont, L. (1985). A modified view of our origins: The Christian beginnings of modern individualism. In M. Carrithers, S. Collins, & S. Lukes (Eds.), *The category of the person* (pp. 93–122). Cambridge, UK: Cambridge University Press.

DuPaul, G. J., Power, T. J., Anastopoulos, A. D., & Reid, R. (1998). *ADHD Rating Scale–IV: Checklists, norms, and clinial interpretation.* New York: Guilford Press.

Eaton, W. W., Neufeld, K., Chen, L.-S., & Cai, G. (2000). A comparison of self-report and clinical diagnostic interviews for depression. *Archives of General Psychiatry, 57,* 217–222.

Edelbrock, C. S., & Costello, A. J. (1988). Structured psychiatric interviews for children. In M. Rutter, A. H. Tuma, & I. S. Lann (Eds.), *Assessment and diagnosis in child psychopathology* (pp. 87–112). New York: Guilford Press.

Edelbrock, C. S., & Rancurello, M. D. (1985). Childhood hyperactivity: An overview of rating scales and their applications [Special Issue]. *Clinical Psychology Review, 5,* 429–445.

Edelbrock, C. S., Rende, R., Plomin, R., & Thompson, L. A. (1995). A twin study of competence and problem behavior in childhood and early adolescence. *Journal of Child Psychology and Psychiatry, 36,* 775–785.

Eley, T. C., Lichtenstein, P., & Moffitt, T. E. (2003). A longitudinal behavioral genetic analysis of the etiology of aggressive and nonaggressive antisocial behavior. *Development and Psychopathology, 15,* 383–402.

Eley, T. C., Lichtenstein, P., & Stevenson, J. (1999). Sex differences in the etiology of aggressive and nonaggressive antisocial behavior: Results from two twin studies. *Child Development, 70,* 155–168.

Endicott, J., & Spitzer, R. L. (1978). A diagnostic interview: The Schedule for Affective Disorders and Schizophrenia. *Archives of General Psychiatry, 35,* 837–844.

Evans, W. R. (1975). The Behavior Problem Checklist: Data from an inner city population. *Psychology in the Schools, 12,* 301–303.

Faraone, S. V., Biederman, J., Keenan, K., & Tsuang, M. T. (1991). Separation of DSM-III attention deficit disorder and conduct disorder: Evidence from a family–genetic study of American child psychiatric patients. *Psychological Medicine, 21,* 109–121.

Feehan, M., McGee, R., & Williams, S. M. (1993). Mental health disorders from age 15 to age 18 years. *Journal of the American Academy of Child and Adolescent Psychiatry, 32,* 1118–1126.

Ferdinand, R. F., Hoogerheide, K. N., van der Ende, J., Heijmens Visser, J. H., Koot, H. M., Kasius, M. C., et al. (2003). The role of the clinician: Three-year predictive value of parents', teachers', and clinicians' judgment of childhood psychopathology. *Journal of Child Psychology and Psychiatry, 44,* 867–876.

Ferdinand, R. F., & Verhulst, F. C. (1995). Psychopathology in Dutch young adults: Enduring or changeable? *Social Psychiatry and Psychiatric Epidemiology, 30,* 60–64.

Ferdinand, R. F., Verhulst, F. C., & Wiznitzer, M. (1995). Continuity and change of self-reported problem behaviors from adolescence into young adulthood. *Journal of the American Academy of Child and Adolescent Psychiatry, 34,* 680–690.

Fergusson, D. M., Horwood, L. J., & Lynskey, M. T. (1993). Prevalence and comorbidity of DSM-III-R diagnoses in a birth cohort of 15 year olds. *Journal of the American Academy of Child and Adolescent Psychiatry, 32,* 1127–1134.

Fleitlich-Bilyk, B., & Goodman, R. (2004). The prevalence of child psychiatric disorders in Southeast Brazil. *Journal of the American Academy of Child and Adolescent Psychiatry, 43,* 727–734.

Fombonne, E. (1992). Parent reports on behaviour and competencies among 6–11-year-old French children. *European Child and Adolescent Psychiatry, 1,* 233–243.

Fonseca, A. C., Simoes, A., Rebelo, J. A., Ferriera, J. A., Cardoso, F., & Temudo, P. (1995). Hyperactivity and conduct disorder among Portuguese children and adolescents: Data from parents' and teachers' reports. In J. Sergeant (Ed.), *Eunethydis: European approaches to hyperkinetic disorder* (pp. 115–129). Zurich: Fotorotar.

Ford, T., Goodman, R., & Meltzer, H. (2003). The British Child and Adolescent Mental Health Survey 1999: The prevalence of DSM-IV disorders. *Journal of the American Academy of Child and Adolescent Psychiatry, 42,* 1203–1211.

Frigerio, A., Cattaneo, C., Cataldo, M., Schiatti, A., Molteni, M., & Battaglia, M. (2004). Behavioral and emotional problems among Italian children and adolescents aged 4 to 18 years as reported by parents and teachers. *European Journal of Psychological Assessment, 20,* 124–133.

Gabel, S., Stadler, J., Bjorn, J., Shindledecker, R., & Bowden, C. (1993). Dopamine-beta-hydroxylase in behaviorally disturbed youth. Relationship between teacher and parent ratings. *Biological Psychiatry, 34,* 434–442.

Gadow, K. D., & Sprafkin, J. (1998). *Adolescent Symptom Inventory–4 Norms Manual.* Stony Brook, NY: Checkmate Plus.

Gadow, K. D., & Sprafkin, J. (1999). *Youth's Inventory–4 Manual.* Stony Brook, NY: Checkmate Plus.

Gadow, K. D., Sprafkin, J., Carlson, G. A., Schneider, J., Nolan, E. E., Mattison, R. E., et al. (2002). A *DSM-IV* referenced, adolescent self-report rating scale. *Journal of the American Academy of Child and Adolescent Psychiatry, 41,* 671–679.

Ghodsian-Carpey, J., & Baker, L. A. (1987). Genetic and environmental influences on aggression in 4- to 7-year-old twins. *Aggressive Behavior, 13,* 173–186.

Gjone, H., & Stevenson, J. (1997). The association between internalizing and externalizing behavior in childhood and early adolescence: Genetic or environmental common influences? *Journal of Abnormal Child Psychology, 25,* 277–286.

Gjone, H., Stevenson, J., & Sundet, J. M. (1996). Genetic influence on parent-reported attention-related problems in a Norwegian general population twin sample. *Journal of the American Academy of Child and Adolescent Psychiatry, 35,* 588–596.

Gjone, H., Stevenson, J., Sundet, J. M., & Eilertsen, D. E. (1996). Changes in heritability across increasing levels of behavior problems in young twins. *Behavior Genetics, 26,* 419–426.

Goodman, R. (1994). A modified version of the Rutter Parent Questionnaire including extra items on children's strengths: A research note. *Journal of Child Psychology and Psychiatry, 35,* 1483–1494.

Goodman, R. (1997). The Strengths and Difficulties Questionnaire: A research note. *Journal of Child Psychology and Psychiatry, 38,* 581–586.

Goodman, R. (1999). The extended version of the Strengths and Difficulties Questionnaire as a guide to child psychiatric caseness and consequent burden. *Journal of Child Psychology and Psychiatry, 40,* 791–799.

Goodman, R. (2001). Psychometric properties of the Strengths and Difficulties Questionnaire. *Journal of the American Academy of Child and Adolescent Psychiatry, 40,* 1337–1345.

Goodman, R., Ford, T., Richards, H., Gatward, R., & Meltzer H. (2000). The Development and Well-Being Assessment: Description and initial validation of an integrated assessment of child and adolescent psychopathology. *Journal of Child Psychology and Psychiatry, 41,* 645–655.

Goodman, R., Ford, T., Simmons, H., Gatward, R., & Meltzer, H. (2000). Using the Strengths and Difficulties Questionnaire (SDQ) to screen for child psychiatric disorders in a community sample. *British Journal of Psychiatry, 177,* 534–539.

Goodman, R., Meltzer, H., & Bailey, V. (1998). The Strengths and Difficulties Questionnaire: A pilot study on the validity of the self-report version. *European Child and Adolescent Psychiatry, 7,* 125–130.

Goodman, R., Meltzer, H., & Bailey, V. (2003). The Strengths and Difficulties Questionnaire: A pilot study on the validity of the self-report version. *International Review of Psychiatry, 15,* 173–177.

Goodman, R., Renfrew, D., & Mullick, M. (2000). Predicting type of psychiatric disorder from Strengths and Difficulties Questionnaire (SDQ) scores in child mental health clinics in London and Dhaka. *European Child and Adolescent Psychiatry, 9,* 129–134.

Gove, P. (Ed.). (1971). *Webster's third new international dictionary of the English language.* Springfield, MA: Merriam.

Goyette, C. H., Conners, C. K., & Ulrich, R. F. (1978). Normative data on revised Conners Parent and Teacher Rating Scales. *Journal of Abnormal Child Psychology, 6,* 221–236.

Graetz, B. W., Sawyer, M. G., & Baghurst, P. (2005). Gender differences among children with DSM-IV ADHD in Australia. *Journal of the American Academy of Child and Adolescent Psychiatry, 44,* 159–168.

Graetz, B. W., Sawyer, M. G., Hazell, P. L., Arney, F., & Baghurst, P. (2001). Validity of *DSM-IV* ADHD subtypes in a nationally representative sample of Australian children and adolescents. *Journal of the American Academy of Child and Adolescent Psychiatry, 40,* 1410–1417.

Griesinger, W. (1867). *Mental pathology and therapeutics* (C. L. Robertson & J. Rutherford, Trans.). London: New Sydenham Society. (Original work published in German as *Die Pathologie und Therapie der psychischen Krankheiten,* 1845)

Hanna, G. L., Yuwiler, A., & Coates, J. K. (1995). Whole blood serotonin and disruptive behaviors in juvenile obsessive–compulsive disorder. *Journal of the American Academy of Child and Adolescent Psychiatry, 34,* 28–35.

Hannesdottir, H., & Einarsdottir, S. (1995). Icelandic Child Mental Health Study: An epidemiological study of Icelandic children 2–18 years of age using the Child Behavior Checklist as a screening instrument. *European Child and Adolescent Psychiatry, 4,* 237–248.

Hartman, C. A., Hox, J., Auerbach, J., Erol, N., Fonseca, A. C., Mellenbergh, G. J., et al. (1999). Syndrome dimensions of the Child Behavior Checklist and the Teacher Report Form: A critical empirical evaluation. *Journal of Child Psychology and Psychiatry, 40,* 1095–1116.

Heimans Visser, J. H., van der Ende, J., Koot, H. M., & Verhulst, F. C. (2000). Predictors of psychopathology in young adults referred to mental health services in childhood or adolescence. *British Journal of Psychiatry, 177,* 59–65.

Hellinckx, W., Grietens, H., & De Munter, A. (2000). Parent-reported problem behavior in 12–16-year-old American and Russian children: A cross-national comparison. In N. N. Singh, J. P. Leung, & A. N. Singh (Eds.), *International perspectives on child and adolescent mental health* (pp. 205–222). Oxford, UK: Elsevier.

Hellinckx, W., Grietens, H., & Verhulst, F. (1994). Competence and behavioral problems in 6- to 12-year-old children in Flanders (Belgium) and Holland: A cross-national comparison. *Journal of Emotional and Behavioral Disorders, 2,* 130–142.

Helstelä, L., & Sourander, A. (2001). Self-reported competence and emotional and behavioral problems in a sample of Finnish adolescents. *Nordic Journal of Psychiatry, 55,* 381–385.

Helstelä, L., Sourander, A., & Bergroth, L. (2001). Parent-reported competence and emotional and behavioral problems in Finnish adolescents. *Nordic Journal of Psychiatry, 55,* 337–341.

Helzer, J. E., Spitznagel, E. L., & McEvoy, L. (1987). The predictive validity of lay DIS diagnoses in the general population: A comparison with physician examiners. *Archives of General Psychiatry, 44,* 1069–1077.

Herjanic, B., & Reich, W. (1982). Development of a structured psychiatric interview for children: Agreement between child and parent on individual symptoms. *Journal of Abnormal Child Psychology, 10,* 307–324.

Hermans, H. J. M., & Kempen, H. J. G. (1998). Moving cultures: The perilous problems of cultural dichotomies in a globalizing society. *American Psychologist, 53,* 1111–1120.

Hermans, H. J. M., & Kempen, H. J. G. (1999). Categorical thinking is the target. *American Psychologist, 54,* 840–841.

Heubeck, B. G. (2000). Cross-cultural generalizability of CBCL syndromes across three continents: From the USA and Holland to Australia. *Journal of Abnormal Child Psychology, 28,* 439–450.

Hewitt, L. E., & Jenkins, R. L. (1946). *Fundamental patterns of maladjustment: The dynamics of their origin.* Springfield: State of Illinois.

Hofstra, M. B., van der Ende, J., & Verhulst, F. C. (2000). Continuity and change of psychopathology from childhood into adulthood: A 14-year follow-up study. *Journal of the American Academy of Child and Adolescent Psychiatry, 39*, 850–858.

Hofstra, M. B., van der Ende, J., & Verhulst, F. C. (2001). Adolescents' self-reported problems as predictors of psychopathology in adulthood: 10-year follow-up study. *British Journal of Psychiatry, 179*, 203–209.

Hofstra, M. B., van der Ende, J., & Verhulst, F. C. (2002). Child and adolescent problems predict *DSM-IV* disorders in adulthood: A 14-year follow-up of a Dutch epidemiological sample. *Journal of the American Academy of Child and Adolescent Psychiatry, 41*, 182–189.

Hudziak, J. J. (1998). *DSM-IV Checklist for Childhood Disorders.* Burlington: University of Vermont, Research Center for Children, Youth, and Families.

Hudziak, J. J., Derks, E. M., Althoff, R. R., Rettew, D. C., & Boomsma, D. I. (2005). The genetic and environmental contributions to attention deficit hyperactivity disorder as measured by the Conners' Rating Scales—Revised. *American Journal of Psychiatry, 162*, 1614–1620.

Hudziak, J. J., van Beijsterveldt, C. E. M., Althoff, R. R., Stanger, C., Rettew, D. C., Nelson, E. C., et al. (2004). Genetic and environmental contributions to the Child Behavior Checklist obsessive–compulsive scale: A cross-cultural twin study. *Archives of General Psychiatry, 61*, 608–616.

Ivanova, M. Y., Achenbach, T. M., Dumenci, L., Rescorla, L. A., Almqvist, F., Bilenberg, N., et al. (2006a). *Testing the 8-syndrome structure of the CBCL in 30 societies.* Manuscript submitted for review.

Ivanova, M. Y., Achenbach, T. M., Rescorla, L. A., Dumenci, L., Almqvist, F., Bathiche, M., et al. (2006b). *Testing the Teacher's Report Form syndromes in 20 societies.* Manuscript submitted for review.

Ivanova, M. Y., Achenbach, T. M., Rescorla, L. A., Dumenci, L., Almqvist, F., Bilenberg, F., et al. (2006c). *The generalizability of the Youth Self-Report syndrome structure in 23 societies.* Manuscript submitted for review.

Jenkins, R. L., & Glickman, S. (1946). Common syndromes in child psychiatry: I. Deviant behavior traits. II. The schizoid child. *American Journal of Orthopsychiatry, 16,* 244–261.

Jensen, A. L., & Weisz, J. R. (2002). Assessing match and mismatch between practitioner-generated and standardized interview-generated diagnoses for clinic-referred children and adolescents. *Journal of Consulting and Clinical Psychology, 70*, 158–168.

Jensen, P., Roper, M., Fisher, P., Piacentini, J., Canino, G., Richters, J., et al. (1995). Test–retest reliability of the Diagnostic Interview Schedule for Children (DISC 2.1): Parent, child, and combined algorithms. *Archives of General Psychiatry, 52,* 61–71.

Jensen, P. S., Rubio-Stipec, M., Canino, G., Bird, H. R., Dulcan, M. K., Schwab-Stone, M. E., et al. (1999). Parent and child contributions to diagnosis of mental disorder: Are both informants always necessary? *Journal of the American Academy of Child and Adolescent Psychiatry, 38*, 1569–1579.

Kalff, A. C., Kroes, M., Vles, J. S. H., Bosma, H., Feron, F. J. M., Hendriksen, J. G. M., et al. (2001). Factors affecting the relation between parental education as well as occupation and problem behaviour in Dutch 5- to 6-year-old children. *Social Psychiatry and Psychiatric Epidemiology, 36*, 324–331.

Kalff, A. C., Kroes, M., Vles, J. S. H., Hendriksen, J. G. M., Feron, F. J. M., Steyaert, J., et al. (2001). Neighbourhood level and individual level SES effects on child problem behaviour: A multilevel analysis. *Journal of Epidemiology and Community Health, 55,* 246–250.

Kashala, E., Elgen, I., Sommerfelt, K., & Tylleskar, T. (2005). Teacher ratings of mental health among school children in Kinshasa, Democratic Republic of Congo. *European Child and Adolescent Psychiatry, 12,* 208–215.

Kasius, M. C., Ferdinand, R. F., van den Berg, H., & Verhulst, F. C. (1997). Associations between different diagnostic approaches for child and adolescent psychopathology. *Journal of Child Psychology and Psychiatry, 38,* 625–632.

Kendler, K. S., Neale, M. C., Kessler, R. C., Heath, A. C., & Eaves, L. J. (1992). Major depression and generalized anxiety disorder: Same genes, (partly) different environments? *Archives of General Psychiatry, 49,* 716–722.

Kendler, K. S., & Roy, M.-A. (1995). Validity of a diagnosis of lifetime major depression obtained by personal interview versus family history. *American Journal of Psychiatry, 152,* 1608–1614.

Klasen, H., Woerner, W., Wolke, D., Meyer, R., Overmeyer, S., Kaschnitz, W., et al. (2000). Comparing the German versions of the Strengths and Difficulties Questionnaire (SDQ-Deu) and the Child Behavior Checklist. *European Child and Adolescent Psychiatry, 9,* 271–276.

Kollins, S. H., Epstein, J. N., & Conners, C. K. (2004). Conners' Rating Scales—Revised. In M. E. Maruish (Ed.), *The use of psychological testing for treatment planning and outcomes assessment: Vol. 2. Instruments for children and adolescents* (3rd ed., pp. 215–233). Mahwah, NJ: Erlbaum.

Koskelainen, M., Sourander, A., & Kaljonen, A. (2000). The Strengths and Difficulties Questionnaire among Finnish school-aged children and adolescents. *European Child and Adolescent Psychiatry, 9,* 277–284.

Koskelainen, M., Sourander, A., & Vauras, M. (2001). Self-reported strengths and difficulties in a community sample of Finnish adolescents. *European Child and Adolescent Psychiatry, 10,* 180–185.

Kovacs, M. (1992). *Children's Depression Inventory manual.* North Tonawanda, NY: Multi-Health Systems.

Kraepelin, E. (1883). *Compendium der Psychiatrie.* Leipzig: Abel.

Kuhlmann, F. (1912). The Binet and Simon tests of intelligence in grading feebleminded children. *Journal of Psycho-asthenics, 16,* 173–193.

Kuo, P.-H., Lin, C. C. H., Yang, H.-J., Soong, W.-T., & Chen, W. J. (2004). A twin study of competence and behavioral/emotional problems among adolescents in Taiwan. *Behavior Genetics, 34,* 63–74.

Lahey, B. B., Flagg, E. W., Bird, H. R., Schwab-Stone, M. E., Canino, G., Dulcan, M. K., et al. (1996). The NIMH Methods for the Epidemiology of Child and Adolescent Mental Disorders (MECA) Study: Background and methodology. *Journal of the American Academy of Child and Adolescent Psychiatry, 35,* 855–864.

Lahey, B. B., Loeber, R., Stouthamer-Loeber, M., Christ, M. A. G., Green, S., Russo, M. F., et al. (1990). Comparison of *DSM-III* and *DSM-III-R* diagnoses for prepubertal children: Changes in prevalence and validity. *Journal of the American Academy of Child and Adolescent Psychiatry, 29*, 620–626.

Laitinen-Krispijn, S., van der Ende, J., Wierdsma, A. I., & Verhulst, F. C. (1999). Predicting adolescent mental health service use in a prospective record-linkage study. *Journal of the American Academy of Child and Adolescent Psychiatry, 38*, 1073–1080.

Lambert, M. C., Knight, F., Taylor, R., & Achenbach, T. M. (1994). Epidemiology of behavioral and emotional problems among children of Jamaica and the United States: Parent reports for ages 6–11. *Journal of Abnormal Child Psychology, 22*, 113–128.

Lambert, M. C., Knight, F., Taylor, R., & Achenbach, T. M. (1996). Comparison of behavioral and emotional problems among children of Jamaica and the United States: Teacher reports for ages 6–11. *Journal of Cross-Cultural Psychology, 27*, 82–97.

Lambert, M. C., Lyubansky, M., & Achenbach, T. M. (1998). Behavioral and emotional problems among adolescents of Jamaica and the United States: Parent, teacher, and self-reports for ages 12 to 18. *Journal of Emotional and Behavioral Disorders, 6*, 180–187.

Landis, J. R., & Koch, G. G. (1977). The measurement of observer agreement for categorical data. *Biometrics, 33*, 159–174.

Landsford, J. E., Dodge, K. A., Malone, P. S., Bacchini, D., Zelli, A., Chaudhary, N., et al. (2005). Physical discipline and children's adjustment: Cultural normativeness as a moderator. *Child Development, 76*, 1234–1246.

Larsson, B., & Frisk, M. (1999). Social competence and emotional/behaviour problems in 6–16 year-old Swedish school children. *European Child and Adolescent Psychiatry, 8*, 24–33.

Leung, P. W. L., Luk, S. L., & Lee, P. L. M. (1989). Problem behaviour among special school children in Hong Kong: A factor-analytical study with Conners' Teacher Rating Scale. *Psychologia, 32*, 120–128.

Lewczyk, C. M., Garland, A. F., Hurlburt, M. S., Gearity, J., & Hough, R. L. (2003). Comparing DISC-IV and clinician diagnoses among youths receiving public mental health services. *Journal of the American Academy of Child and Adolescent Psychiatry, 42*, 349–356.

Lilienfeld, S. O. (2003). Comorbidity between and within childhood externalizing and internalizing disorders: Reflections and directions. *Journal of Abnormal Child Psychology, 31*, 285–291.

Lipsey, M. W., & Wilson, D. B. (2001). *Practical meta-analysis*. Thousand Oaks, CA: Sage.

Liu, X., Guo, C., Okawa, M., Zhai, J., Li, Y., Uchiyama, M., et al. (2000). Behavioral and emotional problems in Chinese children of divorced parents. *Journal of the American Academy of Child and Adolescent Psychiatry, 39*, 896–903.

Liu, X., Kurita, H., Guo, C., Miyake, Y., Ze, J., & Cao, H. (1999). Prevalence and risk factors of behavioral and emotional problems among Chinese children aged 6 through 11 years. *Journal of the American Academy of Child and Adolescent Psychiatry, 38,* 708–715.

Liu, X., Kurita, H., Sun, Z., & Wang, F. (1999). Risk factors for psychopathology among Chinese children. *Psychiatry and Clinical Neurosciences, 53,* 497–503.

Loehlin, J. C. (1998). *Latent variable models: An introduction to factor, path, and structural analysis* (3rd ed.). Mahwah, NJ: Erlbaum.

Loo, S. K., & Rapport, M. D. (1998). Ethnic variations in children's problem behaviors: A cross-sectional, developmental study of Hawaii school children. *Journal of Child Psychology and Psychiatry, 39,* 567–575.

Luk, S. L., Leung, P. W. L., & Lee, P. L. M. (1988). Conners' Teacher Rating Scale in Chinese children in Hong Kong. *Journal of Child Psychology and Psychiatry, 29,* 165–174.

MacDonald, V., Tsiantis, J., Achenbach, T. M., Motto-Stefanidi, F., & Richardson, S. C. (1995). Competencies and problems reported by parents of American and Greek 6- to 11-year-old children. *European Child and Adolescent Psychiatry, 4,* 1–13.

Mann, E. M., Ikeda, Y., Mueller, C. W., Takahashi, A., Tao, K. T., Humris, E., et al. (1992). Cross-cultural differences in rating hyperactive–disruptive behaviors in children. *American Journal of Psychiatry, 149,* 1539–1542.

March, J. (1997). *MASC: Multidimensional Anxiety Scale for Children.* North Tonawanda, NY: Multi-Health Systems.

Marzocchi, G. M., Capron, C., Di Pietro, M., Tauleria, E. D., Duyme, M., Frigerio, A., et al. (2004). The use of the Strengths and Difficulties Questionnaire (SDQ) in Southern European countries. *European Child and Adolescent Psychiatry, 13*(Suppl. 2), 40–46.

Mash, E. J., & Hunsley, J. (2005). Evidence-based assessment of child and adolescent disorders: Issues and challenges. *Journal of Clinical Child and Adolescent Psychology, 34,* 362–379.

McClellan, J. M., & Werry, J. S. (Eds.). (2000). Research psychiatric diagnostic interviews for children and adolescents. *Journal of the American Academy of Child and Adolescent Psychiatry, 39,* 19–27.

McConaughy, S. H., & Achenbach, T. M. (1994). Comorbidity of empirically based syndromes in matched general population and clinical samples. *Journal of Child Psychology and Psychiatry, 35,* 1141–1157.

McConaughy, S. H., & Achenbach, T. M. (2001). *Manual for the Semistructured Clinical Interview for Children and Adolescents* (2nd ed.). Burlington: University of Vermont, Research Center for Children, Youth, and Families.

McConaughy, S. H., & Achenbach, T. M. (2004). *Manual for the Test Observation Form for Ages 2–18.* Burlington: University of Vermont, Research Center for Children, Youth, and Families.

McGee, M. F., Feehan, M., Williams, S., & Anderson, J. (1992). DSM-III disorders from age 11 to age 15 years. *Journal of the American Academy of Child and Adolescent Psychiatry, 31,* 50–59.

Messick, S. (1993). Validity. In R. L. Linn (Ed.), *Educational measurement* (3rd ed., pp. 13–103). Washington, DC: American Council on Education.

Miller, L. C. (1967). Louisville Behavior Checklist for males, 6–12 years of age. *Psychological Reports, 21,* 885–896.

Miller, L. C. (1981). *Louisville Behavior Checklist Manual* (rev. ed.). Los Angeles: Western Psychological Services.

Miller, L. C., Hampe, E., Barrett, C. L., & Noble, H. (1972). Test–retest reliability of parent ratings of children's deviant behavior. *Psychological Reports, 31,* 249–250.

Mish, F. C. (Ed.). (1988). *Webster's ninth new collegiate dictionary.* Springfield, MA: Merriam-Webster.

Montenegro, H. (1983). *Salud mental del escolar. Estandarización del inventario de problemas conductuales y destrezas sociales de T. Achenbach en niños de 6 a 11 años.* Santiago, Chile: Centro de Estudios de Desarrollo y Estimulación Psicosocial.

Morgan, C. J., & Cauce, A. M. (1999). Predicting DSM-III-R disorders from the Youth Self-Report: Analysis of data from a field study. *Journal of the American Academy of Child and Adolescent Psychiatry, 38,* 1237–1245.

Murad, S. D., Joung, I. M. A., van Lenthe, F. J., Bengi-Arslan, L., & Crijnen, A. A. M. (2003). Predictors of self-reported problem behaviours in Turkish immigrant and Dutch adolescents in the Netherlands. *Journal of Child Psychology and Psychiatry, 44,* 412–423.

Muris, P., Meesters, C., Eijkelenboom, A., & Vincken, M. (2004). The self-report version of the Strengths and Difficulties Questionnaire: Its psychometric properties in 8- to 13-year-old non-clinical children. *British Journal of Clinical Psychology, 43,* 437–448.

National Institute of Child Health and Human Development Early Child Care Research Network. (2005). Duration and developmental timing of poverty and children's cognitive and social development from birth through third grade. *Child Development, 76,* 795–810.

Novik, T. S. (1999). Validity of the Child Behavior Checklist in a Norwegian sample. *European Child and Adolescent Psychiatry, 8,* 247–254.

Nunnally, J. C., & Bernstein, I. H. (1994). *Psychometric theory* (3rd ed.). New York: McGraw-Hill.

Obel, C., Heiervang, E., Rodriguez, A., Heyerdahl, S., Smedje, H., Sourander, A., et al. (2004). The Strengths and Difficulties Questionnaire in the Nordic countries. *European Child and Adolescent Psychiatry, 13*(Suppl. 2), 32–39.

Oh, K. J., & Ha, E. H. (1999). Cross-cultural similarities and differences in child behavior problem patterns. *Korean Journal of Psychology, 18,* 87–105.

O'Leary, K. D., Vivan, D., & Nisi, A. (1985). Hyperactivity in Italy. *Journal of Abnormal Child Psychology, 13,* 485–500.

Oppedal, B., Røysamb, E., & Heyerdahl, S. (2005). Ethnic group, acculturation, and psychiatric problems in young immigrants. *Journal of Child Psychology and Psychiatry, 46,* 646–660.

Pike, K. L. (1954). *Language in relation to a unified theory of the structure of human behavior.* Glendale, CA: Summer Institute of Linguistics.

Pike, K. L. (1967). *Language in relation to a unified theory of the structure of human behavior.* The Hague: Mouton.

Ponizovsky, A. M., Ritsner, M. S., & Modai, I. (1999). Suicidal ideation and suicide attempts among immigrant adolescents from the former Soviet Union to Israel. *Journal of the American Academy of Child and Adolescent Psychiatry, 38,* 1433–1441.

Prendergast, M., Taylor, E., Rapoport, J. L., Bartko, J., Donnelly, M., Zametkin, A., et al. (1988). The diagnosis of childhood hyperactivity: A U.S.–U.K. cross-national study of DSM-III and ICD-9. *Journal of Child Psychology and Psychiatry, 29,* 289–300.

Prinz, F. J., & Loney, J. (1986). The hyperactive child grows up: Teachers' descriptions and their predictors. *Advances in Learning and Behavioral Disabilities, 5,* 247–293.

Puig-Antich, J., & Chambers, W. (1978). *The Schedule for Affective Disorders and Schizophrenia for School-Aged Children* (Kiddie-SADS). New York: New York State Psychiatric Institute.

Quay, H. C. (1979). Classification. In H. C. Quay & J. S. Werry (Eds.), *Psychopathological disorders of childhood* (2nd ed., pp. 1–34). New York: Wiley.

Quay, H. C., Morse, W. C., & Cutler, R. L. (1966). Personality patterns of pupils in special classes for the emotionally disturbed. *Exceptional Children, 32,* 297–301.

Quay, H. C., & Peterson, D. R. (1982). *Revised Behavior Problem Checklist.* Coral Gables, FL: University of Miami, Department of Psychology.

Quay, H. C., & Peterson, D. R. (1987). *Manual for the Revised Behavior Problem Checklist.* Coral Gables, FL: University of Miami, Department of Psychology.

Quay, H. C., & Peterson, D. R. (1996). *Manual for the Revised Behavior Problem Checklist–PAR version.* Odessa, FL: Psychological Assessment Resources.

Rapoport, J. L., & Ismond, D. R. (1996). *DSM-IV training guide for diagnosis of childhood disorders.* New York: Brunner/Mazel.

Reich, W. (2000). Diagnostic Interview for Children and Adolescents (DICA). *Journal of the American Academy of Child and Adolescent Psychiatry, 39,* 59–66.

Rescorla, L. A., Achenbach, T. M., Ginzburg, S., Ivanova, M. Y., Dumenci, L., Almqvist, F., et al. (in press). Consistency of teacher-reported problems in 21 countries. *School Psychology Review.*

Rescorla, L. A., Achenbach, T. M., Ivanova, M. Y., Dumenci, L., Almqvist, F., Bilenberg, N., et al. (2006a). *Problems reported by parents of children ages 6 to 16 in 31 countries.* Manuscript submitted for review.

Rescorla, L. A., Achenbach, T. M., Ivanova, M. Y., Dumenci, L., Almqvist, F., Bilenberg, N., et al. (2006b). *Problems reported by adolescents in 24 countries.* Manuscript submitted for review.

Rettew, D. C., Doyle, A. C., Achenbach, T. M., Dumenci, L., & Ivanova, M. Y. (2006). *Meta-analyses of diagnostic agreement between clinical evaluations and standardized diagnostic interviews.* Manuscript submitted for review.

Reynolds, C. R., & Kamphaus, R. W. (1992). *Behavior Assessment System for Children* (BASC). Circle Pines, MN: American Guidance Service.

Reynolds, C. R., & Kamphaus, R. W. (2004). *BASC-2 Behavior Assessment System for Children* (2nd ed.) *Manual.* Circle Pine, MN: AGS Publishing.

Rietveld, M. J. H., Hudziak, J. J., Bartels, M., Van Beijsterveldt, C. E. M., & Boomsma, D. I. (2004). Heritability of attention problems in children: Longitudinal results from a study of twins, age 3 to 12. *Journal of Child Psychology and Psychiatry, 45,* 577–588.

Roberts, R. E., Solovitz, B. L., Chen, Y.-W., & Casat, C. (1996). Retest stability of DSM-III-R diagnoses among adolescents using the Diagnostic Interview Schedule for Children (DISC-2.1C). *Journal of Abnormal Child Psychology, 24,* 349–362.

Robins, L. N. (1985). Epidemiology: Reflections on testing the validity of psychiatric interviews. *Archives of General Psychiatry, 42,* 918–924.

Robins, L. N., Cottler, L., Bucholtz, K., & Compton, W. (1997). *NIMH Diagnostic Interview Schedule for DSM-IV* (version: DIS-IV), written under contract to the NIMH.

Robins, L. N., Helzer, J. E., Croughan, J., & Ratcliff, K. S. (1981). National Institute of Mental Health Diagnostic Interview Schedule: Its history, characteristics, and validity. *Archives of General Psychiatry, 38,* 381–389.

Roid, G. H. (2003). *Stanford–Binet Intelligence Scales* (5th ed.) *Technical manual.* Itasca, IL: Riverside Publishing.

Rønning, J. A., Handegaard, B. H., Sourander, A., & Mørch, W.-T. (2004). The Strengths and Difficulties Self-Report Questionnaire as a screening instrument in Norwegian community samples. *European Child and Adolescent Psychiatry, 13,* 73–82.

Rosenberg, L. A., & Jani, S. (1995). Cross-cultural studies with the Conners Rating Scales. *Journal of Clinical Psychology, 51,* 820–826.

Roussos, A., Karantanos, G., Richardson, C., Hartman, C., Karajiannis, D., Kyprianos, S., et al. (1999). Achenbach's Child Behavior Checklist and Teacher's Report Form in a normative sample of Greek children 6–12 years old. *European Child and Adolescent Psychiatry, 8,* 165–172.

Rutter, M. (1967). A children's behaviour questionnaire for completion by teachers: Preliminary findings. *Journal of Child Psychology and Psychiatry, 8,* 1–11.

Rutter, M., Shaffer, D., & Shepherd, M. (1975). *A multiaxial classification of child psychiatric disorders: An evaluation of a proposal.* Geneva, Switzerland: World Health Organization.

Rutter, M., Tizard, J., & Whitmore, K. (1970). *Education, health and behavior.* New York: Wiley.

Satin, M. S., Winsberg, B. G., Monetti, C. H., Sverd, J., & Foss, D. A. (1985). A general population screen for attention deficit disorder with hyperactivity. *Journal of the American Academy of Child Psychiatry, 24,* 756–764.

Sawyer, M. G., Arney, F. M., Baghurst, P. A., Clark, J. J., Graetz, R. J., Kosky, R. J., et al. (2001). The mental health of young people in Australia: Key findings from the Child and Adolescent Component of the National Survey of Mental Health and Well-Being. *Australian and New Zealand Journal of Psychiatry, 35,* 806–814.

Sawyer, M. G., Mudge, J., Carty, V., Baghurst, P., & McMichael, A. (1996). A prospective study of childhood emotional and behavioural problems in Port Pirie, South Australia. *Australian and New Zealand Journal of Psychiatry, 30,* 781–787.

Sawyer, M. G., Sarris, A., Baghurst P. A., Cornish, C. A., & Kalucy, R. S. (1990). The prevalence of emotional and behaviour disorders and patterns of service utilisation in children and adolescents. *Australian and New Zealand Journal of Psychiatry, 24,* 323–330.

Scerbo, A. S., & Kolko, D. (1994). Salivary testosterone and cortisol in disruptive children: Relationship to aggressive, hyperactive, and internalizing behaviors. *Journal of the American Academy of Child and Adolescent Psychiatry, 33,* 1174–1184.

Schmeck, K., Poustka, F., Döpfner, M., Plück, J., Berner, W., Lehmkuhl, G., et al. (2001). Discriminant validity of the Child Behaviour Checklist CBCL-4/18 in German samples. *European Child and Adolescent Psychiatry, 10,* 240–247.

Schmitz, S., Fulker, D. W., & Mrazek, D. A. (1995). Problem behavior in early and middle childhood: An initial behavior genetic analysis. *Journal of Child Psychology and Psychiatry, 36,* 1443–1458.

Schneiders, J., Drukker, M., van der Ende, J., Verhulst, F. C., van Os, J., & Nicholson, N. A. (2003). Neighbourhood socioeconomic disadvantage and behavioural problems from late childhood into early adolescence. *Journal of Epidemiology and Community Health, 57,* 699–703.

Schwab-Stone, M. E., Shaffer, D., Dulcan, M. K., Jensen, P. S., Fisher, P., Bird, H. R., et al. (1996). Criterion validity of the NIMH Diagnostic Interview Schedule for Children Version 2.3 (DISC-2.3). *Journal of the American Academy of Child and Adolescent Psychiatry, 35,* 878–888.

Sears, R. R. (1977). Sources of life satisfaction of the Terman gifted men. *American Psychologist, 32,* 119–128.

Shaffer, D., Fisher, P., Dulcan, M. K., Davies, M., Piacentini, J., Schwab-Stone, M. E., et al. (1996). The NIMH Diagnostic Interview Schedule for Children Version 2.3 (DISC-2.3): Description, acceptability, prevalence rates, and performance in the MECA study. *Journal of the American Academy of Child and Adolescent Psychiatry, 35,* 865–877.

Shaffer, D., Fisher, P., Lucas, C. P., Dulcan, M. K., & Schwab-Stone, M. E. (2000). NIMH Diagnostic Interview Schedule for Children Version IV (NIMH DISC-IV): Description, differences from previous versions, and reliability of some common diagnoses. *Journal of the American Academy of Child and Adolescent Psychiatry, 39,* 28–38.

Shaffer, D., Gould, M. S., Brasic, J., Ambrosini, P., Fisher, P., Bird, H., et al. (1983). A Children's Global Assessment Scale. *Archives of General Psychiatry, 40,* 1228–1231.

Shweder, R. A., & Bourne, E. J. (1984). Does the concept of the person vary cross-culturally? In R. A. Shweder & R. A. LeVine (Eds.), *Culture theory* (pp. 158–199). Cambridge, UK: Cambridge University Press.

Smedje, H., Broman, J.-E., Hetta, J., & von Knorring, A.-L. (1999). Psychometric properties of a Swedish version of the "Strengths and Difficulties Questionnaire." *European Child and Adolescent Psychiatry, 8*, 63–70.

Sourander, A., Haavisto, A., Rønning, J. A., Multimäki, P., Parkkola, K., Santalahti, P., et al. (2005). Recognition of psychiatric disorders and self-perceived problems: A follow-up study from age 8 to age 18. *Journal of Child Psychology and Psychiatry, 46*, 1124–1134.

Sourander, A., Multimäki, P., Santalahti, P., Parkkola, K., Haavisto, A., Helenius, H., et al. (2004). Mental health service use among 18-year-old adolescent boys: A prospective 10-year follow-up study. *Journal of the American Academy of Child and Adolescent Psychiatry, 43*, 1250–1258.

Sowa, H., Crijnen, A. A. M., Bengi-Arslan, L., & Verhulst, F. C. (2000). Factors associated with problem behaviors in Turkish immigrant children in the Netherlands. *Social Psychiatry and Psychiatric Epidemiology, 35*, 177–184.

Spitzer, R. L., & Cantwell, D. P. (1980). The *DSM-III* classification of the psychiatric disorders of infancy, childhood, and adolescence. *Journal of the American Academy of Child Psychiatry, 19*, 356–370.

Spitzer, R. L., Davies, M., & Barkley, R. A. (1990). The DSM-III-R field trial of disruptive behavior disorders. *Journal of the American Academy of Child and Adolescent Psychiatry, 29*, 690–697.

Stanger, C., Achenbach, T. M., & Verhulst, F. C. (1997). Accelerated longitudinal comparison of aggressive versus delinquent syndromes. *Development and Psychopathology, 9*, 43–58.

Stanger, C., Fombonne, E., & Achenbach, T. M. (1994). Epidemiological comparisons of American and French children: Parent reports of problems and competencies for ages 6–11. *European Child and Adolescent Psychiatry, 3*, 16–29.

Stanger, C., MacDonald, V., McConaughy, S. H., & Achenbach, T. M. (1996). Predictors of cross-informant syndromes among children and youths referred for mental health services. *Journal of Abnormal Child Psychology, 24*, 597–614.

Steinhausen, H. C., Winkler Metzke, C. W., Meier, M., & Kannenberg, R. (1997). Behavioral and emotional problems reported by parents for ages 6 to 17 in a Swiss epidemiological study. *European Child and Adolescent Psychiatry, 6*, 136–141.

Steinhausen, H. C., Winkler Metzke, C. W., Meier, M., & Kannenberg, R. (1998). Prevalence of child and adolescent psychiatric disorders: The Zurich Epidemiological Study. *Acta Psychiatrica Scandinavica, 98*, 262–271.

Stevens, G. W. J. M. (2004). *Mental health in Moroccan youth in the Netherlands.* Rotterdam: Erasmus University.

Stevens, G. W. J. M., Pels, T., Bengi-Arslan, L., Verhulst, F. C., Vollebergh, W. A.

M., & Crijnen, A. A. M. (2003). Parent, teacher and self-reported problem behavior in The Netherlands: Comparing Moroccan immigrant with Dutch and with Turkish immigrant children and adolescents. *Social Psychiatry and Psychiatric Epidemiology, 38*, 576–585.

Stevens, G. W. J. M., Vollebergh, W. A. M., Pels, T., & Crijnen, A. A. M. (in press). Parenting and internalizing and externalizing problems in Moroccan immigrant youth in the Netherlands. *Journal of Youth and Adolescence.*

Stevens, G. W. J. M., Vollebergh, W. A. M., Pels, T., & Crijnen, A. A. M. (2006). *Problem behavior and acculturation in Moroccan immigrant adolescents in the Netherlands: Effects of gender and parent–child conflict.* Manuscript submitted for review.

Stoff, D. M., Pollock, L., Vitiello, B., Behar, D., & Bridger, W. H. (1987). Reduction of 3-H-imipramine binding sites on platelets of conduct disordered children. *Neuropsychopharmacology, 1,* 55–62.

Tackett, J. L., Krueger, R. F., Sawyer, M. G., & Graetz, B. W. (2003). Subfactors of DSM-IV conduct disorder: Evidence and connections with syndromes from the Child Behavior Checklist. *Journal of Abnormal Child Psychology, 31,* 647–654.

Tanaka-Matsumi, J., & Draguns, J. G. (1997). Culture and psychopathology. In J. W. Berry, M. H. Segall, & C. Kagitcibasi (Eds.), *Handbook of cross-cultural psychology. Vol. 3. Social behavior and applications* (pp. 449–491). Boston: Allyn & Bacon.

Taub, N. A., Morgan, Z., Brugha, T. S., Lambert P. C., Bebbington, P. E., Jenkins, R., et al. (2005). Recalibration methods to enhance information on prevalence rates from large mental health surveys. *International Journal of Methods in Psychiatric Research, 14,* 3–13.

Taylor, E., & Sandberg, S. (1984). Hyperactive behavior in English schoolchildren: A questionnaire survey. *Journal of Abnormal Child Psychology, 12,* 143–156.

Terman, L. M. (1916). *The measurement of intelligence.* Boston: Houghton-Mifflin.

Todd, R. D., Huang, H., Smalley, S. L., Nelson, S. F., Willcutt, E. G., Pennington, B. F., et al. (2005). Collaborative analysis of DRD4 and DAT genotypes in population-defined ADHD subtypes. *Journal of Child Psychology and Psychiatry, 46,* 1067–1073.

Triandis, H. C. (1989). The self and social behavior in differing cultural contexts. *Psychological Review, 96,* 506–520.

Trites, R. L., Blouin, A. G., & Laprade, K. (1982). Factor analysis of the Conners Teacher Rating Scale based on a large normative sample. *Journal of Consulting and Clinical Psychology, 50,* 615–623.

Tucker, L. R., & Lewis, C. (1973). A reliability coefficient for maximum likelihood factor analysis. *Psychometrika, 38,* 1–10.

U.S. Public Health Service. (2000). *Report of the Surgeon General's Conference on Children's Mental Health: A national action agenda.* Washington, DC: U.S. Department of Health and Human Services.

Van den Oord, E. J. C. G., Boomsma, D. I., & Verhulst, F. C. (2000). A study of genetic and environmental effects on the co-occurrence of problem behaviors in three-year-old twins. *Journal of Abnormal Psychology, 109*, 360–372.

Van den Oord, E. J. C. G., Verhulst, F. C., & Boomsma, D. I. (1996). A genetic study of maternal and paternal ratings of problem behaviors in three-year-old twins. *Journal of Abnormal Psychology, 105*, 349–357.

Van der Valk, J. C., van den Oord, E. J. C. G., Verhulst, F. C., & Boomsma, D. I. (2001). Using parental ratings to study the etiology of 3-year-old twins' problem behaviors: Different views or rater bias? *Journal of Child Psychology and Psychiatry, 42*, 921–931.

Van der Valk, J. C., van den Oord, E. J. C. G., Verhulst, F. C., & Boomsma, D. I. (2003). Genetic and environmental contributions to stability and change in children's internalizing and externalizing problems. *Journal of the American Academy of Child and Adolescent Psychiatry, 42*, 1212–1220.

Vandiver, T., & Sher, K. J. (1991). Temporal stability of the Diagnostic Interview Schedule. *Psychological Assessment, 3*, 277–281.

Van Widenfelt, B. M., Goedhart, A. W., Treffers, P. D. A., & Goodman, R. (2003). Dutch version of the Strengths and Difficulties Questionnaire (SDQ). *European Child and Adolescent Psychiatry, 12*, 281–289.

Verhulst, F. C. (1985). *Mental health in Dutch children.* Rotterdam, Holland: Sophia Children's Hospital.

Verhulst, F. C., & Achenbach, T. M. (1995). Empirically based assessment and taxonomy of psychopathology: Cross-cultural applications. *European Child and Adolescent Psychiatry, 4*, 61–76.

Verhulst, F. C., Achenbach, T. M., van der Ende, J., Erol, N., Lambert, M. C., Leung, P. W. L., et al. (2003). Comparisons of problems reported by youths from seven countries. *American Journal of Psychiatry, 160*, 1479–1485.

Verhulst, F. C., & Akkerhuis, G. W. (1986). Mental health in Dutch children: (III) Behavioral–emotional problems reported by teachers of children aged 4–12. *Acta Psychiatrica Scandinavica Supplementum, 74*(330), 1–74.

Verhulst, F. C., Akkerhuis, G. W., & Althaus, M. (1985). Mental health in Dutch children: (I) A cross-cultural comparison. *Acta Psychiatrica Scandinavica Supplementum, 72*(323), 1–108.

Verhulst, F. C., Berden, G. F. M. G., & Sanders-Woudstra, J. A. R. (1985). Mental health in Dutch children: (II) The prevalence of psychiatric disorder and relationship between measures. *Acta Psychiatrica Scandinavica Supplementum, 72*(324), 1–45.

Verhulst, F. C., Koot, H. M., & Berden, G. F. M. G. (1990). Four-year follow-up of an epidemiological sample. *Journal of the American Academy of Child and Adolescent Psychiatry, 29*, 440–448.

Verhulst, F. C., Prince, J., Vervuurt-Poot, C., & de Jong, J. B. (1989). Mental health in Dutch children: (IV) Self-reported problems for ages 11–18. *Acta Psychiatrica Scandinavica Supplementum, 80*(356), 1–48.

Verhulst, F. C., & van der Ende, J. (1992a). Six-year developmental course of internalizing and externalizing problem behaviors. *Journal of the American Academy of Child and Adolescent Psychiatry, 31*, 924–931.

Verhulst, F. C., & van der Ende, J. (1992b). Six-year stability of parent-reported problem behavior in an epidemiological sample. *Journal of Abnormal Child Psychology, 20,* 595–610.

Verhulst, F. C., & van der Ende, J. (1997). Factors associated with child mental health service use in the community. *Journal of the American Academy of Child and Adolescent Psychiatry, 36,* 901–909.

Verhulst, F. C., van der Ende, J., Ferdinand, R. F., & Kasius, M. C. (1997). The prevalence of *DSM-III-R* diagnoses in a national sample of Dutch adolescents. *Archives of General Psychiatry, 54,* 329–336.

Visser, J. H., van der Ende, J., Koot, H. M., & Verhulst, F. C. (1999). Continuity of psychopathology in youths referred to mental health services. *Journal of the American Academy of Child and Adolescent Psychiatry. 38,* 1560–1568.

Visser, J. H., van der Ende, J., Koot, H. M., & Verhulst, F. C. (2003). Predicting change in psychopathology in youth referred to mental health services in childhood or adolescence. *Journal of Child Psychology and Psychiatry, 44,* 509–519.

Wadsworth, M. E., & Achenbach, T. M. (2005). Explaining the link between low socioeconomic status and psychopathology: Testing two mechanisms of the social causation hypothesis. *Journal of Consulting and Clinical Psychology, 73,* 1146–1153.

Walker, J. L., Lahey, B. B., Russo, M. F., Frick, P. J., Christ, M. A. G., McBurnett, K., et al. (1991). Anxiety, inhibition, and conduct disorder in children: I. Relations to social impairment. *Journal of the American Academy of Child and Adolescent Psychiatry, 30,* 187–191.

Wechsler, D. (1939). *The measurement of adult intelligence.* Baltimore: Williams & Wilkins.

Wechsler, D. (2003). *WISC-IV Wechsler Intelligence Scale for Children–Fourth Edition. Technical and interpretive manual.* San Antonio, TX: Psychological Corporation.

Weine, A. M., Phillips, J. S., & Achenbach, T. M. (1995). Behavioral and emotional problems among Chinese and American children: Parent and teacher reports for ages 6–13. *Journal of Abnormal Child Psychology, 23,* 619–639.

Weinstein, S. R., Noam, G. G., Grimes, K., Stone, K., & Schwab-Stone, M. (1990). Convergence of DSM-III diagnoses and self-reported symptoms in child and adolescent inpatients. *Journal of the American Academy of Child and Adolescent Psychiatry, 29,* 627–634.

Weisz, J. R. (2004). *Psychotherapy for children and adolescents: Evidence-based treatments and case examples.* Cambridge, UK: Cambridge University Press.

Weisz, J. R., & Addis, M. E. (2006). The research–practice tango and other choreographic challenges: Using and testing evidence-based psychotherapies in clinical care settings. In C. D. Goodheart, A. E. Kazdin, & R. J. Sternberg (Eds.), *Evidence-based psychotherapy: Where practice and research meet* (pp. 179–206). Washington, DC: American Psychological Association.

Weisz, J. R., Rothbaum, F. M., & Blackburn, T. C. (1984). Standing out and standing in: The psychology of control in America and Japan. *American Psychologist, 39,* 955–969.

Weisz, J. R., Sigman, M., Weiss, B., & Mosk, J. (1993). Parent reports of behavioral and emotional problems among children of Kenya, Thailand, and the United States. *Child Development, 64,* 98–109.

Weisz, J. R., Suwanlert, S., Chaiyasit, W., Weiss, B., Achenbach, T. M., & Eastman, K. L. (1993). Behavioral and emotional problems among Thai and American adolescents: Parent reports for ages 12–16. *Journal of Abnormal Psychology, 102,* 395–403.

Weisz, J. R., Suwanlert, S., Chaiyasit, W., Weiss, B., Achenbach, T. M., & Trevathan, D. (1989). Epidemiology of behavioral and emotional problems among Thai and American children: Teacher reports for ages 6–11. *Journal of Child Psychology and Psychiatry, 30,* 471–484.

Weisz, J. R., Suwanlert, S., Chaiyasit, W., Weiss, B., Achenbach, T. M., & Walter, B. R. (1987). Epidemiology of behavioral and emotional problems among Thai and American children: Parent reports for ages 6–11. *Journal of the American Academy of Child and Adolescent Psychiatry, 26,* 890–897.

Weisz, J. R., Weiss, B., Suwanlert, S., & Chaiyasit, W. (2003). Syndromal structure of psychopathology in children of Thailand and the United States. *Journal of Consulting and Clinical Psychology, 71,* 375–385.

Werry, J. S., & Hawthorne, D. (1976). Conners' teacher questionnaire—norms and validity. *Australia and New Zealand Journal of Psychiatry, 10,* 257–262.

Werry, J. S., Sprague, R. L., & Cohen, M. N. (1975). Conners' Teacher Rating Scale for use in drug studies with children: An empirical study. *Journal of Abnormal Child Psychology, 3,* 217–229.

Whiting, J. W. M., & Child, I. L. (1953). *Child training and personality: A crosscultural study.* New Haven, CT: Yale University Press.

WHO World Mental Health Survey Consortium. (2004). Prevalence, severity, and unmet need for treatment of mental disorders in the World Health Organization World Mental Health Surveys. *Journal of the American Medical Association, 291,* 2581–2590.

Wing, J. K., Babor, T., Brugha, T., Burke, J., Cooper, J. E., Giel, R., et al. (1990). SCAN: Schedules for Clinical Assessment in Neuropsychiatry. *Archives of General Psychiatry, 47,* 589–593.

Wittchen, H.-U., Üstün, T. B., & Kessler, R. C. (1999). Diagnosing mental disorders in the community. A difference that matters? *Psychological Medicine, 29,* 1021–1027.

Woerner, W., Becker, A., & Rothenberger, A. (2004). Normative data and scale properties of the German parent SDQ. *European Child and Adolescent Psychiatry, 13*(Suppl. 2), 3–10.

Wolfe, V. V., & Birt, J. H. (1997). Child sexual abuse. In E. J. Mash & L. Terdal (Eds.), *Assessment of childhood disorders* (3rd ed., pp. 569–626). New York: Guilford Press.

World Health Organization. (1978; 1992). *Mental disorders: Glossary and guide to their classification in accordance with the Tenth Revision of the International Classification of Diseases* (9th ed.; 10th ed.). Geneva, Switzerland: Author.

World Health Organization. (1993). *The ICD-10 classification of mental and behavioral disorders: Diagnostic criteria for research.* Geneva, Switzerland: Author.

Yeh, M., & Weisz, J. R. (2001). Why are we here at the clinic? Parent–child (dis)agreement on referral problems at outpatient treatment entry. *Journal of Consulting and Clinical Psychology, 69*, 1018–1025.

Youngstrom, E. A., Findling, R. L., & Calabrese, J. R. (2003). Who are the comorbid adolescents? Agreement between psychiatric diagnosis, youth, parent, and teacher report. *Journal of Abnormal Child Psychology 31*, 231–245.

Yu, C. Y., & Muthén, B. O. (2002). *Evaluation of model fit indices for latent variable models with categorical and continuous outcomes* (Technical Report). Los Angeles: University of California at Los Angeles, Graduate School of Education and Information Studies.

Zukauskiene, R., Ignataviciene, K., & Daukantaite, D. (2003). Subscale scores of the Lithuanian version of CBCL: Preliminary data on the emotional and behavioural problems in childhood and adolescence. *European Child and Adolescent Psychiatry, 12*, 136–143.

Author Index

Achenbach, T. M., 8, 13, 15–29, 35, 36, 37, 39, 40, 42, 49, 62– 65, 70–73, 77, 80–81, 85, 98–104, 111, 118, 125, 127–128, 130, 132–134, 141, 144, 159, 160–162, 165– 169, 171, 177, 203, 221, 235– 239, 241, 248, 256–257, 261, 268, 270–272, 278, 281
Addis, M. E., 280
Akkerhuis, G. W., 36, 100, 125
Al-Awad, A. M. E., 86, 87, 231
Albrecht, G., 163
Althaus, M., 100–101, 125
Althoff, R. R., 43, 134, 136, 142
Ambrosini, P. J., 56
American Psychiatric Association, 14, 47, 49–51, 67, 197, 219, 261, 264, 275
Anderson, J., 181, 187, 189, 193, 211, 213–214, 216, 218
Angold, A., 55–56, 225
Arnett, J. J., 5
Arney, F., 113
Arsenault, L., 137, 145, 146

B

Baghurst, P. A., 97, 102, 113, 214
Bailey, V., 89, 121
Baker, L. A., 38
Barkley, R. A., 219
Baron, G. D., 100–101
Barrett, C. L., 239
Bartels, M., 136, 140–141
Bauermeister, J. J., 249
Bebbington, P. E., 271, 272
Becker, A., 109, 116–117, 174–175, 176
Behar, D., 39
Bengi-Arslan, L., 147–149, 153
Benson, J., 226
Bentler, P. M., 157, 161
Berden, G. F. M. G., 107, 109
Berg, I., 165
Bergeron, L., 60, 235
Bergroth, L., 108, 119
Berkson, J., 220
Bernstein, I. H., 69, 266
Berthiaume, C., 60, 235

Loehlin, J. C., 20
Loney, J., 43
Loo, S. K., 109, 121
Luk, S. L., 87, 172, 231
Lynskey, M. T., 211, 213–214, 216, 225
Lyubansky, M., 71, 81, 102

M

MacDonald, V., 71, 134
Malachowski, B., 242
Mann, E. M., 199
March, J., 65
Marzocchi, G. M., 92, 231
Mash, E. J., 281
McClellan, J. M., 52
McConaughy, S. H., 13, 21, 29, 39, 42, 98, 130, 133–134, 203, 221, 237, 281
McEvoy, L., 239
McGee, M. F., 181, 187, 189, 193, 211, 213–214, 216, 218
McGee, R., 218
McGuire, R., 165
Meehl, P. E., 37, 241, 266
Meesters, C., 175–176
Meier, M., 191
Meltzer, H., 44, 57, 59, 63, 89, 110, 115, 121, 189, 194, 225, 236
Messick, S., 266
Metzke, C. W., 191
Miller, L. C., 15, 239
Mineka, S., 246
Mish, F. C., 8
Modai, I., 151, 153
Moffitt, T. E., 38–39, 40
Monetti, C. H., 43
Montenegro, H., 36
Mørch, W.-T., 91, 175–176
Morgan, C. J., 37, 65
Morse, W. C., 15
Mosk, J., 71
Motto-Stefanidi, F., 71
Mrazek, D. A., 38, 40

Mullick, M., 45, 111, 115, 117
Murad, S. D., 148–149
Muris, P., 175–176
Mustillo, S., 225
Muthén, B. O., 20, 167

N

National Institute of Child Health and Human Development Early Child Care Research Network, 99, 105–106
Neale, M. C., 246
Newcorn, J., 221
Newhouse, P. A., 13
Nisi, A., 88, 171, 173
Noble, H., 239
Novik, T. S., 99, 101
Nunnally, J. C., 69, 266

O

O'Connor, P., 242
O'Leary, K. D., 88, 171, 173
Obel, C., 92
Oh, K. J., 164, 171
Oppedal, B., 151, 153

P

Parker, J. D. A., 15
Pels, T., 150
Peterson, D. R., 8, 15, 43, 104
Phares, V., 261
Phillips, J. S., 77
Pike, K. L., 6
Plomin, R., 38, 40
Pollock, L., 39
Ponizovsky, A. M., 151, 153
Prendergast, M., 198
Prince, J., 36
Prinz, F. J., 43
Puig-Antich, J., 56

Subject Index

Academic problems, 132
Acculturation, 150
ACE genetic model, 138–146
Achenbach System of Empirically
 Based Assessment (ASEBA), 17,
 35–40, 70–86, 118–121, 159, 161–
 170
Adaptive functioning, 18, 118–119
Additive genetic effects, 138
ADE genetic model, 139
ADHD Rating Scale-IV, 58, 61, 64–
 65
Adjustment reaction, 49–51
Adolescent Symptom Inventory–4
 (ASI-4), 58
Affective problems, 85
African Americans, 182
Age, 75–76, 85, 125, 128, 202, 214–
 215, 232, 263
Aggressive behavior, 38–40, 76, 143–
 145, 149, 246, 279
Analyses of covariance (ANCOVAs),
 70
Analyses of variance (ANOVAs), 70

Analytic methods, 204
Anxiety disorders, 51, 246
Anxious/depressed, 145, 147–149,
 170, 246, 279
Arabic, 86
Assessment, 7
Attention problems, 21, 42, 133,
 142–143, 149
Attention-deficit/hyperactivity
 disorder (ADHD), 29, 41–42, 50,
 80, 114, 142
Australia, 70–71, 102, 104, 113, 134,
 165, 169, 183, 211, 215–216, 246,
 278

B

Bangladesh, 44, 115
Base rates of problems, 96, 263
Behavior Assessment System for
 Children (BASC), 15, 38
Belgium, 71, 101
Berkson's bias, 220